Perinatal Epidemiology for Public Health Practice

Melissa M. Adams • Greg R. Alexander
Russell S. Kirby • Martha S. Wingate

Perinatal Epidemiology for Public Health Practice

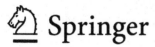 Springer

Authors

Melissa M. Adams, RN, MPH, PhD
1696 Council Bluff Drive NE.,
Atlanta GA 30345-4176
USA
m.melissa1@comcast.net

Greg R. Alexander, RS, MPH, ScD
University of South Florida
Lawton & Rhea Chiles Center for
Healthy Mothers and Babies
3111 E. Fletcher Ave.
Tampa FL 33613
USA

Russell S. Kirby, PhD
University of Alabama at Birmingham
School of Public Health
Department of Maternal & Child Health
Ryals 320
1530 3rd Avenue South
Birmngham, AL 35294-0022
USA
rkirby@uab.edu

Martha S. Wingate, MPH, DrPH
University of Alabama at Birmingham
School of Public Health
Department of Health Care
Organization and Policy
Ryals 330
1530 3rd Avenue South
Birmingham AL 35294-0022
USA
mslay@uab.edu

ISBN 978-1-4419-3478-9   e-ISBN 978-0-387-09439-7
DOI 10.1007/978-0-387-09439-7

9 8 7 6 5 4 3 2 1

springer.com

In February 2007, our coauthor, friend, colleague, and mentor, Dr. Greg Alexander, passed away unexpectedly and was not able to see this book to completion. Greg was a leading scholar and teacher in perinatal epidemiology and maternal and child health. In his quest for knowledge and insight, Greg constantly pushed himself and his colleagues and students to ask, "Why?" and to think beyond the status quo. His questions were not only to make his colleagues and students better, but also to make a better future for tomorrow's children and adults.

This vision was at the core of Greg's passion for his work. It was not just about the papers or the publications on fetal growth curves, prenatal care, racial disparities in birth outcomes, and many other topics. It was about the vision of a world where all children are healthy, safe, and loved. Greg leaves his wonderful wife, Donna, and two amazing daughters, Kerry and Morgan, who were his heart. He knew that life was about more than work and this is evident in his beautiful family. The task of completing this book without Greg's encouragement and prodding has been a long one. We hope that he would be proud of the final product. We are thankful for his ideas and passion that we tried to reflect in this text. Most of all, we are thankful for our friend. We miss you!

Acknowledgements

The contents were enhanced by the generous review and comments that were contributed by William Callaghan, MD; Wendy Hellerstedt, PhD; Mona Lydon-Rochelle, PhD; Mary Ann Pass, MD, MPH; Melissa Romaire, MPH; and Lowell Sever, PhD. This book benefited from the helpful work of Melissa Romaire and Suzanne Roseman, who identified references and data sources. Sheree Boulet, DrPH supported some of the analyses. Students who attended the course "Perinatal Epidemiology" at the School of Public Health, University of Alabama at Birmingham provided helpful comments on several chapters. This book would not have been possible without the longstanding support, practical guidance and patience of William Tucker, Emma Holgren, and Khristine Queja, all of whom are with the publisher, Springer Publishing Company, New York, NY. Donna Petersen provided guidance and encouragement for the promise of a completed textbook. The authors are grateful for all these contributions. The authors take full responsibility, however, for all errors.

MA: Deepest thanks to my loving husband, Philip H. Rhodes, for his on-going multi faceted support throughout the writing of this text. I also extend my appreciation and love to our two children, Jesse and Quinn. To all three of you: please accept my thanks for your many compromises that enabled me to have the time and energy to complete this book.

RK: Many thanks to my wife, Elizabeth, for listening and patience during the protracted gestation time for this book. And to my father, Frank E. Kirby who would have been delighted to see his son carry on a family tradition of book publication and to my mother, Emily Baruch Kirby, also a book author, who can, and to my three daughters, Rachel, Amelia, and Jocelyn who know that my love for them encompasses the totality of their health and well-being and that of their future children.

MW: Much love and thanks to Bill for his patience and understanding during the book process (and during my pregnancy) and his desire to spend time with our daughter during the final stages! To the sweetest reminder of why we do what we do...Mary Hudson; thank you for being our biggest blessing! 3ws

Contents

Chapter 1
Introduction

At the beginning of the twentieth century, women of childbearing age and infants were at a substantial risk of death. In the United States, nearly 1% of women of childbearing age died of pregnancy-related complications and 10% of their babies never celebrated their first birthdays (1–3). During the past century, reductions in maternal and infant mortality were unparalleled historically. The maternal mortality ratio decreased to 15.1 deaths per 100,000 live births in 2005 (4). The infant mortality rate declined more than 90% from 1915 through 2005, decreasing to 6.9 per 1,000 live births.

Improved access to health care, environmental health and sanitation, as well as public health surveillance, increasing levels of education, and other advances contributed to healthier mothers and babies. Improvements in living and environmental conditions in urban areas were a primary focus in efforts to reduce infant mortality. Milk pasteurization contributed to the reduction in milk-borne diseases; improvements in education and economic conditions raised standards of living, thus promoting health; lower fertility rates also contributed to reductions in infant mortality through longer pregnancy spacing, improved nutritional status of mothers, and smaller family size (1, 3). The use of antibiotics further decreased the infant death rate (5). In addition, programs such as Medicaid, Special Supplemental Food Program for Women, Infants, and Children (WIC), and others were implemented to address the underlying issues associated with infant mortality, particularly postneonatal mortality (6). More recently, health promotion campaigns and new medical technologies and therapeutic interventions have been key. One example is the "Back to Sleep" campaign in the 1990s, which encouraged parents to put babies to sleep on their backs and led to a greater than 50% decline in Sudden Infant Death Syndrome (SIDS) (7). The development and use of artificial surfactant to treat and prevent respiratory distress syndrome in premature infants is an example of a clinical therapy that was instrumental in the recent reduction of infant mortality (8).

For mothers, a number of factors contributed to the high rate of death due to pregnancy-related complications. The high number of maternal deaths was due largely to poor obstetric education and delivery practices (2). Obstetrical care was typically provided by poorly or untrained medical practitioners and many unnecessary interventions, such as induction of labor and Cesarean deliveries, occurred. Roughly 40% of maternal deaths resulted from sepsis because of unsafe delivery

M.M. Adams et al., *Perinatal Epidemiology for Public Health Practice.*
doi: 10.1007/978-0-387-09439-7_1; © Springer Science + Business Media, LLC 2009

practices; many of the remaining deaths were due to toxemia and hemorrhage (2). Beginning in the 1930s, a number of initiatives were put in place to help lower the number of maternal deaths in the United States. Hospitals and state public health practitioners initiated maternal mortality reviews to identify practices that caused the deaths. Institutional and physician guidelines were implemented to ensure appropriate training and procedures related to delivery. Deliveries were performed in cleaner environments, leading to fewer infections (9). Legalization of induced abortion began in the 1960s and culminated with Roe V. Wade in 1973. Legalization contributed to decline in deaths from sepsis associated with illegal abortions (10). Of the maternal deaths that occur in the United States today, however, more than half are preventable by the use of existing interventions (11).

Despite these improvements, challenges in the area of maternal and child health in the United States still require attention. Significant disparities by race and ethnicity persist in infant and maternal health, particularly among Blacks and Whites. Black infants are more than twice as likely to die before their first birthday as White infants (12). American Indian/Alaskan Native infants have higher infant death rates compared with White infants, due largely to higher SIDS rates (13). The disparities of maternal mortality existing between Black and White mothers have increased over time. In the early part of the twentieth century, Black women were twice as likely to die of pregnancy-related complications as White women. Today, Black women are 3 times as likely to die from this cause (3).

To address the issues of maternal and infant mortality as well as the other issues facing women and children today, we must understand the factors that contribute to their morbidity and mortality. Strategies to achieve this understanding include researching and intervening on biological, social, economic, psychological, and environmental factors. Epidemiology is one of the effective methods for conducting this research.

Epidemiology is defined as "the study of the distribution and determinants of health-related states or events in specified populations and the application of this study to control health problems" (14). In other words, in a defined population, epidemiology addresses these questions: What is the pattern of a specific disease or outcome? What factors influence this pattern? How can we control this disease or modify this outcome? The purpose of this text is to provide a population-based epidemiologic perspective on maternal, perinatal, and infant health issues with a specific focus on public health interventions that address these issues. This text focuses on perinatal health in the United States. To give perspective to rates in the United States of selected perinatal conditions, we present rates from other countries. The intended audience for this book includes public health practitioners, teachers, and students in public health or other health-related areas, clinicians, advocates, and others interested in these topics.

The textbook has eight chapters. Except for Chapters 1 (Introduction) and 8 (Conclusion), each chapter addresses a topic related to maternal, perinatal, or infant health. The chapters that address these topics follow a similar outline, with variations as needed. Each chapter begins with an overall introduction and definitions of key terms or concepts associated with the overall topic. Specific measures, data sources related to the topic, and measurement issues are presented. The next section focuses on descriptive epidemiology: temporal trends and geographic and demographic variations. Demographic characteristics considered may include age, race, marital status, education, and income. Some chapters discuss attributable risk fractions associated with a specific outcome. The next section describes factors that influence the occurrence of the disease or outcome. This section outlines risk and protective factors as well as the availability, use, and effectiveness of public health interventions. At the end of each chapter, two brief sections list topics for discussion – for those using this text for teaching and a list of important unanswered questions. Additionally, abbreviations and references are included at the end of each chapter.

In writing this text, we assumed that readers understand basic epidemiologic terminology and concepts. We define each problem from a population perspective. We did not plan for this text to provide specific clinical information. We assumed that readers have fundamental knowledge related to clinical conditions. We have included a glossary of terms that may be helpful in learning these concepts. We want our readers to gain a clearer understanding of the plethora of maternal and child health issues that need to be addressed in practice and research. Happy reading!

References

1. Meckel RA. Save the babies: American public health reform and the prevention of infant mortality, 1850–1929. Baltimore, Maryland: The Johns Hopkins University Press, 1990.
2. Loudon I. Death in childbirth: an international study of maternal care and maternal mortality, 1800–1950. New York: Oxford University Press, 1992.
3. Centers for Disease Control and Prevention. Achievements in public health, 1900–1999: Healthier mothers and babies. MMWR, 48:849–858.
4. Kung HC, Hoyert DL, Xu JQ, Murphy SL. Deaths: Final data for 2005. National vital statistics reports; Vol. 56 No. 10. Hyattsville, MD: National Center for Health Statistics. 2008.
5. Public Health Service. Vital statistics of the United States, 1950. Vol. 1. Washington, DC: US Department of Health and Human Services, Public Health Service, 1954:258–259.
6. Pharoah POD, Morris JN. Postneonatal mortality. Epidemiologic Review 1979; 1:170–183.
7. Willinger M, Hoffman H, Wu K, et al. Factors associated with the transition to non-prone sleep positions of infants in the United States: The National Infant Sleep Position Study. JAMA 1998; 280:329–339.
8. Schoendorf KC, Kiely JL. Birth weight and age-specific analysis of the 1990 US infant mortality drop: Was it surfactant? Archives of Pediatric and Adolescent Medicine, 1997; 151:129–134.
9. Children's Bureau. Changes in infant, childhood, and maternal mortality over the decade of 1939–1948: A graphic analysis. Washington, DC: Children's Bureau, Social Security Administration, 1950.
10. National Center for Health Statistics. Vital statistics of the United States, 1973. Vol. II, mortality, part A. Rockville, Maryland: US Department of Health, Education, and Welfare, 1977.
11. Berg CJ, Atrash HK, Koonin LM, Tucker M. Pregnancy-related mortality in the United States, 1987–1990. Obstetrics and Gynecology 1996; 88:161–167.
12. Alexander GR, Wingate MS, Bader D, Kogan MD. The increasing racial disparity in infant mortality rates: Composition and contributors to recent U.S. trends. American Journal of Obstetrics and Gynecology, 2008, 198: 51e1–51e9.
13. Alexander GR, Wingate MS, Boulet S. Pregnancy Outcomes of American-Indians: Contrasts among regions and with other ethnic groups. Maternal and Child Health Journal, 2007, October [Epub ahead of print].
14. Last JM. A dictionary of epidemiology, 2nd ed. New York: Oxford University Press, 1988.

Chapter 2
Reproductive Health Issues

This chapter presents factors that set the context for pregnancy and, ultimately, influence maternal and infant health. We begin with fertility and its opposite, infertility. After briefly discussing the epidemiology of clinical treatment for infertility, we focus on the central theme of this chapter: pregnancy intention. We conclude by exploring a way of ending unintended pregnancy (induced abortion), a way to prevent unintended pregnancy (contraception), and a desirable antecedent of an intended pregnancy (preconception care).

2.1 Fertility

2.1.1 Definition, Measures, Data Sources, and Measurement Issues

Definition: Fertility is the production of live offspring. Mortality and fertility rates can be used to estimate changes in the future growth of a population. The fertility rate also indicates the average number of deliveries per woman. In the United States, *parity* is the number of live-born children that a woman has borne. In the United Kingdom, *parity* is the number of times a woman has delivered a fetus of ≥24 weeks, regardless of whether that fetus was live or stillborn (1). In countries with higher fertility, average parity also tends to be higher. Fertility describes the experience of a population; parity describes the experience of an individual woman. Parity is related to pregnancy outcome, with risks for a range of maternal and fetal adverse outcomes generally highest for first pregnancies and eighth and subsequent pregnancies. When a population's fertility rate is high, women tend to begin childbearing in their teens and continue to their late thirties and early forties. Risks for adverse pregnancy outcomes are highest for young teens and women aged 35 and above.

Fecundity is distinct from fertility. Fecundity is the *ability* of a couple to have children, rather than the actual production of children. Couples may have impaired

M.M. Adams et al., *Perinatal Epidemiology for Public Health Practice.*
doi: 10.1007/978-0-387-09439-7_2; © Springer Science + Business Media, LLC 2009

fecundity if they have difficulty conceiving or carrying a fetus to term. Factors related to the woman, man, or both may impair fecundity (2). Couples may be fecund although they do not bear children.

Measures: General measures of fertility include the crude birth rate, general fertility rate, age-specific fertility rate, total fertility rate, gross reproduction rate, net reproduction rate, and fertility ratio. Many of these rates apply to reproductive-aged women, conventionally defined as women aged 15 through 44 years. These measures are defined in Table 2.1.

The pregnancy rate differs from the other rates in Table 2.1 in that its numerator consists of all pregnancies – regardless of how they end – that occur in a population of reproductive-aged women in a year. Thus the numerator includes live and stillbirths, induced and spontaneous abortions and ectopic pregnancies. The pregnancy rate is informative in studying the magnitude of potential morbidity related to pregnancy. Because the numerator is pregnancies, women who have more than one pregnancy in a year will be counted twice.

The denominator for the crude birth rate is everyone in the population, regardless of their potential to actually bear a child. Because of this inclusiveness, the crude birth rate is influenced by the age distribution in the population. A population with a large portion of persons not in their reproductive years (i.e., children or older adults) relative to the portion of persons aged 15–44 years is likely to have a lower crude birth rate than a population with a large portion of the population aged 15–44 years. This happens because nearly all births occur among women aged 15–44 years.

To minimize the confounding effect of these differences in age distributions when comparing populations, researchers often analyze the general fertility rate. The denominator of the general fertility rate includes only women in their reproductive years. However, confounding effects may still remain if, for example, one population contains a greater portion of women at the peak of their reproductive years (ages 20–29 years) than another population. To address this problem, researchers may examine age-specific rates. These rates are often computed for 5-year intervals of maternal age (quinquennia), e.g., 15–19 years, 20–24 years, etc.

The total fertility rate estimates the number of children a cohort of 1,000 women would bear if they all went through their childbearing years experiencing the age-specific birth rates in effect for a particular time. Thus, it projects the prevailing age-specific fertility rates for women of one age onto those of another age. It is a synthetic, hypothetical rate, usually standardized to a constant age distribution of women. The total fertility rate may be expressed as births per woman or per 1,000 women.

The total fertility rate estimates whether the childbearing population is replacing itself or not. A total fertility rate of about 2,100 per 1,000 women (equal to 2.1 per woman) or above indicates that, on the average, couples are reproducing at a level to replace themselves (replacement fertility). When the total fertility rate exceeds 2,100 for an extended period, the next generation of adults of childbearing age will probably be larger than the present population of that age if all other factors affecting the population, such as death rates and migration, remain constant (3).

Table 2.1 Commonly used measures of fertility (source: (4, 5))

Measure	Definition
Pregnancy rate per 1,000 women aged 15–44 years	$\dfrac{\text{Pregnancies in a population during a year}}{\text{Average or mid - year number of women aged 15–44 years in that year}}$
Crude birth rate per 1,000 people	$\dfrac{\text{Live births in a population during a year}}{\text{Average or mid - year population in that year}} \times 1{,}000$
General fertility rate per 1,000 aged women 15–44 years	$\dfrac{\text{Live births in a population area during a year}}{\text{Mid - year female population aged 15–44 in the same population in the same year}} \times 1{,}000$
Age-specific fertility rate per 1,000 women of a specified age	$\dfrac{\text{Live births among women of specified age in a population during a year}}{\text{Mid - year female population of the specified age in the same population in the same year}} \times 1{,}000$
Total fertility rate per 1,000 women aged 15–44 years	A hypothetical rate computed by summing the age-specific fertility rates in a given period for a hypothetical cohort of women
Gross fertility rate per 1,000 reproductive-age women	$\dfrac{\text{Live - born girls in an population during a year}}{\text{Mid - year female population aged 15–44 years in the same population in the same year}} \times 1{,}000$
Net reproduction rate per 1,000 reproductive-age women	Gross fertility rate, where the denominator is decreased to take into account maternal deaths
Fertility ratio per 1,000 women aged 15–49 years	$\dfrac{\text{Children aged} <5 \text{ years}}{\text{Women aged 15–49 years}} \times 1{,}000$
Cohort fertility rate per 1,000 women born in a year (e.g., 1970) or period of years (e.g., 1970–1974)	Cohort fertility is the sum of the annual age-specific birth rates of women born in a specified year (or period) from ages 15 through 44

The gross fertility rate is similar to the general fertility rate, except that it counts only daughters that a woman bears during her reproductive years. Thus, it is the average number of daughters that a cohort of 1,000 women will bear if they pass through their childbearing years experiencing the age-specific birth rates in effect for a particular time.

The net reproduction rate is the same as the gross fertility rate, but it takes into account age-specific maternal mortality rates. Because of maternal mortality, the net reproduction rate is always less than the gross reproduction rate.

The fertility ratio expresses how many small children a population has in relation to the number of women of reproductive age. Analysts use it when reliable data on the number of births are not available.

A related concept is cohort fertility, which refers to the fertility of women born in a specified interval and followed through their reproductive years. Cumulative birth rates represent the total number of births to women in a birth cohort up to a specified age. For example, the cumulative birth rate for a cohort of women aged 45 years represents completed their family size, since these women are traditionally defined as at the end of their reproductive years.

Data sources: Data for measures of fertility derive from vital records (birth and death certificates), census data, and surveys. Surveys are used in developed countries to estimate the frequency of spontaneous pregnancy losses, induced abortions, and ectopic pregnancies. In countries without reliable registration of births and deaths, surveys measure these outcomes as well as fetal deaths and live births.

Measurement issues: Measurement of fertility is relatively straightforward, provided that reliable data on population size and births are available.

2.1.2   Descriptive Epidemiology

Temporal trends. From 1900 to 2004, the annual general fertility rate (live births per 1,000 women aged 15–44) in the United States changed markedly (Fig. 2.1). Of note is the high general fertility rate during the 1950s (the baby boom), followed by decreases beginning in the 1960s, consistent with the introduction of hormonal contraception. Most recently, the fertility rate declined between 1990 and 1995 (from 71 to 66 per 1,000 women aged 15–44) and thereafter was stable (1999: 65 per 1,000 women aged 15–44). In the United States during the 1990s through the first half of the first decade of the next century, approximately 4 million live births occurred per year.

During the 1990s, the total fertility rate (a hypothetical rate estimating the lifetime total number of births among a group of women aged 15–44 years) never exceeded the replacement rate. The total fertility rate ranged from a high of 2,081 per 1,000 women aged 15–44 in 1990 to a low of 1971 per 1,000 in 1997. In 2004, the total fertility rate was 2,045.5 per 1,000 women (4).

Geographic variability: Consistent with the change in the national general fertility rate, general fertility rates in many states declined from 1990 to 1995 and

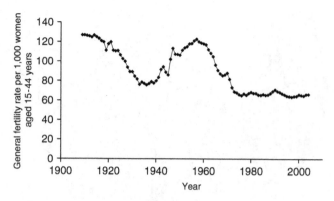

Fig. 2.1 Annual General Fertility Rates, United States, 1909–2004

varied modestly thereafter. By 2004, state-specific general fertility rates varied from a low of 52.1 per 1,000 women aged 15–44 in Maine to a high of 92.3 per 1,000 in Utah. In 2004, states with high general fertility rates included Hawaii (74.0), Alaska (74.4), Idaho (77.3) and the southwestern states of Texas (77.3), New Mexico (71.9), Arizona (79.5), Nevada (72.6), California (70.4), and Utah (92.3) (Fig. 2.2) (4). States with low rates tended to be in the northeast. States with the lowest general fertility rates in 2004 included Vermont (52.1), Maine (52.4), New Hampshire (53.4), Rhode Island (55.0), the District of Columbia (58.2), and West Virginia (58.3). (4) Recent state-specific crude birth rates and total fertility rates showed a similar pattern (5).

Throughout the 1990s and continuing to 2004, the groups of states with the highest and lowest general fertility rates tended to remain the same. Of note is the consistently high rate in Utah, which exceeded the second-ranked state by a considerable amount.

Worldwide, in 2005, total fertility rates ranged from 5,700 live births per 1,000 women aged 15–44 in sub-Saharan African countries and some mid-eastern and Asian countries to 1,300–1,900 live births per 1,000 women in developed countries. In 2005, India and China, the countries with the most annual births, had total fertility rates of 2,900 (India) and 1,700 (China). In 2005, the United States' total fertility rate of 2,000 exceeded that of Canada (1,500), the United Kingdom (1,700), Italy (1,300), France (1,900), Australia (1,700), Japan (1,300), and numerous other developed countries (6).

Demographic variability: In the United States, fertility rates vary by maternal age, marital status, race, ethnicity, country of birth, and cultural and religious orientation. From 1990 through 2004 in the United States, regardless of other factors, general fertility rates were inversely related to age (Table 2.2) (4, 5, 7). The highest rates occurred for women in their late teens and twenties. During the 1990s, age-specific fertility rates decreased for women aged less than 30 and increased for older women, especially those in their late thirties and early forties (Fig. 2.3).

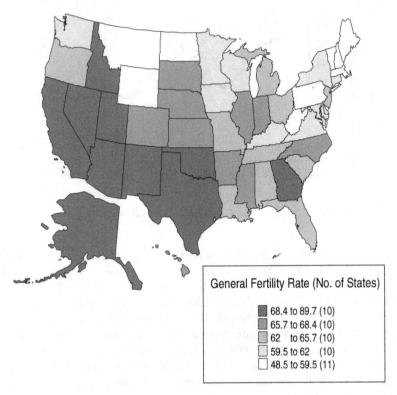

Fig. 2.2 General Fertilty Rates (live births per 1,000 women aged 15–44 years), by state, 2004

Table 2.2 General fertility rates by maternal race and attributes, United States, 2004

Maternal attribute	White	Black	All races
Total	66.1	67.6	66.3
Age (years)			
15–17	19.5	37.2	22.1
18–19	65.0	104.4	70.0
20–24	99.2	127.7	101.7
25–29	118.6	103.6	115.5
30–34	99.1	67.9	95.3
35–39	46.4	34.0	45.4
40–44	8.9	7.9	8.9
Ethnicity			
Hispanic (all races)			97.8
Non-Hispanic	58.4	67.0	
Marital status			
Married	89.2	68.4	87.6
Unmarried	41.6	67.2	46.1

General fertility rates are expressed as live births per 1,000 women aged 15–44 years, except for age-specific rates, which present live births per 1,000 women of the specified age (Source: (4)).

In general, during the 1990s, age-specific fertility rates were highest for married women and for Hispanic women. A notable trend during the 1990s was the increased rate of child-bearing among unmarried women, regardless of age.

Overall, in the United States, compared with White women in their teens and early twenties, Black women of the same age had higher general fertility rates. In contrast, Black women had lower general fertility rates in from their late twenties onward.

Marital status influenced the effect of race on age-specific fertility rates. Among unmarried women in the 1990s, age-specific fertility rates were consistently higher for Black women than for White women. Rates for White women, however, showed

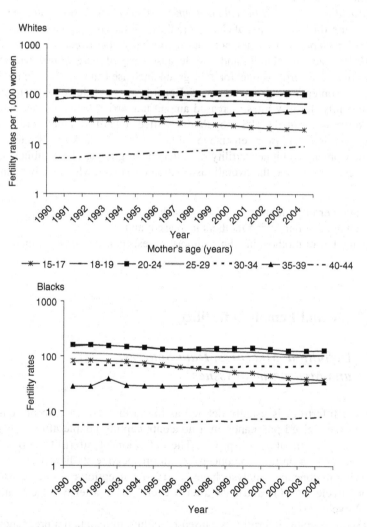

Fig. 2.3 Age-specific fertility rates, by race of mother, United States, 1990–2004

an increasing trend while those for Black women showed a decreasing trend. For example, among unmarried women aged 20–24 years (prime childbearing years), the fertility rate decreased among Black women from 145 live births per 1,000 women in 1990 to 20 in 2004, but increased among White women from 48 in 1990 to 64 in 2004 (4).

During the 1990s, age-specific fertility rates were higher for Hispanic women than for other women, regardless of marital status.

Some religious groups, notably Mormons and old-order Amish either do not limit their fertility or limit it only slightly (8, 9). This tendency among Mormons likely accounts for the consistently high fertility rate in Utah, where ~70% of the population is Mormon.

Characteristics of child-bearing women: The changes in fertility rates during the 1990s occurred in the context of changes in the attributes of women of reproductive age. The large cohort of women born during the baby-boom years of the 1950s and early 1960s aged into their 30s and 40s. Because many of these women had delayed childbearing, the fertility rate for this group increased at the same time as the number of women in the group increased. Regardless of age, fewer women married. Concomitantly, fertility rates increased among unmarried women. The racial and ethnic distribution of the U.S. population shifted toward a higher percentage of Hispanic women and lower percentages of non-Hispanic Black and White women. Hispanic women had higher fertility rates than other groups. The combined impact of these changes altered the overall distribution of women who gave birth in three ways:

- The number of mothers aged 35 increased;
- The number of unmarried mothers increased; and
- The number of mothers in ethnic minorities, especially Hispanics, increased.

2.2 Male and Female Infertility

2.2.1 Definition, Measures, Data Sources, and Measurement Issues

Definition: Infertility is usually defined as the failure to conceive or achieve a clinically recognized pregnancy in a noncontracepting couple after a period of time, usually 12 months (12, p. 63). The definition of infertility derives from observational data on time to conception. In prospective studies of couples who were trying to conceive, analysts have observed conception rates of 31% to 40% after one cycle (10, 11) and 68% after 3 cycles, 81% after 6 cycles, and 92% after 12 cycles (10).

For some couples, infertility is caused by failure to maintain a pregnancy until clinical recognition, rather than failure to conceive (see Sect. 4.2.3 on early pregnancy loss). Infertility is related to male factors in approximately 20% of couples (12). Male factor infertility and tubal infertility have been observed more commonly among younger than older men and women (13).

Infertility is often classified as primary or secondary. *Primary infertility* is infertility that occurs to women who have never had a live birth. *Secondary infertility* occurs to women who have had one or more live births but have difficulty achieving subsequent pregnancies.

Measures: Infertility is measured as the proportion of individuals or couples who report receiving a physician's diagnosis of infertility, the proportion of couples who fail to conceive after a specified period of unprotected intercourse (usually 12 months), or the proportion of couples seeking or using assisted reproductive technology (ART).

Data sources: Diagnoses of infertility can be ascertained from self-report through the National Survey of Family Growth (NSFG), from databases of outpatient care, such as the National Ambulatory Medical Care Survey, both of which are conducted by the National Center for Health Statistics (NCHS), and databases of outpatient care provided by managed care organizations. The number of women using ART can be estimated from annual reports (Assisted Reproductive Technology Surveillance) that are produced by the Centers for Disease Control and Prevention (CDC).

The U.S. 2003 revised model certificate for live births (Appendix 1) asks whether the pregnancy resulted from infertility treatment and distinguishes pharmacologic treatment from ART. A limitation of this information is that it relates only to persons for whom the infertility treatment was successful. One cannot use it to infer rates of use of infertility services in the general population.

Measurement issues. Many individuals and couples with infertility do not seek medical care and thus are not diagnosed with it. A couple's failure to conceive is influenced by frequency and timing of intercourse relative to ovulation. Couples with infrequent intercourse are likely to take longer to conceive than equally fertile couples with more frequent intercourse. Because ART can be expensive and is often not covered by insurance, couples may not seek it. As new, less-invasive and less-expensive types of ART become available, the number of couples willing to seek medical evaluation for infertility and to use ART may increase. Such a change would hinder accurate interpretation of temporal trends.

The validity of the newly introduced item on the live birth certificate concerning use of infertility services is unknown. Probably use will be underreported, as it is for many similar items on the birth certificate (14, 15). Use of infertility services may be more likely to be reported when pregnancy outcomes that are widely known to be associated with infertility treatment occur – such as multiple gestations. Thus, bias may exist in reports of the use of infertility services.

Infertility increases markedly at older ages. Therefore, populations with large numbers of women attempting pregnancy at older ages (e.g., ≥ 35 years) will have higher infertility rates than populations where only a small number of older women attempt pregnancy.

2.2.2   Descriptive Epidemiology

Temporal trends: A generally referenced prevalence of infertility in the Western world is 10–15% (12). Data from the NSFG for 2002 are consistent with this estimate. These data show that for currently married women aged 15–44 years, 34.8% were surgically sterile, 7.4% were infertile, and 57.8% were fertile. Thus, among married women who were not surgically sterile, 11.3% were infertile (16). This prevalence represents a decline the prevalence observed in the 1982 NSFG sample (17). The 2002 prevalence reflects a trend of postponing attempts at childbearing to older ages, when fertility decreases (18). The estimated number of infertile women in the United States in 1995 was 6.2 million (19). During the first quarter of this century, the number of infertile women is projected to increase modestly to approximately 6.4 million in 2025 (19).

Geographic variability. Data on state-specific infertility rates are not available. Comparison of infertility rates among countries is complicated by differences in availability of treatments for infertility as well as cultural attitudes toward infertility.

Demographic variability. Data from the 1995 and 2002 NSFG show that among married women aged 15–44 in the United States who were not surgically sterile, the prevalence of infertility was related to age, parity, education, and ethnicity and race (Table 2.3) (20, 21). The most striking pattern was the increase in the prevalence of infertility associated with advancing maternal age. Paternal age ≥40 years is also an important risk factor for infertility (22).

Data from a follow-back survey of American college graduates, aged 37–70 years at the time of the survey, showed that 17.1% reported infertility. Most (14.0%) had secondary infertility (23).

Characteristics of infertile women. The majority of women who want to have children are in their twenties and have at least a high school education. Paralleling this pattern, the majorities of women who are involuntarily unable to have children are largely younger, nulliparous, and have more than 12 years of education.

2.2.3   Factors Affecting Occurrence, Related Public Health Interventions, and Their Availability and Use

Difficulties in measuring the prevalence of infertility limit our ability to understand the etiology of infertility. The cause of infertility is unidentified for about 5–10% of couples (24). For 8–14% of the women who sought ART in 2003 and 2004, no explanation for their infertility could be found (7, 25).

Factors associated with infertility and longer times to conception among both men and women include advanced age (≥35 years for women and ≥40 years for men), anatomical abnormalities, Chlamydia and other sexually-transmitted infections, and cigarette smoking – either active or passive. Among women, these factors

Table 2.3 Factors associated with infertility among married women who were not surgically sterile, National Survey for Family Growth, 2002 (source: (16))

Age (years) and parity		Percent infertile
Parity = 0	15–29	11.0
	30–34	16.9
	35–39	22.6
	40–44	27.4
Parity ≥ 1	15–29	4.0
	30–34	5.9
	35–39	3.9
	40–44	7.2
Education (years)	<12	10.4
	12	6.5
	13–15	6.6
	≥16	8.4
Race and ethnicity	Hispanic	7.7
	White, non-Hispanic	7.0
	Black, non-Hispanic	11.5

include moderate or heavy alcohol consumption, regular vigorous exercise, prior use of an intrauterine device (IUD), low body mass index, marijuana or cocaine use, ever-use of thyroid replacement hormones, history of preeclampsia, and other factors (12, 22, 26–28). Factors associated with sperm abnormalities or lower sperm counts include occupational exposure to heavy metals (lead, mercury), pesticides, ethylene glycol ethers, and estrogens (29).

Of these factors, the ones most amenable to public health intervention are Chlamydia infection and smoking. Public health efforts to reduce the prevalence of Chlamydia and other sexually transmitted infections include promoting the use of condoms and screening to identify and treat infected persons. Prompt diagnosis and treatment of Chlamydia infections can avert tubal damage, a frequent cause of infertility. A comprehensive Chlamydia prevention program in Wisconsin involved selective or universal screening, depending on the population. An evaluation of this program found that the statewide chlamydial prevalence and incidence declined, as did the rate of complications due to infection (30). Hu et al. computed that annual screening for Chlamydia infection among sexually active women aged 15–29 years in the United States is cost-effective (31).

Both women and men who smoke decrease their fertility. Women who smoke also have poorer responses to infertility treatments (2004 (32)). Because of its many adverse health effects, reducing smoking is a public health priority that is addressed by a range of public health interventions (33).

2.3 Infertility Treatment

2.3.1 Definition, Measures, Data Sources, and Measurement Issues

Definition: Infertility treatment includes a range of pharmacologic, physiologic, and surgical interventions with the aims of promoting conception and maintaining pregnancy. These interventions may be applied to males, females, or both. Two broad categories of treatment for women are the use of ovulation-inducing drugs and assisted reproductive technologies (ART). (We use "ART" to refer to a range of procedures, all of which involve manipulation of an egg or embryo outside the body, followed by transfer to a woman. These procedures may use fresh, frozen, or donated embryos.)

Figure 2.4 presents treatment for infertility in the context of events that may occur to a woman with infertility. The figure begins with the occurrence of infertility, then moves to the possibility that a woman seeks treatment, the success of treatment, and whether treatment results in a single or multiple delivery.

Measures of infertility treatment include the number of ART treatments, success rates for in vitro fertilization (IVF) and related procedures, the proportion of live births resulting from ART, and the rates of use of specific infertility treatments among reproductive-age women.

Data sources: The NSFG retrospectively asks women about lifetime use of infertility treatment (advice, tests on the woman or man), ovulation drugs, surgery to treat blocked tubes, and ART and, more specifically, treatment during the year before the interview.

Since 1996, the CDC, in collaboration with the Society for Assisted Reproductive Technology, has reported the number and outcome of each ART cycle performed by most of the clinics in the United States. A cycle includes administration of ovulation-inducing drugs, harvesting and fertilization of ova, and transfer of resulting embryos to the uterus. ART data collection was mandated by federal legislation, the Fertility Clinic Success Rate and Certification Act of 1992 (Pub. L. 102–493, 42 U.S.C. 263a-1 et seq.). Data are derived from reports submitted by each clinic.

The 2003 revision of the model birth certificate collects data on use of infertility services and type of service used. These data include only women whose treatment was successful and resulted in a viable pregnancy. Thus, they are not informative about the population-wide use of infertility services.

Measurement issues: The infrequent administration of the NSFG limits its ability to provide up-to-date data, which are desirable given the rapid expansion of treatments for infertility. Another limitation of the NSFG is that it does not provide state-specific data.

Data reported by the CDC are limited to ART, which does not comprise the bulk of infertility treatment (20). Although clinic-based data are audited periodically, their accuracy may vary over time. Because clinic-based data lack personal identifiers, one cannot measure the number of women receiving procedures and the woman-specific IVF success rate, but only the number of procedures and the success rate per procedure.

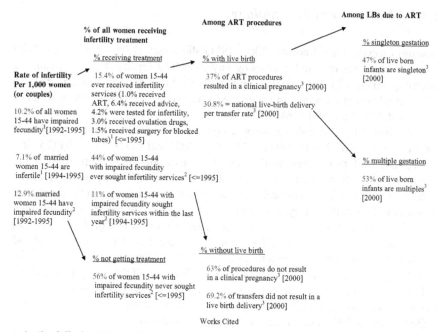

Works Cited

1. Abma J, Chandra A, Mosher W, Peterson L, Piccino L. Fertility, family planning, and women's health: New data from the 1995 National Survey of Family Growth. National Center for Health Statistics. Vital Health Stat 23(19), 1997.

2. Chandra A, Stephen EH. Impaired fecundity in the United States: 1982–1995. Fam Plann Perspect. 1998;30(1):34–42.

3. Wright VC, Shieve LA, Reynolds MA, Jeng G. Assisted reproductive technology surveillance – United States, 2000. MMWR. 52(SS-9):1–20.

Note

Sources 1 and 2 utilize data from the 1995 NSFG. NSFG has specific definitions for infertility and impaired fecundity.

Infertility is assessed in married couples only. "If neither spouse is surgically sterile, a couple is considered infertile if, during the previous 12 months or longer, they were continuously married, had not used contraception, and had not become pregnant." (Abma J p. 107)

Impaired fecundity is assessed for any woman 15–44 years of age. Impaired fecundity is labeled "if she reported that (a) it is impossible for her (or her husband or cohabitating partner) to have a baby for any reason other than a sterilizing operation; (b) it is difficult or dangerous to carry a baby to term; or (c) she and her husband/partner have been continuously married or cohabitating, have not used contraception, and have not had a pregnancy for 3 years or longer." (Abma J p. 108)

Dates: Years in brackets are those in which the data were derived.

Fig. 2.4 Outcomes for infertile women

Although nearly all facilities providing IVF and related treatments are included in CDC's annual report, a few do not provide information. In 2004, 50 (11%) of the 461 facilities known to provide ART services did not report their data (25).

In the United States, characteristics of couples using ART as well as trends in ART use are influenced by insurance coverage. As of 2006, 15 states mandated that health insurance companies operating in their state cover at least some type of infertility treatment (34). Investigators have observed that insurance mandates are associated with greater use of ART (35). Use of ART is likely to increase as more states mandate insurance coverage for it.

The validity of birth certificate data on use of infertility services is unknown.

2.3.2 Descriptive Epidemiology

Temporal trends: Data from the 2002 NSFG show that 11.9% of women (15–44 years) respondents reported ever using any infertility service. Of those using an infertility service, 51.3% received advice, 40.3% had tests (on woman or man), 32.0% used ovulation-inducing drugs, 5.9% had surgery or treatment of blocked tubes, and 2.5% had ART (16).

Data from CDC surveillance show a continuous rise in the annual number of ART cycles from 64,724 in 1996 to 115,392 in 2002 and 127,977 in 2004 (25, 36).

In 2004, ART procedures resulted in 49,458 live-born babies, up from 20,840 live-born babies from ART procedures done in 1996 (25). The increase in the number of live-born infants conceived by ART reflects an increase in the number of cycles as well as in the per-cycle success rate. For cycles that use the woman's own fresh (i.e., nonfrozen) eggs or embryos, the likelihood of a live birth decreases as the woman's age increases. In 2004 in the United States, the per-cycle likelihood of a live birth was 43% for women aged <35, 36% for those aged 35–37, 25% for 38–40, 15% for 41–42, and 6% for ≥42 (25). In 2004, of all the deliveries resulting in live-born infants who were conceived from ART using fresh, nondonor eggs, approximately one-third (33%) were multiple gestations. Of all live infants in the United States in 2004, more than 1% were conceived with ART.

Geographic variability: Data from Europe for 2001 show that, in 23 countries where all clinics reported ART, 289,690 cycles were performed in a population of nearly 106 million. These countries include Belgium, Bulgaria, Denmark, Finland, France, Germany, Greece, Hungary, Iceland, Ireland, Italy, Latvia, The Netherlands, Norway, Poland, Portugal, Russia, Slovenia, Spain, Sweden, Switzerland, United Kingdom, and Ukraine. The number of cycles in these countries exceeds those performed in the United States in 2001 (107,587), a country with more than two-and-half times larger population. The 2001 ART cycles using fresh, nondonor cycles and excluding cycles from France, Iceland, and the Netherlands resulted in 30,609 live births, which represented 1.6% of the births in these European countries. Of live-born infants conceived with IVF and intracytoplasmic sperm injection (ICSI), 75% were singletons (37, 38).

Demographic variability: Data from the NFSG show that, in 2002, use of any service to treat infertility rose with age and was greatest for older, childless women. Receipt of infertility services was more common among childless married women, non-Hispanic White women, and women with higher levels of education and income. Among White women with at least one birth, nearly one out of five received infertility services, a very high level of service receipt compared with other groups (16).

NSFG data from 2002 also show that use of infertility services increased with income. Among women whose income was 0–149% of the poverty level, only 9% had used an infertility service; among those at or above 300% of the poverty level, 18% had used an infertility service (16). This pattern may reflect the absence of insurance coverage for many types of infertility treatment. As a result, most couples must pay out-of-pocket for infertility services. An encouraging observation is that, of couples referred for IVF, ~2–12% conceive spontaneously per year (39).

2.3.3 Public Health Interventions and Their Availability and Use

Public health interventions: No population-based data for the United States are available on adverse outcomes for the woman herself resulting from ART. Thus, nothing is known about interventions to reduce these possible risks.

The most common adverse ART outcome for the infant is multiple gestation. The risk for a multiple gestation, especially a higher-order gestation (three or more fetuses) associated with ART is related to the number of embryos transferred. Because fertility drugs and IVF are expensive and may not be covered by insurance, providers often try to improve success rates at the risk of multiple gestations. For example, instead of transferring only two embryos, which eliminates the risk of higher-order gestations, providers will transfer three or more embryos.

Several analysts have observed that fewer embryos per cycle are transferred in states where insurance coverage for IVF is mandated, compared with states where coverage is not mandated (40, 41). Furthermore, states with insurance mandates have lower rates of multiple deliveries per ART birth (42). Thus, laws that mandate that health insurance cover ART may be an important public health policy intervention to reduce the number of higher-order multiple gestations (43).

Some European providers of ART have eliminated triplet and higher order births by limiting the number of embryos transferred to two (44). American health policy analysts have considered regulating the maximum number of embryos that can be transferred. Consensus on the merit of such a regulation, however, has not been achieved (45). Nonetheless, in 2006, the Society for Assisted Reproductive Technology recommended limiting the number of embryos transferred during in vitro procedures. Cost-effectiveness analysis has shown that, compared with transfer of two embryos, transfer of one embryo costs less, but is also less effective. Analysts conclude that society's choice between single or double embryo transfer depends on society's willingness to pay for an additional successful pregnancy (46, 47).

2.4 Pregnancy Intention

2.4.1 Definition, Measures, Data Sources, and Measurement Issues

Definition: The desirability of conception. Note that *pregnancy* intention differs from *birth* intention: A pregnancy may begin with an unintended conception, but result in an intended and desired birth. Some (but not all) researchers distinguish between an unintended pregnancy and an unplanned pregnancy. They define an unintended pregnancy as a pregnancy that occurs while birth control is used or while the desire to become pregnant is absent (48). An unplanned pregnancy occurs in the absence of a definite plan to conceive a pregnancy (19). As such, it may reflect the ambiguity that many women – especially adolescents – and couples feel toward their pregnancies (49).

Table 2.4 Selected concepts related to unintended pregnancy and related method of measurement in interviews

Concept	Typical interview question
Timing of pregnancy	When you found out you were pregnant, did you want to be pregnant sooner, then, later, or at no time in the future?
Attitude toward pregnancy	When you first found out you were pregnant, were you happy, unhappy, or not sure how to feel about the pregnancy?
	Did you end your pregnancy in an abortion or did you consider having an abortion because you did not want to be pregnant?
Strength of desire to avoid pregnancy	When you first found out you were pregnant, did you definitely not want to be pregnant, were you trying to get pregnant, or were you neither trying to get pregnant nor avoiding pregnancy?
	At the time you conceived (name of child or "this pregnancy"), were you or your partner consistently using contraception, sometimes using it, or never using contraception?

Intention is a qualitative concept with a range of intensity (50). Intention is usually assessed from the perspective of the woman; however, it may also be assessed from the perspective of her partner, their joint perspective or society's perspective. Traditionally, the concept of pregnancy intention has been operationalized as a woman's attitude toward the timing of the pregnancy or birth, with unintended pregnancies often dichotomized as "mistimed" and "unwanted."

Measures: A number of measures of pregnancy intention have been developed (Table 2.4) (17, 48, 51–55). The only measure that has been collected nationally for the past several decades is that regarding timing of pregnancy.

In an in-depth study of measures of pregnancy intention among inner-city, mostly African-American women, analysts identified a single underlying latent construct, "pregnancy desirability" (54). This construct reflected happiness about the pregnancy, effort in achieving the pregnancy, and whether the respondent wanted to have a child with her partner. The generalizability of these findings to other groups of women has not been explored.

Data sources. Intention is usually assessed retrospectively through direct query to the woman. Depending on study design, queries about intention may be made at initiation of prenatal care, late in pregnancy, or days, weeks, or months after delivery. The NSFG collects retrospective national data on pregnancy intention. The Pregnancy Risk Assessment Monitoring System (PRAMS) collects state-specific data from women who are usually 4–6 months postpartum.

Measurement issues: Individual responses to subjective and complex questions regarding pregnancy intention likely vary widely among social groups and individuals and, within an individual, perhaps over time. Ambivalence or insufficient motivation to avoid pregnancy may dominate the attitudes of many women (53).

Results from a recent British study showed that women consistently identified four elements when defining a pregnancy as "planned": (1) intending to become pregnant; (2) stopping contraception; (3) partner agreement; and (4) right time in their life stage (56). This study also showed that women's definitions of an unplanned pregnancy varied widely. Women who report wanting their pregnancies later likely comprise a heterogeneous group, including those for whom the mistimed pregnancy has minor consequences and as well as those for whom it has major deleterious effects. For example, the consequences of a mistimed pregnancy for a woman who wanted to defer pregnancy for a few months to avoid the heat of the summer differs from those for a woman who wanted to defer pregnancy for several years so that she could complete her education. Unfortunately, most of the standard questions about pregnancy intention do not capture this heterogeneity.

A woman's perception of intention may vary during pregnancy and after delivery (57). Women who did not intend to become pregnant may change their views after delivery as they care for their newborn. Women may be reluctant to state that a pregnancy was unintended, especially if they perceive a societal expectation to have children. This reluctance may be more evident in face-to-face interviews, compared with self-administered questionnaires. Rates of unintended pregnancy reported by PRAMS (which collects data primarily by self-administered questionnaire) are higher than those reported by the 1995 NSFG (which primarily used face-to-face interviews for data collection). The concept of planning for the future, including planning pregnancies, may not be salient for all women, especially teens (55). Influenced by religion, culture, or social status, some women may have a fatalistic attitude toward accepting whatever happens in life.

Women who obtain an abortion are considered to have had an unintended and unwanted pregnancy. This assumption is usually correct. It does not hold, however, for the small percentage of abortions that are performed for fetal malformations or maternal health reasons. Women obtaining abortions comprise those with unwanted pregnancies as well as those with mistimed pregnancies.

Use of contraception is a poor measure of intention, because it may be influenced by many factors other than the woman's attitude toward becoming pregnant. These factors include a woman's views about contraception itself as well as about specific contraceptive methods, her ability to pay for contraception, her ability to obtain it (an issue especially important for teens), and her partner's attitude toward use of contraception. Women who use contraception presumably intend to avoid pregnancy. However, some women may use contraception for medical indications. Furthermore, one research report suggests that apparent contraceptive failures may result in intended pregnancies (58).

The role of the partner's view concerning pregnancy intention is an emerging area of study, as are the couple's concordance regarding the pregnancy's intention status and the consequences when the father does not intend the pregnancy (59, 60).

2.4.2 Descriptive Epidemiology

Temporal trends: Overall, in the United States, rates of unintended pregnancies (mistimed and unwanted pregnancies) were stable during the 1980s (54 per 1,000 women) and decreased by the early 1990s (45 per 1,000 women) (Table 2.5) (61). Data from the 2002 NSFG show that, among U.S. women aged 15–44 years in

Table 2.5 Estimated annual rate of unintended pregnancy per 1,000 women aged 15–44, by outcome, United States, 1981–2001

Year	Outcome		Total rate of unintended pregnancy
	Live birth	Abortion	
1981	25.0	29.2	54.2
1987	26.6	26.9	53.5
1994	20.9	24.1	45.0
2001	22.4	24.5	46.9

2001, the rate of unintended pregnancy was 51 per 1,000 (62). In practical terms, this means that, among pregnancies experienced by women aged 15–44 in the United States in 2001, 49% were unintended.

Among unintended pregnancies that result in birth, mistimed pregnancies are more common than unwanted pregnancies. Data from the 2002 NSFG concerning unintended births reveal that most (60%) are mistimed and would occur at a later time; the remaining 40% are unwanted (63).

Among women aged 15–44, the percentage of unintended pregnancies that end in induced abortion has been relatively stable, ranging from 50.3% in 1987, to 54.0% in 1994, and to 42% in 2001 (62). NSFG data for all pregnancies (except spontaneous abortions) that occurred in 2001 show 22% ended in unintended birth and 20% ended in induced abortion (62).

Among adult women in the United States in 1994, nearly half (48%) had experienced one or more unintended pregnancies in their lifetimes, demonstrating the high frequency of these events. Among women aged 15–44 in 1994, at some point in their lives, 26% had had a live birth resulting from an unintended pregnancy. Among this same population of women, 30% had had an abortion related to an unplanned pregnancy. Some women had multiple unintended pregnancies, of which some ended in live births and others in abortion (61). Similar patterns were observed in data collected by the 2002 NSFG (63).

PRAMS provides the only state-specific data for trends in unintended pregnancies resulting in live birth, but available data are limited to the states that conduct PRAMS. In 2002, New York City and 31 states conducted PRAMS, effectively representing 62% of all live births in the United States (64).

Taken in the aggregate, the distribution of state-specific rates has changed little over time, with the median state-specific percent of live births resulting from unintended pregnancies ranging from 42.5% in 1999 to 45.0% in 1997 and 1998 (Fig. 2.5). Data on the percentage of live births resulting from unintended pregnancies for each individual PRAMS state also show very little change from the 1990s through 2002 (65). The exceptions are West Virginia and North Carolina. West Virginia had a modest, but statistically significant decline ($p = 0.05$ and 0.709 for trend) from 42.0% in 1993 to 39.6% in 1999, but subsequently increased to 46.5% in 2001 and dropped to 41.7% in 2002. The percentage of live births resulting from unintended pregnancies in North Carolina declined from 47.6% in 1997 to 41.9% in

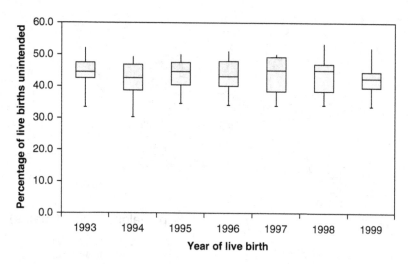

Fig. 2.5 Annual distribution of state-specific percentages of live births that were unintended at conception, PRAMS, 1993–1999 (Box plot of state-specific upper and lower values and 75th, 50th, and 25th percentiles)

1999, but rebounded to 45.3% in 2000 and again declined to 42.6% in 2001 and 40.6% in 2002 (64).

The distribution of the state-specific percentage of live births resulting from unwanted pregnancies showed little change during the 1990s, with median values ranging from 10.9% in 1994 to 12.4% in 1996 and subsequently increasing to 13.3% in 2002 (64).

Compared with data from the NSFG, PRAMS data show higher percentages of unintended pregnancies. This difference may reflect methodologic differences in the way the data were collected. PRAMS data consist mostly of self-reports, collected slightly more than a year after conception. NSFG data were derived from in-person interviews conducted up to 5 years after conception.

Using data from 1979 to 1981, one author estimated that "the typical woman will experience one contraceptive failure for every 2.25 births during her lifetime," concluding that unintended pregnancies are not uncommon relative to live births (68; pp. 222–223). Given lower fertility rates and higher rates for the prevalence of contraceptive use since this study was done, the ratio of the number of live births to unintended pregnancies is likely higher in recent years.

Geographic variability. In 1999, prevalences of unintended pregnancy were available from 17 states (Fig. 2.6 (65)). In general, states with lower general fertility rates tend to have lower prevalences of unintended pregnancy. Utah is an exception: In 1999, it had the lowest prevalence of unintended pregnancy – 33.7% – and the highest general fertility rate – 88.7 live births per 1,000 women aged 15–44. The pattern in Utah is likely due to the pronatalist views of the majority of the population.

High general fertility rates are often accompanied by high percentages of both pregnancies and live births that are unwanted (66). The United States manifests this

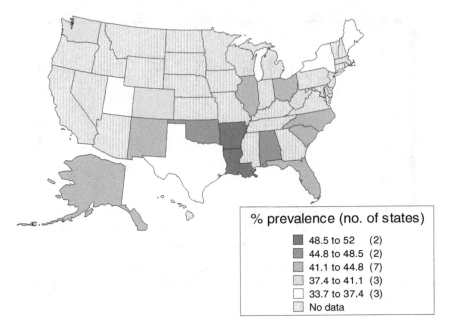

Fig. 2.6 Prevalence of unintended pregnancy among women aged 15–44 who delivered a live birth, by state, 1999

pattern: In addition to having a higher general fertility rate than many other industrialized countries, it has a higher percentage of unwanted pregnancies and live births resulting from unwanted pregnancies. In data compiled by the Global Health Council for 1995–2000, the estimated percent of pregnancies that were unwanted (measured from induced abortions and number of women who did not respond "yes" to the question, "Was your last birth wanted?") was as follows:

- 28% in the United States (accounting for 9.1% of all live births),
- 23% in France (accounting for 11% of all live births),
- 24% in Sweden (accounting for 5.0% of all live births),
- 21% in the United Kingdom (accounting for 6.0% of all live births),
- 50% in the Russian Federation (accounting for 11% of all live births), and
- 27% in Japan (accounting for 4.0% of all live births).

Differences among these countries in the percentage of live births resulting from unwanted pregnancies reflect, in part, differences in the use of induced abortion. The percentages of pregnancies that are unwanted vary widely among developing countries, ranging from 23% in India (accounting for 8.8% of all live births) to 28% in Egypt (accounting for 20.2% of all live births) and 41% in Brazil (accounting for 22.3% of all live births).

Demographic variability. Similar to fertility, pregnancy intention (measured as satisfaction with timing) varies by maternal attributes of age, parity, race and

Table 2.6 Rate of unintended pregnancy, percentage of unintended pregnancies ending in abortion, and percentage of women with a lifetime history of 1 or more unintended pregnancies, by age, NSFG, 2001

Age (years)	Rate of unintended pregnancy per 1,000 women	Percentage of unintended pregnancies ending in abortion	Percentage of women with lifetime history of ≥ 1 unintended pregnancies
15–19	67	40	12.2
20–24	104	49	41.4
25–29	71	50	55.1
30–34	44	49	59.2
35–39	20	60	60.0
≥ 40	6	56	50.4
Total	51	48	47.7

ethnicity, poverty, and marital status. Of these characteristics, age and parity are most consistently associated with pregnancy intention. Women aged less than 30 have higher rates of unintended pregnancy than older women, reflecting their higher overall fertility (Table 2.6) (62).

Older women generally have had more births than have younger women. Data from the 1988 NSFG show that the adjusted odds ratio for having a birth that was unwanted (compared with mistimed or intended) rises sharply with the number of previous births (67).

Non-White women and economically disadvantaged women consistently have higher rates of unintended pregnancy than other women. Among urban poor women in New York City who obtained pregnancy tests at public clinics from 1998 to 2001, a stunning 82% of those found to be pregnant reported that their pregnancies were unintended (68).

Although economic disparities may confound racial comparisons, racial differences persist even after controlling for economic status (61, 65, 67, 69). Black women have higher rates of unintended pregnancy than White women. Data from the 2002 NSFG show that, among births to Black non-Hispanic women aged 20–24 years, 52.9% were unintended. The comparable percentage among White non-Hispanic women was 41.5%. Hispanic women were intermediate at 46.5%. Data from California for 1999 and 2000 showed that, among births to Hispanic women born in the United States, a greater percentage were unintended than among Hispanic women born elsewhere, perhaps reflecting acculturation (69).

Age probably also reflects marital status, with younger women – especially teens – less likely to be married than older women. Data from the NSFG show that, in 2002, currently married women had a lower rate of unintended pregnancy (36.1 per 1,000 women aged 15–44 years) than formerly married, noncohabiting women (50.3 per 1,000) or currently cohabiting women (48.5 per 1,000) (16). Data from the 1994 NSFG showed that, among married women, a substantially lower percentage of unintended pregnancies ended in induced abortion (37.0%) compared with formerly married (65.1%) or never married women (60.1%) (61).

Data from women who responded to PRAMS surveys in 15 states in 1998 showed some differences in demographic attributes between women with unwanted and mistimed pregnancies resulting in live births (70). Risks for unwanted pregnancies were highest for women who were aged ≥ 35, not married, or Black, who had <12 years of education or a parity of ≥ 3, whose prenatal care was paid for by Medicaid, who experienced physical abuse during pregnancy, or who either had no or late initiation of prenatal care. Although many of these attributes were also associated with increased risks for mistimed pregnancies, patterns differed for age and parity. The risk of mistimed pregnancy was highest for women aged <20, with the next highest risk among women aged 20–24. The risk of mistimed pregnancy was *lowest* among women with parities ≥ 1.

. *Characteristics of women with unintended pregnancies*: In general, groups with high pregnancy rates also have a high percentage of pregnancies that are unintended. For example, in the United States in 2001, women aged 15–44 whose income was below the U.S. poverty level had a very high pregnancy rate – 182 per 1,000 – compared with women $\geq 200\%$ above the poverty level – 78 per 1,000. In addition to experiencing higher pregnancy rates than their more economically advantaged peers, women with income at or below the poverty line also had rates of unintended pregnancy (112 per 1,000 women) that were more than 3 times higher than rates for women with incomes that were at least twice the poverty line (62).

Most of the groups with high pregnancy rates include relatively few women and thus account for relatively small portions of the overall number of pregnancies. Exceptions are women aged 20–24 and 25–29 who have high overall pregnancy rates and account for a substantial percentage of all unintended pregnancies. Because of their predominance in the population, White, non-Hispanic, married women in their twenties account for the largest portion of both intended and unintended pregnancies.

2.4.3 Factors Influencing Occurrence, Related Public Health Interventions, and Their Availability and Use

Among sexually active individuals, the availability of contraception is essential for avoiding an unintended pregnancy. Section 2.6 describes factors that influence use of and access to contraception. Among women who conceive, but do not want to continue their pregnancies, the availability of legally induced abortion is essential. The next section addresses this issue.

Among sexually active women, intervals of nonuse of contraception are associated with high risk for pregnancy. Counseling by a health-care professional has been proposed as a factor that influences use of contraception. However, a recent review concluded: "Virtually no experimental or observational literature reliably answers questions about the effectiveness of counseling in the clinical setting to reduce rates of unintended pregnancies in this country" (71).

One study examined the effect of preconception care among women attending health department clinics (72). The authors observed that, in subsequent pregnancies, women who had received preconception care as part of a previous routine family planning visit had a higher percentage of intended pregnancies than those who had not received preconception counseling. Despite this improvement, only 22% of the women in the preconception care group had an intended pregnancy.

2.5   Legal Induced Abortion

2.5.1   Definition, Measures, Data Sources, and Measurement Issues

Definition: Legal induced abortion includes any pharmacologic or surgical treatment with the aim of terminating a pregnancy. In the United States, a legal abortion is one performed by a licensed physician or someone acting under the supervision of a licensed physician. Abortions are usually performed during the first trimester of pregnancy or early in the second trimester of pregnancy. In 2003, only 4.2% of all abortions were performed at 16–20 weeks and 1.4% at ≥ 21 weeks (73). Therapeutic abortions are induced abortions performed to protect the health of the mother. Although abortion is legal in the United States, illegal or self-induced abortions may occur, but probably are rare.

Measures: The legal abortion rate (number of abortions in a year per 1,000 females aged 15–44) estimates the likelihood that a woman of reproductive age will have an abortion within a specified interval, usually a year. In the United States, data are available only on the total number of abortions, not the number of women who have abortions. Because a small number of women have more than one abortion in a year, the legal abortion rate slightly overestimates a woman's likelihood of having at least one legal abortion. The legal abortion rate is influenced by the general fertility rate and the unintended pregnancy rate. Groups with low general fertility rates are likely to have low abortion rates, simply because few pregnancies occur to be at risk of abortion. Groups with high unintended pregnancy rates tend to have high abortion rates.

The abortion ratio (the number of induced abortions per 1,000 live births) reflects the likelihood that, if a pregnancy occurs, it will end in abortion. Because spontaneous abortions are not ascertained, analysts cannot count the total number of pregnancies. Thus, analysts cannot compute the portion of pregnancies that ended by induced abortion.

Data sources: In the United States, legal induced abortions are vital events, subject to registration in most states (74). Although the NCHS collected vital records for abortions from 15 states through 1993, budget constraints curtailed this program. Since then, only the Division of Reproductive Health of the CDC and the Alan Guttmacher Institute have collected national and state-specific abortion data. Although the number of participating areas varies slightly from year-to-year, the CDC annually collects tabulations (i.e., aggregate data, not individual reports) of abortions from nearly all of the states and reporting areas. Data from the largest state, California, are not reported to the CDC. The Alan Guttmacher Institute surveys all abortion providers directly and generally reports a higher (and possibly more accurate) number of abortions than the CDC. Because of privacy concerns, no abortion data include personally identifying information. Thus, repeat abortions obtained by the same woman in one calendar year cannot be identified.

The number of induced abortions as well as the number of women who obtained an abortion can also be estimated from the NSFG, which is conducted periodically by the NCHS. In face-to-face interviews, women report their reproductive events during the preceding 5 years. However, the value of these data are limited, because women report only about half of their induced abortions (75, 76).

The denominator for the abortion rate derives from the mid-year population estimate based on the Current Population Survey. This estimate is available from the Web site for the U.S. Census.

Measurement issues: Abortion providers may underreport the number of legal abortions, especially those performed pharmacologically. The availability and use of pharmacologic means of inducing abortion greatly expanded in the 1990s. Before the 1990s, abortions were performed surgically. Because of temporal differences in completeness of ascertainment of induced abortion, trends in abortion from the 1970s through the 1990s may not be valid.

Underascertainment of induced abortions may result from respondents' failure to disclose past induced abortions (74–76). Thus, data from the NSFG underestimate the true number of induced abortions as well as the number of women who have obtained induced abortions. Aside from data from the NSFG, no data are available to estimate the number of women who have obtained one, two, or multiple induced abortions in a calendar year.

Because abortion providers are not available in all areas, women may travel from their state of residence to another state to obtain abortion services. Abortion rates computed by state of occurrence may overestimate rates for states with higher numbers of abortion providers and underestimate rates for states with few or no abortion providers (81).

2.5.2   Descriptive Epidemiology

Temporal trends: In recent years, the U.S. abortion rate has been stable. Using available data from the United States, the District of Columbia and New York City, the CDC computed a national abortion rate of 17 per 1,000 women aged 15–44 years in 1999, unchanged from 1997 and 1998. The rate declined to 16 per 1,000 in 2003. The CDC computed national abortion ratios of 256 per 1,000 live births in 1999, 245 in 2000, and 241 per 1,000 in 2003, reflecting declines from the peak ratio of 364 per 1,000 in 1984 (73, 77–79).

The Alan Guttmacher Institute, using data from surveys of abortion providers, estimated that 1,287,000 abortions were performed in 2003, representing an annual rate of 20.8 per 1,000 women aged 15–44 (80). In 2003, 23.8% of all pregnancies –

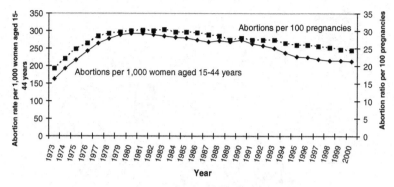

Note: Pregnancies ending in live birth or abortion. Data source: Finer & Henshaw, 2006b

Fig. 2.7 Abortion rate and ratio, United States, 1973–2000

excluding fetal losses – ended in abortion. Data from the Alan Guttmacher institute showed similar trends to those observed by the CDC (Fig. 2.7).

CDC surveillance data show that abortions are not rare. This observation is reinforced by data from the NSFG showing that in 1992 an estimated 43% of women had at least one abortion by age 35–39. This percentage is slightly lower than the estimated 45% of women in this age group who, in 1982, had one or more abortions (61).

Geographic variability: Within the United States for 2001, abortion rates vary widely (Fig. 2.8). For 2003, Idaho, North Dakota, South Dakota, Kentucky, Wyoming, and Utah had low abortion rates of 6–8 per 1,000 resident women aged 15–44. New York had the highest abortion rate of 29 and the District of Columbia had the next highest rate of 24, followed by rates of 19 in Delaware, Nevada, and Washington. Geographic variation in abortion ratios followed a similar pattern to that observed for abortion rates (73).

Access to abortion services may influence abortion rates. Between 1992 and 2000 in the United States, the number of abortion providers declined 24% from 2,380 to 1,819. By 2000, 34% of women aged 15–44 lived in a county without an abortion provider (81). U.S. abortion providers who were surveyed in 2001–2002 estimated that approximately 25% of women who had abortions in non-hospital facilities traveled more than 50 miles to the facility (82).

Data for 2003 for three related measures – the abortion, unintended pregnancy, and general fertility rates – for selected states (Table 2.7) suggest that the relationships between abortion, pregnancy intention, and fertility vary among states. For example, Maine has relatively low rates of abortion, unintended pregnancy, and general fertility. Despite its very high fertility rate, Utah also has low rates of abortion and unintended pregnancy. Colorado has a low abortion rate despite a mid-range rate of unintended pregnancy and Washington has a high abortion rate, despite mid-range unintended pregnancy and general fertility rates.

International comparisons: During the 1990s, the United States had higher abortion rates than nearly all comparable industrialized countries (83). In 1996,

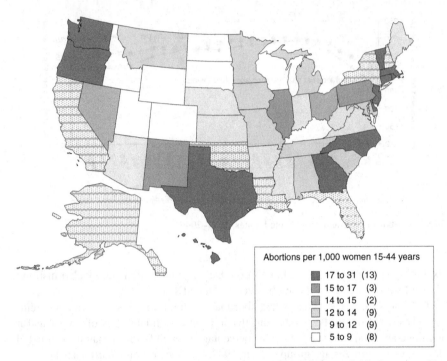

Fig. 2.8 Abortion rates and ratios, by state, United States, 2001. Data unavailable for states with horizontal lines and stippling. Source: (79)

Table 2.7 Abortion,[a] unintended pregnancy, and general fertility rates, selected states, 2003

State	Abortion rate (abortions per 1,000 women aged 15–44 years)	Unintended pregnancy rate (%)	General fertility rate (live births per 1,000 women aged 15–44 years)
Colorado	9	39.7	68.8
West Virginia	NA	39.6	58.3
Utah	6	33.7	92.3
Maine	9	34.0	52.4
Arkansas	10	49.6	68.3
Alabama	11	47.4	62.4
South Carolina	13	44.4	63.6
Ohio	14	41.3	62.7
New Mexico	16	43.6	71.9
Illinois	15	44.5	66.7
North Carolina	15	41.9	66.0
Washington	19	38.0	61.7

[a] Abortions counted by woman's state of residence. NA: not available.

when the U.S. abortion rate was 22.9 per 1,000 women aged 15–44, abortion rates in other selected countries were:

Australia – 22.2
Canada – 16.4
Denmark – 16.5
England and Wales – 15.6
Germany – 7.6
Holland – 6.5
Sweden – 18.7

European countries have used mifepristone for early medical abortions for more than a decade. This contrasts with the United States, where the Food and Drug Administration approved mifepristone much more recently in 2000. In the United States and France, it is approved for use up to 49 days from the onset of a woman's last menstrual period. In Great Britain and Sweden, this period extends to 63 days. Experience from Europe shows wide variation in its use. In 2000 in England and Wales, clinicians used mifepristone for slightly less than 20% of eligible abortions; the comparable percentage in Scotland was 60%. Mifepristone appears not to have influenced the overall rate of abortions in the United States (84).

Demographic variability: Abortion rates and ratios vary by the woman's age, marital status, and race (Table 2.8) (73). In 2003, abortion rates were highest for women in their twenties, reflecting their overall high fertility. In comparison, rates were lower for younger women and much lower for older women.

Table 2.8 Abortion rates and ratios by attributes of the woman, selected states, 2003 (source: (73))

Maternal attribute		Abortions per 1,000 women	Abortions per 1,000 live births
Age (years)	15–19	16	374
	20–24	31	300
	25–29	23	195
	30–34	14	144
	35–39	7	173
	$\geq$40	3	293
Race	White	10	165
	Black	29	491
Ethnicity	Hispanic	23	228
	Non-Hispanic	14	234
Marital Status	Married	–	63
	Unmarried	–	538
Number of previous live births	0	–	227
	1	–	190
	2	–	271
	3	–	283
	$\geq$4	–	234

In contrast to abortion rates, abortion *ratios* were highest at the extremes of maternal age. Thus, although fewer women in these age groups became pregnant, those who became pregnant were more likely to end their pregnancies in abortion than were women of other ages.

In 2003, the abortion ratio was more than eight times higher for unmarried women (i.e., women who were never married, divorced, or widowed) than for married women.

Abortion rates and ratios also vary strikingly by race. In 2003, the abortion ratio for Black women was nearly 3 times greater than that for White women.

The abortion ratio varies modestly by the woman's number of previous live births, being lowest for women with either one previous live birth or more than three previous births and highest for women with no, two, or three previous live births (73).

Characteristics of women having abortions: Available surveillance show that, from the late 1990s through 2003 in the United States, women aged 25 and above obtained approximately half of all legal abortions (21, 79). In 2003, 16% of the women who obtained abortions were teens. More than half of the women who obtained abortions from 1995 to 1999 were White, more than 80% of whom were unmarried. In 1999, 41% of women obtaining abortions had no live births and 28% had one live birth.

Abortions performed at shorter gestations have a lower risk for complications than those performed at longer gestations, especially after 15 weeks (85). In the United States, the percentage of women obtaining abortion at 8 or fewer weeks of gestation has increased steadily from 52% in 1990 to 59% in 2003 (21). CDC data for 2003 show that 19% of abortions occurred at 9–10 weeks, and 10% at 11–12 weeks. Less than 2% occurred after 20 weeks of gestation. In recent years, nearly all abortions (96%) were performed by suction curettage (78, 79).

A survey of a nationally representative sample of 10,683 women who received abortions in 2000 showed that more than half (54%) used contraception in the cycle they conceived. Among demographic subgroups, the percentage of women not using contraception when they conceived was highest for women who were <25-years old, not married, and Black or Hispanic as well as those whose income was ≤300% of the poverty level, and who had ≤12 years of education. Overall, 14% of respondents indicated that they conceived despite perfect contraceptive use (86).

2.5.3 Risk Factors, Related Public Health Interventions, and Their Availability and Use

The key to preventing abortion is preventing unintended pregnancy. Public health interventions to reduce unintended pregnancy are discussed in Section 2.6.

Promoting early recognition of pregnancy and insuring access to legal abortion are essential for reducing morbidity and mortality associated with abortion. No public health interventions aimed at promoting early recognition of pregnancy have been assessed rigorously. The widespread availability of over-the-counter home test kits to detect pregnancy has doubtless increased early recognition.

The importance of maintaining legal access to abortion has been demonstrated empirically by the marked drop in abortion-related mortality that followed national legalization of abortion in 1974 (78). In 1972, 65 abortion-related deaths occurred, of which 39 were attributed to illegal abortion. Of the 47 abortion-related deaths in 1973, 19 were attributed to illegal abortions. During the 1990s, 5–12 abortion-related deaths occurred per year in the entire United States. Nearly all of these deaths resulted from legal abortions, suggesting that mortality associated with illegal abortions has been virtually eliminated.

Access to first trimester abortion, when the procedure is safest, can be limited by procedural and financial barriers as well as a shrinking number of abortion providers. Minimizing these barriers promotes early abortions. A study in Mississippi examined the effect of the introduction of a legal requirement for a 24 hour delay in abortion after the initial request. This requirement increased the percentage of abortions performed after 12 weeks of gestation (87). Reductions in federal and state funding for abortion have limited the ability of low-income women to obtain abortions. A study of health professionals who provided abortion in 2001 and 2002 noted that 56% reported experiencing anti-abortion harassment in 2000 (82). Such harassment can deter providers from beginning or continuing to perform abortions. Fewer providers can result in delays in obtaining abortions.

Figure 2.9 depicts the circumstances under which pregnancies originate and relates these circumstances to ways that pregnancies can resolve. The distribution of pregnancies by origin as well as the distribution of pregnancies by resolution change over time, reflecting medical interventions and societal norms.

Why should public health practitioners care about contraception?

Lack of use of contraception is the single most important preventable factor in the occurrence of unintended pregnancies. The risks for both maternal and infant morbidity and mortality are higher for women whose pregnancies are unintended than for women whose pregnancies are intended.

Unintended pregnancies resulting from lack of use of contraception are not rare. Among active duty women in the U.S. Air Force during 2001, an estimated 3.5% had an unintended pregnancy secondary to nonuse (88). In California, from 1998 to 2001, approximately 4.5% of women of reproductive age were at risk of unintended pregnancy, due to lack of use of contraception (89).

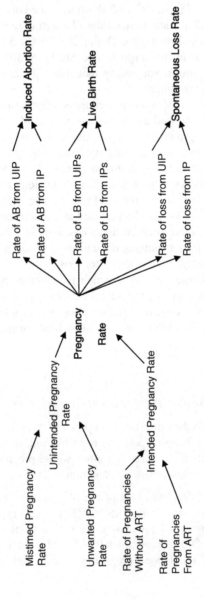

All rates per 1,000 pregnancies

Abbreviations: AB – abortion, IP – intented pregnancy, UIP – unitendend pregnancy, ART – assisted reproductive technology

Fig. 2.9 Summary diagram of pregnancy origins and outcomes

2.6   Contraception

2.6.1   Definition, Measures, Data Sources, and Measurement Issues

Definition: Any intervention that has the goal of preventing conception or implantation of a fertilized egg. Methods may be behavioral (e.g., coitus interruptus), pharmacological (e.g., hormonal control of ovulation or prevention of implantation), mechanical (e.g., intrauterine device, diaphragm, condom), or surgical (e.g., tubal ligation, vasectomy). Contraception is often categorized as either reversible or permanent (i.e., sterilization). One or both partners may use contraception.

In practice, studies consider the use of contraception among persons who are sexually active, at risk of pregnancy (e.g., not currently pregnant or sterile), and not desiring pregnancy. For a given interval, individuals may use contraception all of the time, some of the time, or never. The manner in which they use contraception may be correct always, some of the time, or never. "Ideal" use assumes consistent and correct use. Because ideal use rarely occurs, most analysts refer to "typical" use, which incorporates the concept of inconsistent and/or incorrect use some of the time.

Measures: The most relevant measure is the percentage of sexually active individuals not desiring pregnancy and at risk of pregnancy who consistently and correctly use (or whose partner uses) one or more contraceptive methods during a specified time interval. Measures of contraceptive use that include persons not at risk for pregnancy will underestimate relevant contraceptive use because the denominator will be inflated incorrectly.

Data sources: Use of a method is usually ascertained by questioning the respondent about her or his current or past practices and the concurrent practices of her or his partner. When asking about past practices, responses may be more accurate when respondents first use a calendar to recall their life situation (e.g., where they lived, their major activities, the people who were important in their lives, and their health insurance). Researchers can then ask questions about contraceptive use in the context of that situation.

The only nationally-representative survey to collect data on contraceptive use is the NSFG, most recently conducted in 1995 and 2002. No comparable population-wide, state-specific data are available. Survey data for selected states are available, however, for their subpopulations of women who have recently had a live birth (through CDC's Pregnancy Risk Assessment Monitoring System, (PRAMS)) and high school students (through CDC's Youth Risk Behavioral Surveillance System (YRBSS)).

Sales information (e.g., condom sales) and administrative records (e.g., prescriptions for oral contraceptives, surgical sterilization procedures) provide data for estimating rates of contraceptive use. However, these data are frequently difficult to interpret.

Measurement issues: For social or religious reasons, respondents may not disclose contraceptive practices. Furthermore, a respondent may not be aware of the true contraceptive status of her or his partner.

For contraceptive methods that are temporary, technique and consistency of use may alter efficacy. Information about these aspects of use, however, is difficult to obtain retrospectively. A respondent may not be knowledgeable about her or his partner's consistency of use or technique of use.

Although sterilization data provide a numerator, a corresponding denominator equal to the number of persons eligible to be sterilized (i.e., persons who have not already been sterilized or whose partner has not been sterilized) is unknown. Thus, a true sterilization rate cannot be determined. Although an individual may fill a prescription, she may not use it consistently, which, in the case of oral contraceptives, can greatly reduce efficacy. Family planning programs that use federal Title X funds collect data on the annual number of visits and selected characteristics of persons served and their attributes (96). Analysts cannot use these data to compute rates, however, because they cannot be linked to a denominator of people eligible for and needing services.

2.6.2   Descriptive Epidemiology

Temporal trends: Data from the NSFG provide the only source of long-term national trends in contraceptive use. State-specific data on trends in contraceptive use are not available. During the past two decades, the percentage of all women aged 15–44 using contraception during the 3 months before interview increased from 56% (1982) to 64% (1995), subsequently declining to 62% (2002) (90). Among sexually active women at risk of pregnancy, the percentage not using contraception during the 3 months before interview decreased from 12% (1982) to 7.5% (1995), but increased again to 11% (2002). In contrast, use of contraception at first premarital intercourse has steadily increased during the past two decades. Among women whose first intercourse occurred during the 1980s, 61% used contraception. This percentage increased to 73% by 1995–1998 and 79% by 1999–2002.

Geographic variability: Although variations in survey methods preclude precisely quantifying differences in contraceptive use among countries, general patterns emerge. International data show wide variation in the prevalence of contraceptive use, with rates generally – but not always – highest in developed countries. For example, among developed countries, recent (1997–2003) prevalence rates of contraceptive use (6) among women aged 15–44 are:

China – 87%
Egypt – 59%
India – 47%

Japan – 56%
Mexico – 74%
Peru – 71%
Philippines – 49%
South Africa – 60%
UK – 84%
USA – 76%

For many developing countries, rates range from less than 10% (e.g., Angola, Ethiopia, Sierra Leone) to mid-range prevalences of 20–50% (e.g., Haiti – 28%, Kenya – 39%, Malawi – 33%). Prevalence rates in less-developed countries vary widely, ranging from 40–65% (e.g., India – 47%) to ≥70% (e.g., Brazil – 77%, China – 87%, Columbia – 78%, Mexico – 74%, Viet Nam – 77%).

Demographic variability. In the United States in 2002, the prevalence of contraceptive use among sexually active women aged 15–44 who were at risk of unintended pregnancy increased modestly with age from a low of 82.0% for women aged 15–19 to 89.5% for those aged 25–29 and 90.2% for those aged 35–29 (90). Contraceptive use also varied modestly by marital status (lowest among never married non-cohabitating women – 83.8%, and highest among married women – 92.0%), race and ethnicity (lowest for non-Hispanic Blacks – 84.9%, intermediate for Hispanics – 88.4, and highest for non-Hispanic Whites – 90.6), and intention to have more children (lowest among those intending to have more children – 85.7%, and highest among those not intending to have more children – 91.7%). Contraceptive use varied negligibly by education or income (90).

Patterns of contraceptive use. Data from the NSFG show that, of all women aged 15–44 who used contraception in 2002, the distribution of women by primary method was:

- 30.6% – contraceptive pills,
- 27.0% – female sterilization,
- 18.0% – condoms,
- 9.2% – male sterilization,
- 5.3% – 3-month injectables (Depo-Provera), and
- 9.9% – other methods.

The percentages of women using contraceptive pills and female sterilization differed little between 1982 and 2002 (90). Specific information about postcoital contraception (so-called "emergency contraception") has not been reported from the 2002 NSFG.

2.6.3 Factors Influencing Use and Related Public Health Interventions, and Their Use and Availability

All methods of contraception, including emergency contraception, are cost-effective in reducing unintended pregnancies (91–94). Although evidence to support the efficacy of counseling by health professionals to prevent unintended pregnancy is inconsistent (71), in 1996 the U.S. Task Force on Clinical Preventive Services recommended "periodic counseling about effective contraceptive methods" for all men and women at risk of unintended pregnancy (101).

Among the myriad factors influencing use of contraception among women not desiring pregnancy are occurrence of side effects as well as fears about potential side effects, partner's attitudes, availability, cost, awareness of contraceptive options, and the woman's own ability to use a method correctly and consistently. Public health interventions have largely focused on decreasing financial barriers to contraception and increasing knowledge of it. Nonetheless, a study of services provided by publicly funded family planning agencies from 1995 through 2003 documented persistent increases in costs for services (95). Two studies examining the impact of publicly-funded family planning services concluded that the widespread availability of these services decreases the rates of unintended pregnancy and its sequelae: abortion and unintended birth (96, 97). No comparable studies have examined the impact of insurance coverage for contraception among privately insured women. One can expect that by decreasing financial barriers to contraception, insurance coverage for it would be associated with greater rates of use and lower rates of unintended pregnancy.

In 2001, seventeen states required private insurers to provide comprehensive coverage for contraception (105). These mandates are often referred to as "contraceptive equity" laws. A study conducted in 2001–2002 compared insurance coverage for contraceptives between states with and without contraceptive equity laws. The results showed that, in states with such laws, the percentage of insurance plans covering contraception was significantly higher (with coverage ranging from 87% to 92%, depending on type of insurance plan) than in states without these laws (contraceptive coverage ranging from 47% to 61% of plans) (98).

Most public health interventions to increase contraceptive use among persons not desiring pregnancy have focused on preventing teen pregnancy, with emphasis on school-based sex education and youth development. Data from the 2002 NSFG show that, among adolescents aged 15–19, 66.2% of boys and 69.9% of girls had received formal instruction on methods of birth control (99). A trend toward "abstinence only" sex education (i.e., education that presents only abstinence as a way to prevent pregnancy) (100) and laws requiring parental notification before minors can receive contraceptives may hinder public health efforts to increase contraceptive use among sexually active youth (101, 102).

Providing postcoital (emergency) contraceptive services is an intervention that is relevant regardless of a woman's age. Emergency contraception involves treatment with pills containing hormones. It is available in the United States by prescription only. Many public health professionals judge that the general population's knowledge of emergency contraception is limited. The question of whether increasing the public's knowledge will increase their use of it, with a concomitant reduction in unintended pregnancy, is unanswered. As a first step in addressing this issue, in 1997 and 1998, researchers examined whether a media campaign could increase the public's knowledge of emergency contraception (103). Using a pre–post evaluation design, they observed an increase in knowledge of emergency contraception as well as an increase in calls to emergency contraception hot-lines. Equally important, television advertisements for postcoital contraception did not spark public controversy.

However, experience in Scotland suggests that attempts at widespread advance distribution of emergency contraception may not reduce rates of unintended pregnancy – as long as emergency contraception is available by prescription only. During 2000–2001, when emergency contraception was available by prescription only, investigators conducted widespread media campaigns encouraging women to request emergency contraception – which was available for free – from their health-care providers. The investigators used the rate of induced abortions as a surrogate measure of the rate of unintended pregnancy. They observed no difference in the rate of abortion between the target area and other areas in Scotland. Qualitative investigation showed that, despite the media campaigns, both providers and women were reluctant to discuss emergency contraception (104, 105).

From these observations, one can conclude that the benefits of emergency contraception are unlikely to be realized unless access to it is less restricted. This conclusion is especially relevant to regulatory decisions in the United States. In 2004, the U.S. Food and Drug Administration (FDA) considered whether emergency contraception should be available "over the counter", i.e., without prescription. Although a nongovernmental advisory group recommended over the counter availability, the FDA opted not to accept this recommendation (106).

2.7 Preconception Care

2.7.1 Definition, Measures, Data Sources, and Measurement Issues

Definition: Care that is provided before conception and that has the aim of improving maternal and/or infant health during and after pregnancy. This care includes a broad range of behavioral, pharmacological, and counseling interventions (107–112). Interventions may include treating acute and chronic maternal diseases (e.g., hypertension, diabetes, or anemia); assessing immunization status; supporting smoking cessation; providing folic acid supplementation; and counseling. Counseling may inform prospective parents of pregnancy-related risks for the mother or fetus (e.g., advanced maternal age).

Measures: Perhaps the best measure is receipt of indicated components of preconception care. Note that some of the components vary among couples, reflecting variations in health status. For example, a woman with diabetes would be asked if, before her pregnancy, she received care for her diabetes with the aim of improving the outcome of her pregnancy for herself and her baby. Thus, investigators must obtain sufficient information about the respondent's preconception health status to determine the components of preconception care that she should have received. Using this information, an investigator can ask whether each component was received.

In addition to ascertaining treatment for medical conditions, measures of preconception care should also assess receipt of counseling to optimize maternal health, for example, counseling to achieve optimal body weight and stop tobacco and alcohol use. Measures should assess components of preconception care that are universally recommended (e.g. use of folic acid supplements).

Data sources: In general, data are sparse. Receipt of preconception care (including periconceptional use of folic acid supplements) is usually ascertained retrospectively by inquiry to pregnant or postpartum women. Some of the states participating in PRAMS may collect limited data on preconception counseling. Internationally, data are collected from periodic surveys.

Measurement issues: Accurate measurement is difficult because a uniform definition of preconception care does not exist. In addition, respondents may not recognize or remember that they received preconception care. Some aspects of preconception care must be tailored to the woman's preconception health status. Without information about this status, the adequacy of preconception care cannot be fully assessed. Recollection of preconception care is especially problematic when the interval between receipt of preconception care and conception is long. For example, a long interval may occur for women with infertility.

Use of administrative data to measure receipt of preconception care is limited by the lack of a Current Procedural Terminology (CPT) code distinguishing visits for this reason (CPT codes are industry-wide codes used for billing and insurance reimbursement for outpatient health care). To measure the impact of preconception care, investigators must ascertain the extent to which the respondent followed the recommendations or treatment plan that she received.

2.7.2   Descriptive Epidemiology

Temporal trends: Except for information about periconceptional use of folic acid supplements, data on preconception care are sparse. Data from the National Health and Nutrition Examination Surveys (NHANES) show marked increases in the median serum and red blood cell folate concentrations for women aged 15–44 from 1988–1994 to 1999–2000 (113). Most of this increase probably reflects food fortification and so is independent of preconception counseling. According to nationally representative surveys by the March of Dimes, the percentage of non-pregnant women aged 18–45 who took a daily vitamin supplement containing folic acid increased from 25% in 1995 to 32% in 2000 and 31% in 2002. Many of these women may take the supplement to maintain general good health. This possibility is consistent with the low level of awareness of the U.S. Public Health Services' recommendation for folic acid supplementation among child-bearing women. In 2002 only 10% of such women knew that folic acid should be taken before pregnancy (2002).

Data from the national Behavioral Risk Factor Surveillance System for 2004 show that, among women aged 18–44 who were not pregnant, more than half had behaviors that increased their risks for an adverse pregnancy outcome. Nearly half of the nonpregnant reproductive-age women from 12 selected states in 2004 said that they "didn't know about folic acid for birth defects prevention" (114).

Geographic variability. In the absence of a uniform definition of preconception care, comparisons among states or countries are difficult to interpret. Because periconceptional supplementation with folic acid is universally recommended, it provides a crude measure of at least one component of preconception care. Data for 1998 from 12 states participating in the Pregnancy Risk Assessment Monitoring System show a relatively modest range in the percentage of new mothers who were aware of folic acid and its benefits: 66.4%–83.4% (115). Most but not all of these states showed an increasing trend in awareness.

Demographic variability: Recent reports have shown wide variation in awareness of the benefits of folic acid supplementation (115, 116). In general, awareness is lowest for women who are unmarried, aged less than 30, or in a minority group, or who have less than 12 years of education, a low income, or an unintended pregnancy (117).

2.7.3 Public Health Interventions and Their Availability and Use

Nearly all public health interventions related to preconception health have sought to increase periconceptional folic acid intake, either by fortifying foods (primarily cereals and breads) with folic acid or promoting intake of vitamin supplements that contain folic acid. The benefits of food fortification have been marked. Investigators observed a 31% reduction in the United States in the prevalence of spina bifida from 1995–1996 (pre-folic acid fortification) to 1998–1999 (post-folic acid fortification) (118). Investigators reported a similar impact in Canada of food fortification with folic acid (119).

In 1992, the U.S. Public Health Service recommended that women of reproductive age at risk of pregnancy take supplements that include folic acid (1992). A report issued in 2003 by the Association of State and Territorial Health Officials ("State Efforts to Increase Folic Acid Consumption and Reduce Neural Tube Defects") reviewed public health approaches to increasing periconceptional supplementation with folic acid. These approaches include into those focusing on women and those focusing on their health-care providers.

A study conducted in 1999–2000 in California evaluated the impact of mailing multivitamin supplements containing folic acid to members of a health-care organization. After an initial increase in supplement use, the prevalence of use returned to prestudy levels, showing no impact of the intervention (120). In the same study, investigators also failed to observe an impact of education about the benefits of folic acid supplementation that was administered by providers to female patients.

State health departments have established media campaigns and school education programs aimed at increasing women's knowledge of the importance of folic acid supplementation. Mass mailings to health-care providers have been implemented to educate them about the need to counsel women regarding folic acid supplementation. An assessment of an educational campaign aimed at health-care providers in Florida showed improvements in their knowledge of periconceptional folic acid and the self-reported frequency with which they recommended it to patients (35).

A Danish study examined the cost-effectiveness of preconception care aimed at smoking cessation and folic acid supplementation. The researchers concluded that preconception care was not cost effective when only smoking-related morbidity and neural tube defects were considered. The researchers suggested that preconception care may have a net positive benefit if prevention of other adverse pregnancy outcomes is taken into account (121).

Discussion Topics

1. What factors likely influence whether an individual or couple seeks medical care for infertility? How prevalent are they?
2. How could increased availability of treatment for infertility influence pregnancy outcomes?
3. What factors account for differences in fertility among developing countries?
4. What are the implications of the fertility rate for pregnancy outcome?
5. Can demographic attributes account for state-specific differences in fertility, unintended pregnancy, and abortion rates? If not, what other factors are important?
6. What factors could explain a discrepancy between the percentage of women with infertility, as measured from population-based surveys, and the percentage of women who have ever sought infertility services (as measured from the NSFG)?
7. Why are data on sales of contraceptives and prescriptions for contraceptives difficult to interpret when considering (a) prevalence of contraceptive use and (b) trends in contraceptive use?

Promising Areas for Future Research

1. Development of methods to measure population-wide adverse effects to the women of infertility treatment.
2. Surveys of male views on pregnancy intention.
3. Development of methods to measure population-wide provision and impact of preconception care.

Abbreviations

ART   Assisted reproductive technology
CDC   Centers for Disease Control and Prevention
CPT   Current procedural terminology
IVF   In vitro fertilization
NCHS   National Center for Health Statistics
NSFG   National Survey of Family Growth

References

1. Patient Plus. (15 April 2007). Gravidity and partiy in pregnancy.
2. National Center for Health Statistics. National Survey of Family Growth. (15 April 2007). Fecundity Status.
3. Pennsylvania Department of Health. (15 April 2007). Tools of the trade. Definitions used in public health assessment.
4. Hamilton, B. E. (2004). Reproduction rates for 1990–2002 and intrinsic rates for 2000–2001: United States. *Natl. Vital Stat. Rep., 52(17),* 1–12.
5. Last, J. M., et al. (2001). *A Dictionary of Epidemiology* (4th ed.). New York: Oxford University Press.
6. Martin, J. A., Hamilton, B. E., Sutton, P. D., Ventura, S. J., Menacker, F., & Kirmeyer, S. (2006). Births: final data for 2004. *Natl. Vital Stat. Rep., 55,* 1–101.
7. Hamilton, B. E., Sutton, P. D., & Ventura, S. J. (2003). Revised birth and fertility rates for the 1990s and new rates for Hispanic populations, 2000 and 2001: United States. *Natl. Vital Stat. Rep., 51(12),* 1–94.
8. UNICEF (2006). *The state of the world's children 2007.* New York, NY: UNICEF House.
9. Ventura, S. J., Abma, J. C., Mosher, W. D., & Henshaw, S. (2004). Estimated pregnancy rates for the United States, 1990–2000: an update. *Natl. Vital Stat. Rep., 52(23),* 1–9.
10. Conley, L. J. (1990). Childbearing and childrearing practices in Mormonism. *Neonatal Netw., 9,* 41–48.
11. Greksa, L. P. (2002). Population growth and fertility patterns in an Old Order Amish settlement. *Ann. Hum. Biol., 29,* 192–201.
12. Chandra A. (1994). Infertility. In Wilcox LS, Marks JS, Editors. From Data to Action: CDC's Public Health Surveillance for Women, Infants, and Children. Atlanta: Centers for Disease Control and Prevention.
13. Gnoth, C., Godehardt, D., Godehardt, E., Frank-Herrmann, P., & Freundl, G. (2003). Time to pregnancy: results of the German prospective study and impact on the management of infertility. *Hum. Reprod., 18,* 1959–1966.
14. Wang, X., Chen, C., Wang, L., Chen, D., Guang, W., & French, J. (2003). Conception, early pregnancy loss, and time to clinical pregnancy: a population-based prospective study. *Fertil. Steril., 79,* 577–584.
15. Evers, J. L. (2002). Female subfertility. *Lancet, 360,* 151–159.
16. Wright, V. C., Chang, J., Jeng, G., & Macaluso, M. (2006b). Assisted reproductive technology surveillance – United States, 2003. *MMWR Surveill. Summ., 55,* 1–22.
17. Northam, S. & Knapp, T. R. (2006). The reliability and validity of birth certificates. *J. Obstet. Gynecol. Neonatal Nurs., 35,* 3–12.
18. Roohan, P. J., Josberger, R. E., Acar, J., Dabir, P., Feder, H. M., & Gagliano, P. J. (2003). Validation of birth certificate data in New York State. *J Community Health, 28,* 335–346.

19. Chandra, A., Martinez, G. M., Mosher, W. D., Abma, J. C., & Jones, J. (2005). Fertility, family planning, and reproductive health of U.S. women: data from the 2002 National Survey of Family Growth. *Vital Health Stat., 23,* 1–160.

20. Stanford, J. B., Hobbs, R., Jameson, P., DeWitt, M. J., & Fischer, R. C. (2000). Defining dimensions of pregnancy intendedness. *Matern. Child Health J., 4,* 183–189.

21. Chandra, A. & Stephen, E. H. (1998). Impaired fecundity in the United States: 1982–1995. *Fam. Plann. Perspect., 30,* 34–42.

22. Stephen, E. H. & Chandra, A. (1998). Updated projections of infertility in the United States: 1995–2025. *Fertil. Steril., 70,* 30–34.

23. Abma, J. C., Chandra, A., Mosher, W. D., Peterson, L. S., & Piccinino, L. J. (1997). Fertility, family planning, and women's health: new data from the 1995 National Survey of Family Growth. *Vital Health Stat., 23,* 1–114.

24. Stephen, E. H. & Chandra, A. (2006b). Declining estimates of infertility in the United States: 1982–2002. *Fertil. Steril., 86,* 516–523.

25. de La Rochebrochard, E. & Thonneau, P. (2003). Paternal age > or =40 years: an important risk factor for infertility. *Am. J Obstet. Gynecol., 189,* 901–905.

26. Wyshak, G. (2001). Infertility in American college alumnae. *Int. J. Gynaecol. Obstet., 73,* 237–242.

27. Adamson, G. D. & Baker, V. L. (2003). Subfertility: causes, treatment and outcome. *Best. Pract. Res. Clin. Obstet. Gynaecol., 17(2),* 169–185.

28. Wright, V. C., Chang, J., Jeng, G., Chen, M., & Macaluso, M. (2007). Assisted reproductive technology surveillance – United States, 2004. *MMWR Surveill. Summ., 56,* 1–22.

29. Alderete, E., Eskenazi, B., & Sholtz, R. (1995). Effect of cigarette smoking and coffee drinking on time to conception. *Epidemiology, 6,* 403–408.

30. Basso, O., Weinberg, C. R., Baird, D. D., Wilcox, A. J., & Olsen, J. (2003). Subfecundity as a correlate of preeclampsia: a study within the Danish National Birth Cohort. *Am. J. Epidemiol., 157,* 195–202.

31. Buck, G. M., Sever, L. E., Batt, R. E., & Mendola, P. (1997). Life-style factors and female infertility. *Epidemiology, 8,* 435–441.

32. Sheiner, E. K., Sheiner, E., Hammel, R. D., Potashnik, G., & Carel, R. (2003). Effect of occupational exposures on male fertility: literature review. *Ind. Health 41(2),* 55–62.

33. Hillis, S. D., Nakashima, A., Amsterdam, L., Pfister, J., Vaughn, M., Addiss, D., et al. (1995). The impact of a comprehensive chlamydia prevention program in Wisconsin. *Fam. Plann. Perspect., 27,* 108–111.

34. Hu, D., Hook, E. W., III, & Goldie, S. J. (2004). Screening for *Chlamydia trachomatis* in women 15 to 29 years of age: a cost-effectiveness analysis. *Ann. Intern. Med., 141,* 501–513.

35. Kmietowicz, Z. (2004). Smoking is causing impotence, miscarriages, and infertility. *BMJ, 328 (7436),* 364.

36. Robbins, H., Krakow, M., & Warner, D. (2002). Adult smoking intervention programmes in Massachusetts: a comprehensive approach with promising results. *Tob. Control, 11(suppl 2),* ii4–ii7.

37. Bitler, M. & Schmidt, L. (2006b). Health disparities and infertility: impacts of state-level insurance mandates. *Fertil. Steril., 85,* 858–865.

38. Hauser, K. W., Lilly, C. M., & Frias, J. L. (2004). Florida health care providers' knowledge of folic acid for the prevention of neural tube defects. *South Med. J., 97(5),* 437–439.

39. Wright, V. C., Schieve, L. A., Reynolds, M. A., & Jeng, G. (2005). Assisted reproductive technology surveillance – United States, 2002. *MMWR Surveill. Summ., 54(2),* 1–24.

40. Andersen, A. N., Gianaroli, L., Felberbaum, R., de Mouzon, J., & Nygren, K. G. (2005). Assisted reproductive technology in Europe, 2001. Results generated from European registers by ESHRE. *Hum. Reprod., 20,* 1158–1176.

41. Gleicher, N., Weghofer, A., & Barad, D. (2006). A formal comparison of the practice of assisted reproductive technologies between Europe and the USA. *Hum. Reprod., 21,* 1945–1950.

42. Van Voorhis, B. J. (2007). In vitro fertilization. *N. Engl. J. Med., 356,* 379–386.

43. Jain, T., Harlow, B. L., & Hornstein, M. D. (2002). Insurance coverage and outcomes of in vitro fertilization. *N. Engl. J. Med., 347,* 661–666.

44. Reynolds, M. A., Schieve, L. A., Jeng, G., & Peterson, H. B. (2003). Does insurance coverage decrease the risk for multiple births associated with assisted reproductive technology? *Fertil. Steril., 80,* 16–23.

45. Henne, M. B. & Bundorf, M. K. (2008). Insurance mandates and trends in infertility treatments. *Fertil. Steril. 89,* 66–73.

46. Bitler, M. & Schmidt, L. (2006). Health disparities and infertility: impacts of state-level insurance mandates. *Fertil. Steril., 85,* 858–865.

47. Roest, J., van Heusden, A. M., Verhoeff, A., Mous, H. V., & Zeilmaker, G. H. (1997). A triplet pregnancy after in vitro fertilization is a procedure-related complication that should be prevented by replacement of two embryos only. *Fertil. Steril., 67,* 290–295.

48. Little, S. E., Ratcliffe, J., & Caughey, A. B. (2006). Cost of transferring one through five embryos per in vitro fertilization cycle from various payor perspectives. *Obstet. Gynecol., 108,* 593–601.

49. Fiddelers, A. A., van Montfoort, A. P., Dirksen, C. D., Dumoulin, J. C., Land, J. A., Dunselman, G. A., et al. (2006). Single versus double embryo transfer: cost-effectiveness analysis alongside a randomized clinical trial. *Hum. Reprod., 21,* 2090–2097.

50. Fiddelers, A. A., Severens, J. L., Dirksen, C. D., Dumoulin, J. C., Land, J. A., & Evers, J. L. (2007). Economic evaluations of single- versus double-embryo transfer in IVF. *Hum. Reprod. Update, 13,* 5–13.

51. Santelli, J., Rochat, R., Hatfield-Timajchy, K., Colley Gilbert, B., Curtis, K., Cabral, R., Hirsch, J., Schieve, L., (2003). The measurement and meaning of unintended pregnancy: a review and critique. *Perspect. Sex. Reprod. Health, 35(2),* 94–101.

52. Zabin, L. S., Astone, N. M., & Emerson, M. R. (1993). Do adolescents want babies? The relationship between attitudes and behavior. *J. Res. Adolesc., 3,* 67–86.

53. Bachrach, C. A. & Newcomer, S. (1999). Intended pregnancies and unintended pregnancies: distinct categories or opposite ends of a continuum? *Fam. Plann. Perspect., 31,* 251–252.

54. Campbell, A. A. & Mosher, W. D. (2000). A history of the measurement of unintended pregnancies and births. *Matern. Child Health J., 4,* 163–169.

55. Kaufmann, R. B., Morris, L., & Spitz, A. M. (1997). Comparison of two question sequences for assessing pregnancy intentions. *Am. J. Epidemiol., 145,* 810–816.

56. Piccinino, L. (1999). Ambivalent attitudes and unintended pregnancy. Peterson LS. *Adv. Popul., 3,* 337–349.

57. Speizer, I. S., Santelli, J. S., Afable-Munsuz, A., & Kendall, C. (2004). Measuring factors underlying intendedness of women's first and later pregnancies. *Perspect. Sex. Reprod. Health, 36,* 198–205.

58. Stevens-Simon, C., Beach, R. K., & Klerman, L. V. (2001a). To be rather than not to be – that is the problem with the questions we ask adolescents about their childbearing intentions. *Arch. Pediatr. Adolesc. Med., 155,* 1298–1300.

59. Barrett, G. & Wellings, K. (2002). What is a 'planned' pregnancy? Empirical data from a British study. *Soc. Sci. Med., 55,* 545–557.

60. Poole, V. L., Flowers, J. S., Goldenberg, R. L., Cliver, S. P., & McNeal, S. (2000). Changes in intendedness during pregnancy in a high-risk multiparous population. *Matern. Child Health J., 4,* 179–182.

61. Trussell, J., Vaughan, B., & Stanford, J. (1999). Are all contraceptive failures unintended pregnancies? Evidence from the 1995 National Survey of Family Growth. *Fam. Plann. Perspect., 31,* 246–247, 260.

62. Korenman, S., Kaestner, R., & Joyce, T. (2002). Consequences for infants of parental disagreement in pregnancy intention. *Perspect. Sex. Reprod. Health, 34,* 198–205.

63. Leathers, S. J. & Kelley, M. A. (2000). Unintended pregnancy and depressive symptoms among first-time mothers and fathers. *Am. J. Orthopsychiatry, 70,* 523–531.

64. Henshaw, S. K. (1998). Unintended pregnancy in the United States. *Fam. Plann. Perspect., 30*, 24–29, 46.
65. Finer, L. B. & Henshaw, S. K. (2006). Disparities in rates of unintended pregnancy in the United States, 1994 and 2001. *Perspect. Sex. Reprod. Health., 38*, 90–96.
66. Trussell, J. (2007). The cost of unintended pregnancy in the United States. *Contraception., 75*, 168–170.
67. Williams, L., Morrow, B., Shulman, H., Stephens, R., D'Angelo, D., & Fowler, C. (2006). PRAMS 2002 Surveillance Report. Atlanta, GA: Centers for Disease Control and Prevention.
68. Hatcher, R. A., Editor (1998). Contraceptive Technology, 17th Ed. NewYork: Irvington Publishers.
69. Beck, L. F., Morrow, B., Lipscomb, L., et al. (2002). Prevalence of selected maternal behaviors and experiences, Pregnancy Risk Assessment Monitoring System (PRAMS), 1999. *MMWR CDC Surveill. Summ., 51(2)*, 1–26.
70. Daulaire, N., Leidl, P., Mackin, L., Murphy, C., & Stark, L. (2002). Promises to Keep: the toll of unintended pregnancies on women's lives in the developing world. Washington, DC: Global Health Council.
71. Kost, K. & Forrest, J. D. (1995). Intention status of U.S. births in 1988: differences by mothers' socioeconomic and demographic characteristics. *Fam. Plann. Perspect., 27*, 11–17.
72. Besculides, M. & Laraque, F. (2004). Unintended pregnancy among the urban poor. *J. Urban Health, 81*, 340–348.
73. Cubbin, C., Braveman, P. A., Marchi, K. S., Chavez, G. F., Santelli, J. S., & Gilbert, B. J. (2002). Socioeconomic and racial/ethnic disparities in unintended pregnancy among postpartum women in California. *Matern. Child Health J., 6*, 237–246.
74. D'Angelo, D. V., Gilbert, B. C., Rochat, R. W., Santelli, J. S., & Herold, J. M. (2004). Differences between mistimed and unwanted pregnancies among women who have live births. *Perspect. Sex. Reprod. Health, 36*, 192–197.
75. Moos, M. K., Bartholomew, N. E., & Lohr, K. N. (2003). Counseling in the clinical setting to prevent unintended pregnancy: an evidence-based research agenda. *Contraception, 67*, 115–132.
76. Moos, M. K., Bangdiwala, S. I., Meibohm, A. R., & Cefalo, R. C. (1996). The impact of a preconceptional health promotion program on intendedness of pregnancy. *Am. J. Perinatol., 13*, 103–108.
77. Strauss, L. T., Gamble, S. B., Parker, W. Y., Cook, D. A., Zane, S. B., & Hamdan, S. (2006). Abortion surveillance – United States, 2003. *MMWR Surveill. Summ., 55(11)*, 1–32.
78. Saul, R. (1998). Abortion reporting in the United States: an examination of the federal–state partnership. *Fam. Plann. Perspect., 30*, 244–247.
79. Fu, H., Darroch, J. E., Henshaw, S. K., & Kolb, E. (1998). Measuring the extent of abortion underreporting in the 1995 National Survey of Family Growth. *Fam. Plann. Perspect., 30*, 128–133, 138.
80. Jones, E. F. & Forrest, J. D. (1992). Underreporting of abortion in surveys of U.S. women: 1976 to 1988. *Demography, 29*, 113–126.
81. Gober, P. (1994). Why abortion rates vary: a geographical examination of the supply and demand for abortion. Services in the United States in 1988. *Annals, Amer. Assoc. Geogr, 84*, 230–250.
82. Elam-Evans, L. D., Strauss, L. T., Herndon, J., Parker, W. Y., Bowens, S. V., Zane, S., et al. (2003). Abortion surveillance – United States, 2000. *MMWR Surveill. Summ., 52(12)*, 1–32.
83. Elam-Evans, L., Strauss, L. T., Herndon, J., Parker, W. Y., Whitehead, S., & Berg, C. J. (2002). Abortion surveillance – United States, 1999. *Surveill. Summ. MMWR, 51(9)*, 1–28.
84. Strauss, L. T., Herndon, J., Chang, J., Parker, W. Y., Levy, D. A., Bowens, S. B., et al. (2004). Abortion surveillance – United States, 2001. *MMWR Surveill. Summ. 53(9)*, 1–32.
85. Finer, L. B. & Henshaw, S. K. (2006). Estimates of U.S. abortion incidence, 2001–2003. New York: Alan Guttmacher Institute.
86. Finer, L. B. & Henshaw, S. K. (2003). Abortion incidence and services in the United States in 2000. *Perspect. Sex. Reprod. Health, 35*, 6–15.

87. Henshaw, S. K. & Finer, L. B. (2003). The accessibility of abortion services in the United States, 2001. *Perspect. Sex. Reprod. Health, 35,* 16–24.

88. Henshaw, S. K., Singh, S., & Haas, T. (1999). The incidence of abortion worldwide. *Int. Fam. Plann. Perspect., 25(Suppl),* S30–S37.

89. Jones, R. K. & Henshaw, S. K. (2002). Mifepristone for early medical abortion: experiences in France, Great Britain and Sweden. *Perspect. Sex. Reprod. Health, 34,* 154–161.

90. Lawson, H. W., Frye, A., Atrash, H. K., Smith, J. C., Shulman, H. B., & Ramick, M. (1994). Abortion mortality, United States, 1972 through 1987. *Am. J. Obstet. Gynecol., 171,* 1365–1372.

91. Jones, R. K., Darroch, J. E., & Henshaw, S. K. (2002). Contraceptive use among U.S. women having abortions in 2000–2001. *Perspect. Sex. Reprod. Health, 34,* 294–303.

92. Joyce, T., Henshaw, S. K., & Skatrud, J. D. (1997). The impact of Mississippi's mandatory delay law on abortions and births. *JAMA, 278,* 653–658.

93. Robbins, A. S., Chao, S. Y., Frost, L. Z., & Fonseca, V. P. (2005). Unplanned pregnancy among active duty servicewomen, U.S. Air Force, 2001. *Mil. Med, 170,* 38–43.

94. Foster, D. G., Bley, J., Mikanda, J., Induni, M., Arons, A., Baumrind, N., et al. (2004). Contraceptive use and risk of unintended pregnancy in California. *Contraception, 70,* 31–39.

95. Mosher, W. D., Martinez, G. D., Chandra, A., Abma, J. C., & Wilson, S. J. (2004). Use of contraception and use of family planning services in the United States: 1982–2002. *Adv. Data, 350,* 1–36.

96. Alan Guttmacher Institute (2002). Family Planning Report: 2001 Summary. NewYork: Alan Guttmacher Institute.

97. Trussell, J., Leveque, J. A., Koenig, J. D., London, R., Borden, S., Henneberry, J., et al. (1995). The economic value of contraception: a comparison of 15 methods. *Am. J. Public Health, 85,* 494–503.

98. Trussell, J. & Calabretto, H. (2005). Cost savings from use of emergency contraceptive pills in Australia. *Aust. NZ J. Obstet Gynaecol., 45,* 308–311.

99. Trussell, J., Koenig, J., Ellertson, C., & Stewart, F. (1997). Preventing unintended pregnancy: the cost-effectiveness of three methods of emergency contraception. *Am. J. Public Health, 87,* 932–937.

100. Yuskiv, N., Honein, M. A., & Moore, C. A. (2005). Reported multivitamin consumption and the occurrence of multiple congenital anomalies. *Am. J. Med. Genet. A, 136,* 1–7.

101. U.S. Preventive Services Task Force. (1996). Guide to Clinical Preventive Services, 2nd Edition. Washington, DC: U.S. Department of Health and Human Services.

102. Lindberg, L. D., Frost, J. J., Sten, C., & Dailard, C. (2006). The provision and funding of contraceptive services at publicly funded family planning agencies: 1995–2003. *Perspect. Sex. Reprod. Health, 38,* 37–45.

103. Forrest, J. D. & Samara, R. (1996). Impact of publicly funded contraceptive services on unintended pregnancies and implications for Medicaid expenditures. *Fam. Plann. Perspect., 28,* 188–195.

104. Mitchell, J. B. & McCormack, L. A. (1997). Access to family planning services: relationship with unintended pregnancies and prenatal outcomes. *J. Health Care Poor Underserved, 8,* 141–152.

105. NARAL Foundation (2001). Emergency contraception (EC): an important and underutilized contraceptive option. http://www.prochoiceamerica.org/assets/files/Birth-Control-EC-EC-underutilized.pdf (accessed October 15, 2008).

106. Sonfield, A., Gold, R. B., Frost, J. J., & Darroch, J. E. (2004). U.S. insurance coverage of contraceptives and the impact of contraceptive coverage mandates, 2002. *Perspect. Sex. Reprod. Health, 36,* 72–79.

107. Abma, J. C., Martinez, G. M., Mosher, W. D., & Dawson, B. S. (2004). Teenagers in the United States: sexual activity, contraceptive use, and childbearing. *Vital Health Stat. 23(24),* 1–48.

108. Landry, D. J., Darroch, J. E., Singh, S., & Higgins, J. (2003). Factors associated with the content of sex education in U.S. public secondary schools. *Perspect. Sex. Reprod. Health, 35*, 261–269.
109. Reddy, D. M., Fleming, R., & Swain, C. (2002). Effect of mandatory parental notification on adolescent girls' use of sexual health care services. *JAMA 288*, 710–714.
110. Tanne, J. H. (2007). Abstinence education has no effect on US teenagers' sexual activity. *BMJ, 334(7599)*, 867.
111. Trussell, J., Koenig, J., Vaughan, B., & Stewart, F. (2001). Evaluation of a media campaign to increase knowledge about emergency contraception. *Contraception, 63*, 81–87.
112. Fairhurst, K., Ziebland, S., Wyke, S., Seaman, P., & Glasier, A. (2004). Emergency contraception: why can't you give it away? Qualitative findings from an evaluation of advance provision of emergency contraception. *Contraception, 70*, 25–29.
113. Glasier, A., Fairhurst, K., Wyke, S., Ziebland, S., Seaman, P., Walker, J., et al. (2004). Advanced provision of emergency contraception does not reduce abortion rates. *Contraception, 69*, 361–366.
114. Grimes, D. A. (2004). Emergency contraception: politics trumps science at the U.S. Food and Drug Administration. *Obstet. Gynecol., 104*, 1104.
115. Brundage, S. C. (2002). Preconception health care. *J S.C. Med. Assoc., 98*, 253–254.
116. Frey, K. A. (2002). Preconception care by the nonobstetrical provider. *Mayo Clin. Proc., 77*, 469–473.
117. Grubbs, S. & Brundage, S. C. (2002). Preconception management of chronic diseases. *J SC Med. Assoc., 98*, 270–276.
118. Korenbrot, C. C., Steinberg, A., Bender, C., & Newberry, S. (2002). Preconception care: a systematic review. *Matern. Child Health J., 6*, 75–88.
119. Morrison, E. H. (2000). Periconception care. *Prim. Care, 27*, 1–12.
120. Rucquoi, J. K. (2002). Genetic counseling in preconception health care. *Am. Fam. Physician, 66*, 2206.
121. Erickson, J. D., Mulinare, J., Yang, Q., Johnson, C. L., Pfeiffer, C., Gunter, E. W., et al. (2002). Folate status in women of childbearing age, by race/ethnicity – United States, 1999–2000. *MMWR, 51*, 808–810.
122. Anderson, J. E., Ebrahim, S., Floyd, L., & Atrash, H. (2006). Prevalence of risk factors for adverse pregnancy outcomes during pregnancy and the preconception period – United States, 2002–2004. *Matern. Child Health J., 10*, S101–S106.
123. Ahlywalia I. & Daniel K (2001). Are women with recent live births aware of the benefits of folic acid? *MMWR, 50*, 3–4.
124. de Walle, H. E., Cornel, M. C., & de Jong-van den Berg, L. T. (2002). Three years after the Dutch folic acid campaign: growing socioeconomic differences. *Prev. Med., 35*, 65–69.
125. de Jong-van den Berg, L. T., Hernandez-Diaz, S., Werler, M. M., Louik, C., & Mitchell, A. A. (2005). Trends and predictors of folic acid awareness and periconceptional use in pregnant women. *Am. J. Obstet. Gynecol., 192*, 121–128.
126. Williams, L. J., Mai, C. T., Edmonds, L. D., Shaw, G. M., Kirby, R. S., Hobbs, C. A., et al. (2002). Prevalence of spina bifida and anencephaly during the transition to mandatory folic acid fortification in the United States. *Teratology, 66*, 33–39.
127. De Wals, P., Tairou, F., Van Allen, M. I., Uh, S. H., Lowry, R. B., Sibbald, B., et al. (2007). Reduction in neural-tube defects after folic acid fortification in Canada. *New Eng. J. Med., 357*, 135–142.
128. Lawrence, J. M., Watkins, M. L., Ershoff, D., Petitti, D. B., Chiu, V., Postlethwaite, D., et al. (2003). Design and evaluation of interventions promoting periconceptional multivitamin use. *Am. J. Prev. Med., 25*, 17–24.
129. de Weerd, S., Polder, J. J., Cohen-Overbeek, T. E., Zimmermann, L. J., & Steegers, E. A. (2004). Preconception care: preliminary estimates of costs and effects of smoking cessation and folic acid supplementation. *J. Reprod. Med., 49*, 338–344.

Chapter 3
Maternal Morbidity

Despite the popular notion that pregnancy is a time of heightened well-being for women, the opposite is often true. The absolute risk of death from pregnancy is low in developed countries. Risks for pregnancy-related mortality, however, continue to be high for women in developing countries, who often have limited ability to control their fertility and limited access to emergency obstetrical services. The persistent loss of productivity as well as the suffering associated with maternal morbidity and mortality justify the study of these problems. Recent clinical and public health focus has been mostly on the infant, rather than on the mother.

This chapter presents pregnancy-related health conditions, which are of interest not only by their own importance, but also because of their repercussions for fetal and infant health. We emphasize the risk of a specific morbidity in each of a woman's pregnancies, rather than the risk of that morbidity for a woman in any of her pregnancies. We focus on pregnancy-related conditions that occur most frequently or that most severely compromise maternal health in the USA. We begin by examining definitions of maternal morbidity in general, and then consider specific conditions. We conclude by discussing public health interventions. In Chap. 4, we apply the same format to maternal mortality.

3.1 Definitions, Measures, and Measurement Issues

Definition: Last defines morbidity as "any departure, subjective or objective, from a state of physiologic or psychological well-being" (1). Table 3.1 presents our definition of maternal morbidity, which parallels the currently most widely used definition of maternal mortality (Sect. 4.1). Morbidity may have its onset during pregnancy and delivery or an unlimited time after pregnancy termination. It may resolve or result in long-term disability. For morbidities with onset during pregnancy, the length of gestation at onset often indicates disease severity, with earlier onset often corresponding to more severe disease (2).

Measuring all maternal morbidity is difficult. Severe, *near-miss* maternal morbidity has emerged as a measure of importance in its own right as well as a sentinel

M.M. Adams et al., *Perinatal Epidemiology for Public Health Practice.*
doi: 10.1007/978-0-387-09439-7_3; © Springer Science + Business Media, LLC 2009

Table 3.1 Definitions of maternal morbidity

1. Condition that is directly caused by pregnancy, regardless of whether it manifests during or after pregnancy termination; or
2. Condition that existed before pregnancy, but is exacerbated by pregnancy; or
3. Condition whose causal relationship to pregnancy is undetermined.

for the level of general maternal morbidity (3–10). Near-miss morbidity comprises acute conditions related to pregnancy that, if untreated or inadequately treated, could result in death. Near-miss morbidity is a slight misnomer, because it actually refers to a death (not a morbidity) that was nearly missed. Although researchers have not established a standard, widely accepted definition of near-miss morbidity, they use a combination of diseases (e.g., eclampsia), morbid events (e.g., stroke), and procedures (e.g., transfusion) to identify it (4). Causes of near-miss morbidity are diverse and include uterine atony, sepsis, severe hypotension, uterine rupture, placenta accreta, pulmonary edema, and hypertensive disease. Empirical data demonstrating a relationship between near-miss morbidity and either overall maternal morbidity or overall mortality have not been published.

Near-miss morbidity comprises acute conditions related to pregnancy that, if untreated or inadequately treated, could result in death.

Person-time combines the concepts of persons and time. It accounts for variability in the length of observation among persons. An individual's person-time is the amount of time for which she is observed. Observation may end when the event of interest occurs, the person is lost to follow-up, or the study ends. For example, in a study of the occurrence of postpartum depression during 8 weeks after delivery, a woman with onset of depression at 3 weeks postpartum contributes 3 weeks of person-time. A woman followed to the end of the study without developing depression contributes 8 weeks of person-time.

Measures: Analysts may compute the *risk* or *rate* of morbidity. When an entire population is followed throughout pregnancy, the *morbidity risk* is computed as the proportion of pregnancies complicated by the morbidity. Note that this definition uses the *pregnancy*, rather the woman, as the unit of observation. Alternatively, an analyst may compute the *incidence rate* for a morbidity, using the number of events in the numerator and the number of weeks (or months) of person-time in the denominator. If person-time is very short, such as the few hours or days surrounding delivery, analysts may compute the rate as a risk, counting the denominator as the number of pregnancies under observation. For example, the proportion of women delivering by cesarean section in a given interval of time adequately describes the rate of cesarean delivery.

When computing incidence rates for an event that may recur, such as urinary tract infections (UTI), analysts use its first occurrence in the numerator and person-time in the denominator. For the incidence rate of second events, the numerator is the number of second events and the denominator is the person-time *of women who have already had one event,* beginning to count time from the onset of the first event. This approach insures that only women who have the potential for being in the numerator are included in the denominator.

Data from administrative sources, such as hospital discharge summaries, are usually coded numerically using the *International Classification of Diseases* (ICD), which is maintained by the WHO.

International Classification of Disease (ICD)

The ICD is a numerical coding system for all causes of morbidity and mortality. The ICD is maintained by the WHO and reflects input from its member countries. To reflect changes in knowledge, the WHO has revised the ICD ten times since its inception in 1893.

The ICD-9 has been used since 1979. The ICD-10 became available in 1998. The ICD-9 continues to be widely used in the USA. Codes in the ICD-10 use a letter and numbers; those in the ICD-9 use numbers only. Information about ICD-9 and ICD-10 is available from the WHO's web site. The NCHS' web site lists modifications of the ICD codes that are used in the USA. Regardless of the ICD version, the ICD modification, ICD-CM (clinical modification) is used widely.

Revisions in ICD codes complicate interpretation of disease trends, notably when conditions previously lumped into a catch-all category (e.g., other) are moved into a specific category. For example, for pregnancy-related hypertension, the ICD-10 is considerably more detailed than the ICD-9.

Data Sources: Potential sources for morbidity data include medical examination, abstraction of medical records, electronic clinic or administrative databases (e.g., hospital discharge summaries), pharmacy and laboratory data, surveys of hospitals or women, and certificates for fetal deaths or live births (Table 3.2).

Medical examinations prospectively ascertain morbidity. They are typically performed on a convenience sample of women, such as those receiving prenatal care at a clinic. They may be performed during and after pregnancy, when women are likely to receive obstetrical services. For example, contact occurs at enrollment for prenatal care and hospitalization for delivery. Medical examinations differ from routine care, because they use a standard protocol for collecting data needed to determine the presence or absence of morbidity. Medical examinations may also provide data on postpartum morbidities.

Medical records abstraction requires review of records to identify diagnoses, treatments, and their relevant dates. Hospital records for delivery usually include a summary of prenatal care that lists diagnoses and procedures. These delivery-related hospital records do not include outpatient postpartum care unless the outpatient requires hospitalization and the hospitalization occurs at the same

Table 3.2 Sources of data on maternal morbidity

Data source	Strengths	Limitations	Comments
Medical examination	• Consistent diagnostic criteria can be applied.	• Ascertainment completeness depends on use of antepartum and postpartum care. • Single exams provide data for prevalence, not incidence. • Repeat exams needed to estimate incidence. • Costly, especially if exams repeated antepartum and postpartum. • Usually not population-based.	• Usually performed for special studies.
Medical record abstraction	• Usually provides data on morbidity from start of prenatal care through final postpartum visit, permitting estimation of incidence and prevalence.	• Ascertainment completeness depends on use of antepartum and postpartum care. • Data needed to confirm or rule out a diagnosis may be absent. • For women receiving care at different sites from different providers, data will be incomplete if records from all providers are not available. • Costly. • Usually not population-based. • Confidentiality concerns may preclude use for research.	• Usually performed for special studies.
Clinic databases	• Often automated and detailed. • Usually provide data on morbidity from start of prenatal care through final postpartum visit, permitting estimation of incidence and prevalence. • May include repeat pregnancies for the same woman, permitting longitudinal study of morbidity for that woman. • If data are gathered over time, useful for assessing temporal changes in practice patterns. • May permit longitudinal assessment of morbidity if women received all their care at one institution.	• Ascertainment completeness depends on use of antepartum and postpartum care. • Not population-based. • Data needed to confirm or rule out a diagnosis may be absent. • Costly to implement data collection and monitor its quality. • Access often restricted to clinic staff. • Confidentiality concerns may preclude use for research.	• Found most often at academic medical centers.

	Advantages	Limitations	Availability
Administrative databases	• Automated. • Low-cost. • Often available for large numbers of gravidas. • Usually use standard codes for diagnoses and procedures.	• Ascertainment completeness depends on use of antepartum and postpartum care. • Not population-based. • Usually limited range of data. • Data usually collected for another purpose; limited or no quality control. • Access often restricted to clinic staff. • Confidentiality concerns may preclude use for research.	• Typically available from insurance companies, health care organizations and hospitals.
Pharmacy and laboratory databases	• Automated. • Low-cost. • Often available for large numbers of gravidas. • May be linked to administrative or clinic data, providing a more complete understanding of morbidity.	• Ascertainment completeness depends on use of antepartum and postpartum care. • Not population-based. • Range of data often limited. • Access often restricted to clinic staff. • Confidentiality concerns may preclude use for research. • Data usually collected for another purpose; limited or no quality control. • For pharmacy data, reason for use is unknown (a single drug may be used to treat multiple conditions).	• Typically available from insurance companies and health care organizations.
Surveys of hospital-discharges summaries	• Most comprehensive source for morbidities that are present at delivery. • If population-based, useful for surveillance. • Usually use standard codes for diagnoses and procedures.	• Costly. • Not useful for antepartum and postpartum conditions that do not require hospitalization. • Trends in practice patterns may hamper interpretation of findings. • Demographic data are usually limited. • Usually not possible to identify repeat hospitalizations for the same woman.	• National Hospital Discharge Survey provides national data. • The State Inpatient Databases (SID) provide state-wide hospital discharges in a uniform format from approximately 28 states. • Several states link hospital discharge data with birth certificates, permitting detection of repeat hospitalizations for an individual woman.

(continued)

Table 3.2 (continued)

Data source	Strengths	Limitations	Comments
Surveys based on self-report	• Usually population-based, thus providing generalizable data. • Ascertains morbidity, regardless of whether woman hospitalized for it. • Useful for surveillance.	• Costly. • Bias due to non-response. • Bias due to respondent's inability or reluctance to give accurate information.	• PRAMS and BRFSS are examples.
Fetal death and birth certificates	• Available in electronic format. • Available for all women whose pregnancies end in a delivery. • Low-cost.	• Underascertainment and probably bias. • Not useful for postpartum conditions. • Not useful for morbidity associated with pregnancies that do not end in delivery. • Delay in availability.	• May be linked with hospital discharge data, providing more comprehensive understanding of morbidity.

place as the delivery. Thus, postpartum morbidity must be obtained from outpatient records. Complete ascertainment of morbidity usually requires review of inpatient and outpatient records. Wider use of electronic medical records likely will provide a readily accessible source of data on outpatient care.

Clinic databases are typically found at large academic medical centers. They generally are collected for research purposes and include a standard set of detailed data for all the women for whom the medical center provided obstetrical care. These data are collected and managed in an electronic format suitable for analysis.

Electronic administrative databases are often developed for insurance reimbursement. Healthcare insurers may accrue databases that include ante-, intra-, and postpartum care diagnoses and treatments. Using standard forms for each patient encounter, clinicians select diagnoses and treatments from a form that lists them and their respective codes. The codes are then transformed to an electronic format. Insurers typically maintain separate databases for outpatient and hospital care. For billing and other purposes, hospitals maintain electronic databases of each patient's diagnoses and treatments (i.e., procedures). Most administrative databases use standard ICD and CPT (Current Procedural Terminology) codes for diagnoses and treatments, respectively.

Insurers and large health care providers maintain electronic databases of medicines that are dispensed to patients. Laboratories maintain electronic databases of results of laboratory tests. A single drug may be prescribed for a variety of conditions and a laboratory test may be used to monitor or diagnose many conditions. Thus, the utility of pharmacy and laboratory databases often depends on success in linking them to clinic and hospital databases that include patients' diagnoses. With such linkage, researchers can use pharmacy and laboratory data to categorize disease severity. Electronic medical records typically include data on medicines that are prescribed as well as laboratory results.

Hospital surveys may include partial or 100% samples of hospital discharge summaries. The National Hospital Discharge Survey (NHDS) is a national probability sample of discharges from nonfederal, short-stay hospitals. The National Center for Health Statistics (NCHS) conducts it annually and includes hospital discharges for approximately 31,000 deliveries. Data include hospital characteristics, discharge diagnoses, procedures, demographic and payment information, and status at discharge. Because the survey samples hospitalizations rather than individuals, an individual may be sampled for an antepartum hospitalization as well as the hospitalization for her delivery. This potential double sampling limits the usefulness of the NHDS for measuring morbidity, except for conditions that are present at delivery. For these morbidities, all deliveries serve as an unduplicated denominator. Although the NHDS contains nearly complete data on hospital attributes and payment source, a substantial portion of records lacks data for marital status and race, diminishing the validity of analyses based on these variables. Over more than three decades that the NHDS has been conducted, researchers have maintained the overall representativeness of the sample by deleting or adding hospitals. The hospital sample was most recently updated in 1991, 1994, 1997, and 2000. Rate changes in these years may be due partly to changes in the composition of the hospital sample.

The State Inpatient Databases (SID) are part of the Health Care Cost and Utilization Project sponsored by the federal Agency for Healthcare Quality and

Research (AHRQ). The SID include statewide hospital discharge data, prepared in a uniform format, for approximately 28 states (http://www.hcup-us.ahrq.gov/sidoverview.jsp. Accessed December 20, 2007). Variables include principal and secondary diagnoses, principal and secondary procedures, admission and discharge status, patient demographics, expected payment source, total charges, length of stay and, for selected states, hospital and county identifiers that permit linkage to the American Hospital Association Annual Survey file.

Several states obtain data for all hospital discharges in the state and link them to birth and fetal death certificates, permitting assessment of antepartum and delivery-related hospitalizations for individual women.

Self-reported data derive from surveys, which ask women about illness before pregnancy and/or after delivery. The state-based Pregnancy Risk Assessment Monitoring System (PRAMS) exemplifies such a survey (http://www.cdc.gov/prams. Accessed December 20, 2007). The analysts who conduct PRAMS sample new mothers from birth certificates. Mothers are contacted by mail or telephone and asked about their experiences during and after pregnancy. The National Survey of Family Growth (http://www.cdc.gov/nchs/nsfg.htm. Accessed December 20, 2007) and the Medical Expenditure Survey (http://www.meps.ahrq.gov/mepsweb/ accessed December 20, 2007) also ascertain self-reported pregnancy-related illness.

The 1988 National Maternal and Infant Health Survey used a national, population-based sample of more than 13,000 women whose pregnancies ended in live births or late fetal deaths (11, 12). This survey obtained data from fetal death and birth certificates, maternal questionnaires, and records for prenatal care and hospitalization for delivery. The low response rate for clinical data has limited the generalizability of this one-time survey.

Self-reported data offer the potential for completely ascertaining the full scope of mild to severe antepartum, intrapartum, and postpartum morbidities for an individual woman. Attaining this potential depends on the respondent's completeness and accuracy of recall. Apart from data collected by health care organizations, no single source provides data on the continuum of maternal experience from the antepartum through the postpartum periods.

Population-based data for morbidity experienced by an individual woman across her pregnancies are limited and available for a few populations. Working with a state's birth and fetal death certificates for 5 or more years, researchers have linked successive deliveries. Birth and fetal death certificates, however, generally grossly underascertain maternal morbidity. Hospital discharge summaries ascertain maternal morbidity much more completely (13). Analysts in at least one state have linked maternal hospital discharge summaries to birth and fetal death certificates, which were linked across pregnancies. These linkages produce the best available population-based data on maternal morbidity across pregnancies.

Certificates for fetal deaths or live births collect a wide range of information about maternal conditions occurring during pregnancy and delivery (Table 3.3). In some instances, severe morbidity, whose diagnosis is unspecified, is indicated by provision of unanticipated care, such as admission to an intensive care unit. Methods for completing birth certificates vary widely. The birth attendant, a clerk

Table 3.3 Maternal morbidity data collected on the U.S. Standard Certificate of Birth, 2003

1. Prepregnancy: diabetes, hypertension
2. Gestational: diabetes, hypertension
3. Infections present during gestation: gonorrhea, syphilis, herpes simplex virus, chlamydia, hepatitis B, hepatitis C
4. Prolonged labor
5. Clinical chorioamnionitis
6. Maternal transfusion
7. 3rd or 4th-degree laceration
8. Ruptured uterus
9. Unplanned hysterectomy
10. Admission to intensive care unit
11. Unplanned operating room procedure following delivery

Birth attendants check boxes to indicate which conditions are present (*Source*: http://www.cdc.gov/nchs/vital_certs_rev.htm, accessed December 20, 2007)

who reviews the hospital record, or other personnel, may provide information for these certificates.

Measurement Issues: Table 3.2 summarizes strengths and limitations of the range of data on maternal morbidity. No source provides high-quality data on antepartum, intrapartum, and postpartum pregnancy-related morbidity that is suitable for surveillance. The only exception is population-based maternal hospital discharge data for deliveries, which provide information on intrapartum morbidity and the small set of morbidities that persist until delivery, such as preeclampsia and gestational diabetes. Transient morbidities as well as those for which most women are treated as outpatients, such as nausea and vomiting, urinary tract infection, or preterm labor remain difficult to ascertain accurately. No population-based surveillance data are available about long-term pregnancy-related disabilities, such as urinary incontinence.

When ascertainment is based on self-report, self-recognition of illness and willingness to reveal illnesses may hinder ascertainment. This may be particularly true for conditions that carry social stigma, for example, sexually transmitted diseases and psychiatric conditions, such as depression.

A final challenge relates to temporal changes in diagnostic criteria, treatment practices, and healthcare insurance, which may complicate interpretation of trends. For example, the increased emphasis on cost containment that occurred during the 1990s resulted in lower hospitalization rates for many maternal morbidities, although the underlying incidence of these conditions may not have changed. Another apparent trend during the 1990s is the increasing number of diagnoses on hospital summaries. Scrutiny of hospitals' and clinicians' charges by managed care organizations may have encouraged these providers to justify their charges by recording diagnoses more completely.

This discussion focuses on morbidity occurring in pregnancies that result in delivery. Very little data exist for morbidity related to ectopic pregnancy (14) and spontaneous and induced abortion. Only small portions of women with these conditions are hospitalized. Population-based outpatient data for the remaining majority of women are not widely available.

Measuring Maternal Morbidity Internationally: Developed countries with national systems of health care and unique personal identifiers (e.g., Denmark, Norway, Sweden) are virtual gold mines of information on maternal morbidity. These countries often have large electronic databases that permit researchers to identify women with specific morbidities and to observe recurrence patterns within individual women. In contrast, many developing countries lack an infrastructure for providing health care as well as the capacity to develop an electronic database to track such care. In consequence, aside from special studies, ascertaining maternal morbidity is very difficult.

Healthy People 2010 Objectives for Maternal Morbidity (15):

- 16-5a: Reduce maternal illness and complications during hospitalized labor and delivery to 24 per 100 deliveries.
- 16-5b: Reduce ectopic pregnancies.
- 16-5c: Reduce postpartum complications, including postpartum depression.

The Healthy People 2010 Objectives comprise more than 400 health-related objectives for the USA. They were developed and are monitored by federal agencies with broad public consultation.

3.2 Overall Maternal Morbidity

Overall Occurrence: The baseline for Health People 2010 Objective 16-5a provides the best current measure of overall maternal morbidity prevalence. It is measured from the NHDS. Because this measure includes only pregnancy-related morbidities that persist until delivery (e.g., gestational diabetes, preeclampsia, etc.) and none that occurs after delivery, it grossly underestimates total maternal morbidity. In 1998, 31.2 complications occurred during every 100 hospitalizations for labor and delivery and this is the baseline rate (http://www.healthypeople.gov/document/html/objectives/16-05.htm. Accessed December 20, 2007). The rate increased in 1999 (31.4/100) and 2000 (32.2/100), then dropped slightly in 2001 (31.8/100). By 2002, the rate was 4% below the baseline rate. Data for geographic variability are not available. African-American women consistently have a higher rate than white women. For example, in 2001, the rate for African-American women was 39.0 per 100 deliveries, but for white women it was 30.0 per 100 deliveries. The complication rate is modestly lower for women in their twenties, compared with older or younger women.

Diverse, etiologically heterogeneous conditions contribute to maternal morbidity. To better understand these constituents of morbidity, we examine the most frequently occurring ones. We begin with antepartum conditions, continue with complications of labor and delivery, and end with postpartum illnesses.

3.3 Antepartum Conditions

As judged by hospitalization rates, antepartum morbidity is common. A study of maternal hospitalization during pregnancy among 46,179 women who were enrolled in managed care in 1997 showed that 8.7% were hospitalized (16). Of these women, 12.5% had more than one hospitalization during pregnancy. Nearly a quarter of all hospitalizations were related to pregnancy loss. Among women whose pregnancies ended in a live birth, 5.8% were hospitalized and discharged while still pregnant and 0.8% were hospitalized for ≥4 days before delivery. This study did not include hospitalization for ectopic pregnancy, which is an important cause of severe morbidity and mortality.

Computing the ratio of hospitalizations during pregnancy to deliveries for 1999 and 2000 in the USA, Bacek and colleagues reported a ratio of 12.8 per 100 deliveries. These analysts used data from the NHDS (17). Studying the ratio of hospitalization during pregnancy per 100 deliveries in Canada from 2002 to 2003, analysts reported a rate of 13.6. They observed variations among provinces/territories (30 per 100 in Yukon) and by maternal age (27.1 per 100 women aged <20 years) (18).

3.3.1 Ectopic Pregnancy

Occurrence: During the 1990s, clinical management of ectopic pregnancy switched from predominately inpatient care to outpatient care. In the absence of reliable data on outpatient care, accurate estimation of the rate of ectopic pregnancy in the USA during the 1990s is virtually impossible (14). US data from the 1970s, 1980s, and early 1990s show a consistent rise in the number of ectopic pregnancies (Fig. 3.1) (19). Data from women in Northern California who were insured by Kaiser Permanente from 1997 to 2000 show an annual rate of 20.7 ectopic pregnancies per 1,000 reported pregnancies and a ratio of 1.03 per 1,000 women aged 15–44 years (20). These data are similar to the incidence of ectopic pregnancy observed nationally during the early 1990s.

Data from a district in London show a decline in the rate of ectopic pregnancy from 2.4 per 1,000 deliveries in 1990 to 1.6 per 1,000 in 1999 (21). Researchers have observed declines during the 1990s of smaller magnitudes in France (22) and New South Wales, Australia (23). A hospital-based study in Sweden reported decreases in ectopic pregnancy from 1985 through 1995 (24).

More recent data from central France for 1992–2002 showed a 2% decrease in the ratio of ectopic pregnancy per 1,000 women aged 15–44 years to 0.953 (25).

Demographic Variability and Characteristics of Women with Ectopic Pregnancies: The characteristics of women who have ectopic pregnancies reflect the

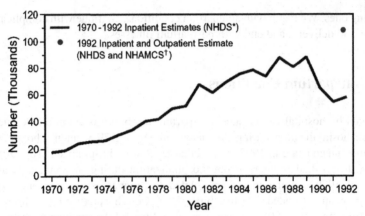

*National Hospital Discharge Survey.
†National Hospital Ambulatory Medical Care Survey.

Fig. 3.1 Number of ectopic pregnancies – United States, 1970–1992 (*Source*: (18))

demographic distribution of women, variations in fertility among women, and attributes associated with the underlying etiologies of ectopic pregnancy. Variability in risks associated with demographic attributes mirrors the underlying etiologies of ectopic pregnancy in a specific population. For example, ectopic pregnancy is associated with tubal ligation (26). In the USA, a greater proportion of older women are likely to have completed their childbearing and had tubal ligations. Thus, older women in the USA are likely to have a higher risk of ectopic pregnancy than younger women. Because fertility rates are highest among women in their twenties, and women currently in their twenties have a higher likelihood of having had a chlamydia infection (a risk factor for ectopic pregnancy) than older women, a large portion of women with ectopic pregnancies are likely to be in this age group.

"The U.S. Preventive Services Task Force (USPSTF) recommends screening for chlamydial infection for all sexually active nonpregnant young women aged 24 and younger and for older nonpregnant women who are at increased risk."
(http://www.ahrq.gov/clinic/uspstf/uspschlm.htm. Accessed December 20, 2007)

Risk Factors and Related Public Health Interventions: Ectopic pregnancy is etiologically associated with cigarette smoking; tubal ligation; current or past use of an intrauterine device; vaginal douching; ovulation induction; congenital malformations of the fallopian tubes, often secondary to the women's in-utero exposure to diethylstilbestrol; and history of pelvic inflammatory disease, chlamydia infection, interrupted pregnancies or pelvic surgery (25, 27–32).

Public health interventions include reducing cigarette smoking among women, promoting targeted screening for sexually transmitted infections, especially chlamydia, and discouraging vaginal douching.

Availability and Use of Public Health Interventions: Public health workers have identified effective interventions to reduce cigarette smoking (33). Health workers have implemented some – but not all – of these interventions (34, 35). No public health interventions to discourage vaginal douching have been tested. Public health activities to promote screening for sexually transmitted infections include recommendations by the US Task Force for Clinical Preventive Services for screening. The National Committee for Quality Assurance, which accredits managed care organizations, uses an organization's rate of chlamydia screening as a health care quality measure. These actions encourage providing chlamydia screening and insurance coverage for screening as well as measuring screening rates.

3.3.2 Nausea and Vomiting (Hyperemesis of Pregnancy)

Occurrence: Nausea and vomiting occur initially at 4–8 weeks gestation and spontaneously abate by 20–22 weeks (36, 37). Although frequent vomiting – hyperemesis – is not life-threatening, it sometimes results in dehydration severe enough to require hospitalization. Studies from the USA, Nova Scotia, Canada, and Sweden have reported that approximately 1% of women with deliveries were hospitalized for hyperemesis (16, 38, 39). The study from the USA was from a managed care population. In this study, hospitalizations for hyperemesis represented 9.3% of all hospitalizations among women who had a live birth. In the Swedish cohort, the overall rate of nausea and vomiting was 79%. Thus, many women experienced nausea and vomiting, but very few required hospitalization.

Factors Influencing Occurrence: Although nausea and vomiting are nearly ubiquitous during pregnancy, several factors modify its occurrence. The rate of nausea and vomiting is lower among women who smoke, those who take multivitamins early in pregnancy, and those aged >30 years. It is higher among multiparous women, those with hyperthyroid disorders, psychiatric illness, previous molar pregnancy, preconception diabetes, gastrointestinal disorders, and asthma as well as those with multiple gestations or a female fetus (38, 40, 41). Little is known about trends in occurrence or preventive measures.

3.3.3 Urinary Tract Infections

UTI occur frequently during pregnancy, delivery, and the postpartum period. Bacteriuria, bacteria in the urine, often precedes UTI. A study of women with "untreated group B streptococcal bacteriuria in early pregnancy" showed that, compared with uninfected women, they had an increased risk for "chorioamnionitis at delivery" (42). Investigators have reported a prevalence of bacteriuria at entry to prenatal care of 2.7% among women who delivered at three hospitals in North Carolina (43). Among Canadian women who were tested repeatedly in the first, second, and third trimesters, 4.7% had asymptomatic bacteriuria (44). A hospital-based study of pregnant Irish women reported prevalences of 4.7% for bacteriuria and 3.2% for symptomatic UTI (45). A study of enrollees in a managed care plan reported that, among women whose pregnancies ended in a live birth, 3.5% were hospitalized during pregnancy at least once for UTI (16).

Trends: Data from the NHDS show an increase in the percentage of delivery-associated discharges with a code for "infections of genitourinary tract in pregnancy" (ICD 9 646.61 or 646.62) from 1.8% of discharges in 1990 to a peak of 3.7% in 1998, declining to 2.6% in 2000 and 2.5% in 2001. The increasing trend should be interpreted cautiously, because it may reflect improved ascertainment or more complete coding of diagnoses.

Geographic Variability: Data from the NHDS show that during the 1990s, the West had the lowest percentage of delivery-associated discharges with diagnoses coded as ICD-9 646.61 or 646.62. In most years during this decade, the highest percentage was in the Northeast.

Demographic Variability: NHDS data also show that, throughout the 1990s among delivery-associated discharges, a lower percentage of married women than single women had diagnoses coded as IC9-9 646.61 or 646.62 (Fig. 3.2). This pattern held across all maternal age groups. The impact of maternal race on the association between marital status and UTI could not be assessed because race was missing for a substantial proportion of women.

Factors Influencing Occurrence: Medical factors that increase the risk for UTI after 20 weeks of gestation include a history of UTI, either before pregnancy or earlier in pregnancy, a history of chlamydia infection, and preeclampsia (46, 47).

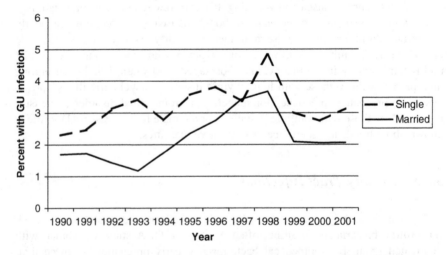

Fig. 3.2 Annual rate of GU infection at delivery, by marital status, NHDS, US, 1990–2001

A study found that ingesting supplements that included Vitamin C during pregnancy substantially reduced the risk of UTI (48).

Influenza: Observations from the 1918 and 1957 influenza pandemics show that pregnant women have increased risk for influenza-related morbidity (48). Investigators have estimated that, during an average influenza season lasting 2.5 months, 25 of 10,000 third-trimester women will be hospitalized with influenza-related morbidity (49). This rate is substantially higher than that for first-trimester or postpartum women. Because of this increased risk for influenza-related hospitalization, the Advisory Committee on Immunization Practices recommends inactivated influenza vaccine for women who will be in their second or third trimesters of pregnancy during influenza season (50). To minimize risk to the fetus, immunization should occur after the first trimester.

3.3.4 Gestational Diabetes

Gestational diabetes mellitus is defined as "the presence of carbohydrate intolerance of varying degrees of severity with onset or first recognition during pregnancy" (52). Screening for gestational diabetes is not recommended by the United States Task Force on Clinical Preventive Services, because of the absence of documented maternal or fetal benefits (53–56). Nonetheless, screening routinely occurs, usually between 24 and 28 weeks of gestation.

In 2000, the American Diabetes Association decreased the plasma glucose threshold for diagnosing gestational diabetes (57). Investigators observed that this change increased the rate of gestational diabetes detected through screening from 3.2% (using the previous threshold) to 4.8%. Groups with low baseline rates of gestational diabetes showed the greatest increase. For example, the detected rate increased 70% for women <25 years of age and 58% for white women (58). The change in diagnostic criteria will complicate interpretation of trends in gestational diabetes. Increasing levels of preconception overweight and obesity as well as increases in the proportion of women aged ≥35 who are bearing children are likely to raise the rate of gestational diabetes.

Women with gestational diabetes have increased risks for preeclampsia, premature rupture of membranes, and cesarean section delivery (59). Their infants have increased risks for macrosomia and preterm delivery (59, 60). Compared with women without gestational diabetes, those who develop it face a 10–50% risk of developing type 2 diabetes during the 5 years after they deliver (61).

Occurrence: Among women who received their prenatal care through a managed care organization in California, 5.1% were diagnosed with gestational diabetes in 1991. This percentage rose to 7.4% in 1997 and dropped to 6.9% in 2000 (62). Among women in Colorado who also received care from a managed

care organization, the percentage diagnosed with gestational diabetes rose from
2.1% in 1994 to 4.1% in 2002 (63). Both of these studies used a consistent
diagnostic standard for gestational diabetes throughout the years of observation.
A study using the newer 2000 plasma glucose threshold for diagnosing gestational
diabetes found a prevalence of 4.8% among a cohort of more than 26,000 women
who were screened at a mean gestation of 27 weeks (58).

Trends: Data from the NHDS show that, during the 1990s, the percentage of
women diagnosed with gestational diabetes at delivery increased from 1.9% in
1990 and 1991 to 3.5% in 2000 and 3.7% in 2001. The increasing trend was evident
in strata defined by region of the USA and maternal age, race, and marital status.

Geographic Variability: NHDS data for the 1990s showed that the rate of
gestational diabetes at hospitalization for delivery was consistently higher in the
Northeast United States than in other regions.

Demographic Variability: The risk for gestational diabetes is highest among
women who are 35 years or older (64), have a low socioeconomic status, or are
Native American, Asian, or from the Indian subcontinent or Middle East (58, 59,
65–67). Data from the NHDS show consistently elevated rates of gestational
diabetes at hospital discharge among women aged 30 years and older (Fig. 3.3).
Relative to older women, women aged 19 years or younger have the lowest rates of
gestational diabetes. Of note are the high prevalences observed in Native Americans, such as Zunis (15.3%) (68), Cree (11.4%) (69), and those in Saskatoon,
Canada (11.5%) (70).

Factors Influencing Occurrence: Risk for gestational diabetes is increased
among women who are obese before conception, infrequently are physically active,
have a family history of gestational diabetes, or have a history of infertility,
gestational diabetes, cesarean delivery, or neonatal death (59, 65–67, 71). The
risk of recurrence of gestational diabetes ranges from 30 to 69%. One study
observed that women who experienced gestational diabetes in two preceding
pregnancies had a recurrence risk of 72% (72). A higher maternal preconception

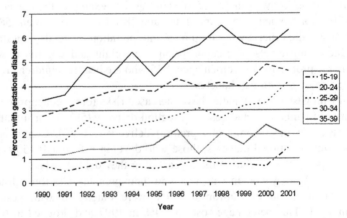

Fig. 3.3. Annual rate of gestational diabetes at delivery by maternal age, NHDS, US, 1990–2001

weight increases the risk for recurrence. The effectiveness of preconception weight loss in lowering the recurrence risk is unknown. The recurrence pattern is consistent with the possibility that some women have a strong inherent predisposition for gestational diabetes.

> ### Overweight, Obesity, and Maternal Morbidity
>
> Preconception obesity increases the risk for a range of morbidities, with the degree of increase relative to the extent of the obesity. Compared with normal-weight women, obese women have increased risks for gestational diabetes, pregnancy-induced hypertension, preeclampsia, labor induction, unsuccessful attempted vaginal birth after cesarean delivery, nonelective cesarean delivery, postcesarean infections, and endometritis (58, 72–76). The length of perineal lacerations is positively associated with maternal body mass index (BMI), after adjusting for infant head circumference (77). Infants of overweight or obese women are more likely to be macrosomic and require admission to a neonatal intensive care unit (58, 72, 75, 76). National trends show an increasing prevalence of overweight and obesity and younger ages at their occurrence (79–81). These trends will increase potentially preventable maternal and infant morbidity. Preventing overweight and obesity is an important target for public health interventions.

3.3.5 Pregnancy-Related Hypertensive Disorders

We consider hypertensive disorders that are etiologically related to pregnancy including transient gestational hypertension, mild and severe preeclampsia, and eclampsia. Preeclampsia and eclampsia may occur before or after delivery and may be superimposed on hypertension that existed before pregnancy. These disorders likely have multiple etiologies. At least one investigator has suggested dividing preeclampsia into early ($\leq$34 weeks' gestation) and late onset, a suggestion supported by differences in fetal growth among preterm and term infants delivered to preeclampic women (82, 83). Hypertensive disorders are associated with increased risk for placental abruption and associated hemorrhage, acute renal dysfunction, disseminated intravascular coagulation, HELLP syndrome (hemolysis, elevated liver enzymes, and low platelets), maternal death, and fetal and infant morbidity and mortality (84, 85). Women who experience preeclampsia subsequently have higher risks for thromboembolism, hypertension, and death from cardiovascular disease (86–89).

Occurrence: Inconsistencies in diagnostic criteria may account for at least part of the temporal, geographic, and demographic variability in the occurrence of hypertensive disorders. Pregnancy-associated hypertensive disorders are relatively common. In a cohort of women who had a live birth in 1997 and were enrolled in a managed care organization during their pregnancies, 9.1% were hospitalized at least once for a

pregnancy-associated hypertensive disorder (16). The cohort's prevalence of pregnancy-associated hypertensive disorders was undoubtedly higher than this hospitalization rate, because not all women with these disorders are hospitalized.

Among hypertensive disorders, transient hypertension of pregnancy is the most
prevalent and eclampsia the least prevalent. The most current and informative
American study of the occurrence of hypertensive disease associated with
pregnancy followed 4,302 nulliparae from the second trimester to delivery (90).
In this cohort, 16.6% developed mild pregnancy-associated hypertension, 5% mild
preeclampsia, 0.7% severe pregnancy-associated hypertension, and 2.5% severe
preeclampsia (85). Because nulliparae have a higher risk of hypertensive disorders
than multiparae, the incidences observed in this study are higher than one would
expect among all women who give birth.

Trends: NHDS data show that, during the 1990s, the combined prevalence of
hypertensive disorders at delivery increased, largely driven by increases in transient
hypertension of pregnancy (ICD-9 code 642.31), severe preeclampsia (ICD-9 code
642.51), and preeclampsia or eclampsia superimposed on preexisting hypertension
(ICD-9 code 642.71) (Fig. 3.4).

Geographic Variability: During the 1990s, the combined rate of preeclampsia
and eclampsia observed in NHDS data was highest in the South and lowest in the
West, with the Midwest and Northeast in between.

Data from the Medical Birth Register of Norway for 1967 through 1998 showed
that preeclampsia occurred among 3.9% of first pregnancies, 1.7% of second
pregnancies, and 1.8% of third pregnancies (91). Data from the Swedish Medical
Birth Registry for 1991–1992 showed a prevalence during pregnancy of eclampsia
of 0.03% (92). Data from the South East Thames region of England showed an
incidence of 0.4% for severe preeclampsia and 0.02% for eclampsia (93). Data for
the United Kingdom in 2005 and 2006 showed an incidence of 0.03% (94). Data

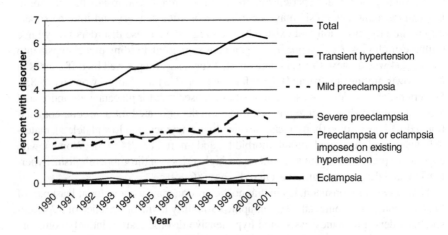

Fig. 3.4. Annual rate of preghancy-related hypertensive disorders at delivery, NHDS, USA,
1990–2001

from the NHDS for the USA from 1990 through 2001 show a similarly low prevalence of eclampsia at hospitalization for delivery of 0.09%.

Demographic Variability. NDHS data also showed that during most years from 1990 through 2001, the rate of mild preeclampsia at hospitalization for delivery was highest for women aged 15–19 years. The high proportion of women aged 15–19 years who were having their first birth likely contributes to their elevated rate. From 1990 through 2001, the NHDS rates for preeclampsia or eclampsia imposed on existing hypertension were highest for women aged 35 years and older, most likely reflecting a higher background rate of existing hypertension in these women compared with younger women. Analyses of women in California in 1995 showed that, compared with younger women, those aged ≥35 years had modestly increased risks for severe preeclampsia, eclampsia, gestational hypertension, or mild pre-eclampsia (64). These age-related risks were consistently higher across racial groups (Blacks, Hispanics, Whites, and others).

Valid data on racial differences in the prevalence of pregnancy-related hypertensive disorders are sparse, due either to incompleteness or inaccuracy of ascertainment (e.g., birth certificates), or because race is unknown for a notable portion of the study sample (e.g., NHDS). One study, based on birth certificate data, reported a lower risk for black women than white women (95).

Factors Influencing Occurrence: The etiology of pregnancy-related hypertensive disorders is poorly understood. Nonetheless, researchers have identified numerous factors that influence their occurrence (Table 3.4). Genetic factors clearly play a role, but their exact nature is unknown (87, 96). Abnormal placentation and endothelial dysfunction may be the underlying problems leading to preeclampsia or eclampsia (97, 98).

3.4 Peripartum Conditions

Peripartum morbidities occur immediately before or after delivery. They include UTI, surgical infections, hemorrhage, perineal lacerations, uterine rupture, pre-eclampsia and eclampsia, stroke, Bell's palsy, and lumbosacral spine and lower extremity nerve injuries (99, 100). He we focus on three conditions that occur frequently and are associated with severe maternal morbidity: hemorrhage, perineal lacerations, and operative delivery.

3.4.1 Hemorrhage

Severe maternal hemorrhage can result in an obstetrical emergency that leads to *near-miss* or *severe* maternal morbidity (6, 101). Placenta previa, placental abruption, retained placenta, uterine rupture, and atonic uterus are the most frequent causes of maternal hemorrhage. Among managed care enrollees who delivered a live birth in 1997, 3.1% were hospitalized one or more times during pregnancy for placenta previa and another 1.2% were hospitalized for abruption (102).

Table 3.4 Factors that influence the occurrence of pregnancy-related hypertension and preeclampsia, by consistency of findings

Relationship with occurrence of hypertensive disorder	Factor
Consistently increases risk	Abnormal placentation (97)
	Preeclampsia in a previous pregnancy (97)
	Maternal obesity (75, 112, 222)
	Prepregnancy diabetes, hypertension, or systemic lupus (223)
	Multiple gestation (97, 224, 225)
	Male fetal sex (224)
	History of preeclampsia in a first-degree relative (226, 227)
Increases risk, as demonstrated in one or a small number of studies	Paternal age ≥35 years (228)
	Low level of consumption of vitamin C (229)
	Positive IgG seroprevalence to *Chlamydia pneumoniae* (230–232)
	History of hypertension and/or type 2 diabetes in a first-degree relative (233)
	Maternal periodontal disease (234)
	Lengthy time to first pregnancy or interpregnancy interval (possibly secondary to subfecundity) (90, 235)
Increases risk in some, but not all studies	Maternal thrombophilias (236–239)
	Brief preconception exposure to paternal sperm or change of partner between pregnancies. The association with partner change may be confounded by interpregnancy interval (94, 240–242).
Decreases risk, as demonstrated in one or a small number of studies	Folic acid supplementation during pregnancy (231)
	Previous induced or spontaneous abortion (243)
Decreases risk in some, but not all studies	Maternal cigarette smoking (94, 244–248)
	Aspirin for women with prepregnancy risk (225, 249)
Decreases risk, as supported by strong evidence	Calcium supplementation for women with low baseline calcium intake or high risk for preeclampsia (250)

Data from the NHDS for 1990 through 2001 showed that the prevalence of hemorrhage during the 24 h after delivery increased more than twofold during the 1990s (Fig. 3.5). By the late 1990s, it was the most prevalent type of peripartum hemorrhage. The prevalence of third-stage postpartum hemorrhage declined modestly. The prevalences of other causes of hemorrhage at delivery were stable. The numbers of admissions for both antepartum and postpartum hemorrhage associated with coagulation defects were too small for meaningful analysis.

Geographic Variability: Sample sizes in the NHDS were sufficient to assess regional differences for the two most frequent causes of hemorrhage. Although the rate of immediate postpartum hemorrhage increased in all regions during the 1990s, it was consistently highest in the West, with little difference among the rates for other regions. NHDS data for premature separation of the placenta show similar, fairly stable rates for all regions through the 1990s.

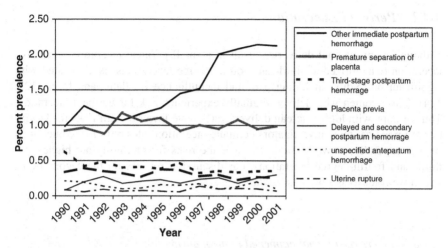

Fig. 3.5. Prevalence of hemorrhage at delivery, NHDS, USA, 1990–2001

Among almost 49,000 women delivering during 1997–1998 in the South East Thames region in England, 0.7% had severe postpartum hemorrhage and 0.02% had uterine rupture (93). Comparable data for the USA are not available for the rate of severe postpartum hemorrhage, but the rate of uterine rupture is much lower than NHDS annual rates during the late 1990s, which ranged from 0.10 to 0.20%.

Factors Influencing Occurrence: The risk for placental abruption increases with high maternal parity, maternal smoking, maternal experience of physical violence during pregnancy, abdominal injury, maternal prepregnancy hypertension, HELLP syndrome, and pregnancy-associated hypertensive disorders (103–109). An increased risk for uterine rupture is associated with attempted vaginal birth after cesarean delivery (110, 111) especially for births occurring after interpregnancy intervals of 6 months or less (112). Among the factors that increase the risk for postpartum hemorrhage are maternal obesity, postterm delivery, a second stage of labor lasting ≥120 min, leiomyoma, previous postpartum hemorrhage, and maternal age ≥35 years (93, 113–116). In one study, prepregnancy type 2 diabetes increased the risk for postpartum hemorrhage sixfold (117). Lydon-Rochelle observed that, in Washington state, assisted vaginal delivery increased the risk for postpartum rehospitalization due to hemorrhage (118).

Where are babies born and who delivers them? (no, it's not the stork!)

In 2004 in the USA, 99.1% of births occurred in hospitals, a percentage that has been stable throughout the 1990s through 2004 (119–122). The percentage of births attended by physicians declined from 95.4% in 1989 to 91.7% in 2000 and 91.3% in 2001–2004. Concomitantly, the percentage of births delivered by midwives (who were nearly all certified nurse midwives) more than doubled from 3.4% in 1989 to 7.4% in 2000, 8.1% in 2002, and 7.9% in 2004. During the 1990s, Hispanic women were more likely to have a midwife at their delivery than non-Hispanic white or black women.

3.4.2   Perineal Laceration

Although many vaginal deliveries result in a small perineal laceration, extensive laceration (categorized as third- and fourth-degree lacerations) is associated with significant morbidity, including pain and incontinence for flatus and feces (123, 124). Only women who deliver vaginally experience risk for perineal laceration. Thus, groups with high cesarean delivery rates have lower overall risks for laceration. In practice, most investigators compute laceration rates only for women who deliver vaginally, as we do here. Because the risks for morbidity are highest for third- and fourth-degree lacerations, our discussion focuses on these conditions, which we refer to as *severe lacerations*.

Can mothers recall what happened to them during labor?

Researchers interviewed women approximately two and half months after delivery regarding the medicine (oxytocin), procedures (artificial rupture of membranes, episiotomy, forceps, vacuum, perineal sutures, cesarean), and morbidity (external anal sphincter laceration). Seventy-one percent of women correctly recalled having an operative delivery, 32% correctly recalled having a external anal sphincter laceration, 77% correctly recalled having an episiotomy, and 95% correctly recalled repair of a laceration. Twenty-three percentage of women incorrectly said that they had repair of a laceration, when no repair had occurred. Parity, length of time since delivery, and ethnicity were associated with accuracy of recall (124).

Occurrence: Domestically and internationally, hospital-based rates of severe laceration vary widely over place and time (Table 3.5). This variation may reflect differences in obstetric practices, such as the background rates of cesarean delivery, episiotomy, and vacuum- or forceps-assisted delivery.

Temporal Trends: Data from the NHDS show that the rate of severe lacerations declined from 7.4% of vaginal deliveries in 1990 to 5.2% in 1998 to 5.0% in 2001 (126). The decline occurred for third- and fourth-degree lacerations, women aged ≤34 years, and all regions (Fig. 3.6). For women aged ≥35 years, sparse data limit the ability to assess trends.

Factors Influencing Occurrence: Investigators have identified a range of risk factors for severe perineal laceration (Table 3.6) (78, 127–140). Of particular interest are factors related to obstetrical care, which may be more amenable to change than maternal-, infant-, or labor-related factors. The relationship between epidural anesthesia and severe laceration may be explained by the increase of forceps-assisted delivery among women who receive epidural anesthesia (129).

Trends in Episiotomy and Repair of Perineal Lacerations:

In the USA among women who delivered vaginally, the episiotomy rate has steadily declined from 63.9% in 1980 to 55.4% in 1990 and 39.2% in 1998 (125). The decrease in the 1990s was most pronounced among women with first- and second-degree lacerations. During the 1990s, as the episiotomy rates dropped, the rate of repair of perineal lacerations increased, largely due to an increase in the rate of repair of first- and second-degree lacerations. By 2000, repair of a perineal laceration followed 39.2% of vaginal deliveries (140).

NHDS data show that episiotomy rates in 1998 were highest for white women (43.0%) and those with private insurance (43.7%) (125, 141). Rates were lowest in the West (31.9%) and for women whose hospitalizations were paid by Medicaid (33.3%), another government source (31.2%), or the woman herself (30.5%). In these data, among women who delivered vaginally, the severe laceration rate was 7.8% for women who had an episiotomy and 3.6% for those without episiotomies.

Similarly, a hospital-based study found that women with episiotomies had significantly longer perineal tears (median = 4.9 cm) than those without episiotomy (median = 1.1 cm) (78).

Table 3.5 Hospital-based rates of severe perineal laceration

Location and years	Severe laceration rate	References
USA		
Miami, FL, 1989–1995 (academically affiliated hospital)	2.24%	(126)
Michigan, 1996–1998 (academically affiliated hospital)	Primiparas, aged ≥18 yrs, gestation ≥35 weeks Black women – 10.4% White women – 19.9%	(127)
Kansas, 1996–2000 (community-based hospital)	6.38%	(128)
18 of the largest hospitals in Philadelphia, 1994–1998	Primiparas without prolonged labor or obstructed presentation with infants weighing 2,500–4,000 g Hospital range: 4–13%	(129)
International		
England, 1991–1993	Third-degree laceration: 0.86%	(219)
Sweden, 1995–1997	Third-degree laceration: 3.05% Fourth-degree laceration: 0.24% Total severe: 3.29%	(220)
Austria, 1999	Third-degree laceration: 2.9%	(221)

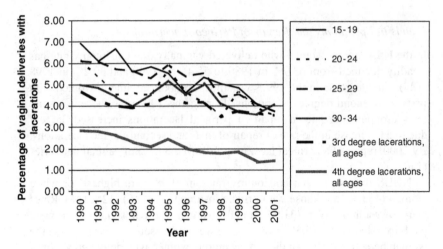

Fig. 3.6 Annual percent of vaginal deliveries with severe perineal lacerations, by maternal age and laceration type, NHDS, USA, 1990–2001

Table 3.6 Common risk factors for severe perineal laceration

Maternal attributes
White race
Older maternal age
Nulliparity
History of severe laceration in a preceding pregnancy
Maternal circumcision
Infant attributes
Nonvertex presentation
Occiput posterior position
Birthweight ≥3,000 g
Labor attributes
Shoulder dystocia
Second stage of labor ≥120 min
Obstetrical care
Operative vaginal delivery (forceps or vacuum extraction)
Failed attempted vaginal operative delivery
Episiotomy (midline)
Epidural anesthesia
Delivery by an obstetrician rather than a midwife

3.4.3 Operative Delivery

Operative vaginal delivery procedures include forceps and vacuum extraction. Operative abdominal delivery involves cesarean section. Operative delivery, whether vaginal or cesarean, is associated with a decreased sense of postpartum well-being as well as increased risks for maternal morbidity and, for cesarean delivery, maternal mortality (118, 127, 143–147). Operative vaginal delivery also increases the risk for infant morbidity and mortality, severe maternal perineal laceration, and postpartum fecal incontinence (124, 138, 139, 148). Data for 28 states from the Agency for Healthcare Research and Quality's Nationwide Inpatient Sample (NIS) show that, in 2000, 24.5% of women who had an operative vaginal delivery experienced obstetric trauma, compared with 8.6% of women who had vaginal deliveries without instrumentation (Care of Women in US Hospitals, 2000. HCUP Fact Book No. 3. AHRQ Publication No. 02–0044, October 2002. Agency for Healthcare Research and Quality, Rockville, MD. http://www.ahrq.gov/data/ hcup/factbk3/factbk3.htm). Women who have operative deliveries have an increased risk for rehospitalization during the 60 days after delivery (118).

A recent systematic literature review concluded that, compared with forceps deliveries, vacuum deliveries are associated with less perineal trauma, less regional and general anesthesia, and less likelihood of cesarean delivery (149). In contrast, forceps deliveries were associated with less risk for neonatal cephalhematoma and retinal hemorrhage.

Morbidities associated with cesarean delivery include postpartum depression, UTI, surgical site infection, peripartum and postpartum stroke and intracranial venous thrombosis, and puerperal fever and hemorrhage (100, 150–152). Cesarean delivery involves longer hospital stays and is more costly than vaginal delivery (Care of Women in US Hospitals, 2000. HCUP Fact Book No. 3. AHRQ Publication No. 02-0044, October 2002. Agency for Healthcare Research and Quality, Rockville, MD. http://www.ahrq.gov/data/hcup/factbk3/factbk3.htm).

Over time, the rates of each type of operative delivery are related to each other, with the rate rising for one type as it falls for another. For example, rates of vacuum delivery tend to rise as those for forceps delivery fall (135, 141) and rates of primary cesarean delivery rise as those for forceps delivery fall (153). Thus, studying all types of operative delivery simultaneously is more informative than considering each in isolation.

Information about the primary or repeat nature of cesarean delivery as well as information on attempted vaginal delivery before cesarean section facilitates interpretation of cesarean section trends. Women with previous cesarean deliveries have an increased risk in subsequent deliveries for uterine rupture at the site of their cesarean scar (absolute risk of approximately 1–2%) (154, 155), especially if the scar is vertical rather than low horizontal or labor is induced (110, 154). Many women with past cesarean deliveries opt for a repeat cesarean section delivery rather than face the risk of uterine rupture associated with attempted vaginal delivery. Among those who attempt vaginal delivery, reported success rates range from 35–70% (155, 156). When comparing the cesarean delivery rates among populations, ideally researchers would like to compare primary cesarean section delivery rates (i.e, the rate among women without a previous cesarean section delivery) and repeat cesarean section delivery rates (i.e, the rate among women with a previous cesarean section delivery). Unfortunately, accurate population-based information on history of cesarean section is often unavailable (157).

Temporal Trends: Data from the NHDS show that the rate of forceps delivery steadily decreased during the 1990s (1990 – 8.6% of vaginal deliveries, 1995 – 5.8%, 2000 – 4.0%), while the rate of vacuum extraction steadily increased through the late 1990s and dropped thereafter (1990 – 6.1% of vaginal deliveries, 1995 – 9.2%, 2000 – 8.4%) (Table 3.7) (141). Both trends extend patterns that began in the 1980s.

Data from birth certificates for the USA show that the rates of primary cesarean section delivery as well as total cesarean section delivery declined during the first part of the 1990s and increased thereafter. The rate of vaginal birth after previous cesarean had the opposite pattern, increasing during the first half of the 1990s and decreasing thereafter (Fig. 3.7) (122). In 1991, the total cesarean section delivery rate was 22.6%. It decreased to a low of 20.7% in 1996 and then rebounded to 22.9% in 2000. Comparable percentages for primary cesarean section delivery were 1991 – 15.9%, 1996 – 14.6%, and 2000 – 16.0%.

Geographic Variability: Data from the NHDS show that, during the 1990s, overall rates of operative delivery were lowest in the Northeast and West. Although all regions followed the same patterns throughout the 1990s as observed nationally, the South consistently had the highest rates of forceps delivery and the lowest rates of vacuum delivery, whereas the reverse was true for the West. During the 1990s, both NHDS and birth certificate data show that the total cesarean section delivery rate was generally lowest in western states, except for California and highest in California and Southern states (Table 3.7 and Fig. 3.8) (141, 158).

International data on vaginal operative deliveries are sparse. Data from Australia show similar pattern as observed in the USA. During the 1990s in New South Wales, Australia, among all operative vaginal deliveries, the percentage involving forceps declined from 58.1% in 1990 to 33.8% in 1997, when it nearly equaled the rate of vacuum deliveries (159).

Cesarean section delivery rates in many developed as well as developing countries are lower than in the USA. In Wales, Scotland, England, and Northern Island during the mid-1990s, rates of cesarean section delivery steadily increased, from a range of 14.3–16.6% in 1993 to 18.2–19.0% in 1997–1998 (160). Using a stratified analysis of cesarean section delivery rates in Denmark during 1996, researchers reported rates ranging from 13.2 to 15.2% (161). Swedish researchers similarly reported a cesarean section delivery rate of 15% in 2000 (162). The national rate of cesarean section delivery in Italy in 1996 was 22.4% (163), comparable to the US rate. In Taiwan during 2000, 32.3% of pregnancies ended in cesarean section delivery (164), markedly higher than the US rate.

Australian researchers studied the rates of operative deliveries during 1996–1997 among low-risk women, defined as those who were 20–34 years of age, had no medical or obstetric complications, had a singleton of normal size presenting in cephalic position, and delivered at 37–41 weeks' gestation (165). They observed that women with private insurance who delivered in private hospitals had higher rates of operative interventions.

Data from the Demographic and Health Surveys show that the percentage of cesarean deliveries during the late 1990s varied widely among regions and, within regions, among countries (Table 3.8). Rates were lowest in sub-Saharan Africa,

Table 3.7 Percentage of deliveries by year, operative method, region and hospital type, NHDS, United States, 1990–2001

| | Method of delivery | | | | | | | | | | | |
| | Cesarean section delivery | | | | Forceps | | | | Vacuum | | | |
Region Year	Northeast	Midwest	South	West	Northeast	Midwest	South	West	Northeast	Midwest	South	West
1990–1992	22.8	22.1	27.1	20.2	3.3	5.4	7.8	3.7	4.2	5.0	4.0	7.9
1992–1995	21.3	21.0	24.6	18.9	2.6	4.3	6.2	3.0	5.9	6.4	4.9	9.9
1996–1998	22.4	20.4	24.0	20.0	2.4	3.2	5.2	1.9	6.1	7.7	5.4	10.3
1999–2001	24.9	21.3	25.2	21.4	2.0	2.4	3.8	1.3	5.1	6.9	4.9	8.4

| | Method of delivery | | | | | | | | |
| | Cesarean section delivery | | | Forceps | | | Vacuum | | |
Hospital type Year	Proprietary	Government	Nonprofit	Proprietary	Government	Nonprofit	Proprietary	Government	Nonprofit
1990–1992	29.2	21.4	23.1	9.2	4.3	5.2	3.7	3.0	5.9
1992–1995	26.4	21.1	21.3	6.0	4.6	4.1	5.4	5.1	7.1
1996–1998	26.7	21.8	21.2	3.7	5.3	3.2	7.6	5.4	7.5
1999–2001	27.6	23.2	22.8	3.0	3.3	2.5	6.4	5.3	6.3

Cesarean deliveries include all deliveries performed by cesarean section, with or without unsuccessful attempted operative vaginal delivery (i.e., forceps or vacuum extraction); forceps deliveries include deliveries with forceps, with or without vacuum extraction; vacuum deliveries include deliveries with vacuum extraction only

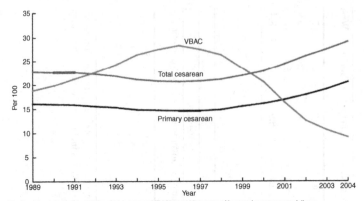

Top line: Number of vaginal births after cesarean (VBAC) per 100 woman with a previous cesarean delivery.
Middle line: Percentage of all births by cesarean delivery.
Bottomline: Number of primary cesarean deliveries per 100 live births to woman who have not had a previous cesarean.
NOTE: Due to changes in data collection from implementation of the 2003 revision of the U.S. Standard Certificate of Live Birth, there may be small discontinuities in rates of primary cesarean delivery and VBAC In 2003 and 2004.

Fig. 3.7. Cesarean section delivery rates, by type, USA, 1989–2004 (*Source*: (121))

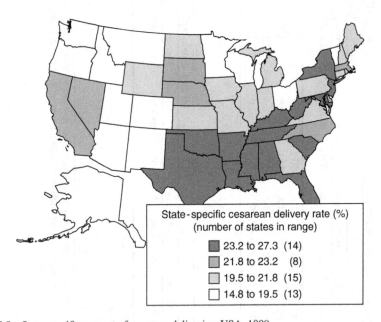

Fig. 3.8. State-specific percent of cesarean deliveries, USA, 1999

except for South Africa (range 0.7–5.6%; South Africa – 15.5%) and South and Southeast Asia (range 0.8–5.7%). Although rates in Latin America and the Caribbean were as low as 1.6% (Haiti), other countries in the region had rates that exceeded those in the USA (Columbia – 23.6%; Dominican Republic – 27.9%).

Other researchers have reported exceedingly high cesarean section delivery rates in Mexico (national rate, 1996 – 24.1%; rate for in-hospital deliveries, 1997 – 31.3%), Argentina (national rate, 1996 – 25.4%), Brazil (national rate, 1994 – 27.1%; rate for in-hospital deliveries, 1997 – 31.3%), and Chile (national rate, 1997 – 40.0%) (166).

Demographic Variability: NHDS data show that, during the 1990s, all maternal age groups had the same pattern of decreasing rates of forceps delivery and

What is an optimal rate of cesarean section?

The optimal cesarean delivery rate has been discussed since at least 1978 (166, 167). Controversy stems from tradeoffs between maternal and neonatal health, with concerns that lower cesarean rates will increase maternal morbidity related to vaginal operative delivery and, for repeat cesarean delivery, uterine rupture (168). Cesarean delivery of term, singleton breech pregnancies markedly reduces the risk of neonatal adverse outcomes and modestly increases the likelihood of maternal adverse outcomes (169). Cesarean delivery is very effective in reducing mother-to-child transmission of HIV (170). Evidence supporting cesarean delivery for many other clinical presentations is sparse or contradictory (171–174).

Variations in practitioner-specific and hospital-specific cesarean delivery rates suggest opportunities for reducing rates (175, 176). Evidence-based methods to reduce cesarean rates include external cephalic version, vaginal birth after cesarean, and individual psychological support for the mother during labor (177). In the USA in 1995, 28 health care organizations collaborated in a demonstration project intended to reduce cesarean delivery rates safely (178). Their approach included these elements: (1) preventing cesarean deliveries for failed induction of labor, (2) avoiding hospital admissions for false labor, and (3) managing pain more effectively to help women tolerate labor. More than half of the participating hospitals reduced their cesarean rates.

Use of a standard treatment protocol at a tertiary hospital in Italy reduced cesarean rates from 26.4% (1982) to 12% (1996), with no increase in neonatal mortality. Rates of vaginal operative delivery in 1996 were low at 1.5% (162). Through active management of labor, a hospital in Washington state lowered the primary cesarean delivery rate from 9.2% in 1989 to 7.1% in 1998 and the repeat cesarean delivery rate from 7.4% to 3.8%. Neonatal morbidity and mortality rates were stable (179, 180).

Despite the Year 2010 health objective for 15% of full-term, singleton, vertex deliveries by cesarean, no clear evidence points to an organized national effort to achieve this goal. The Year 2010 objective for women with a prior cesarean is 63%. (www.healthypeople.gov/document/html/objectives/16-09.htm). If current concerns persist regarding uterine rupture associated with attempted vaginal birth after cesarean delivery, the percentage of cesarean delivery will not decrease and may increase.

Table 3.8 Percentage of cesarean deliveries, by country

Country and date of survey	Cesarean delivery rate during the 5 years before the survey
Sub-Saharan Africa	
Benin 2001	3.3
Burkina Faso 1998/99	1.1
Cote d'Ivoire 1998/99	2.5
Ethiopia 2000	0.7
Gabon 2000	5.6
Ghana 1998	4
Guinea 1999	2
Malawi 2000	2.8
Mali 2001	1.1
Mauritania 2000/01	3.2
Rwanda 2000	2.1
South Africa 1998	15.5
Tanzania 1999	2.9
Uganda 2000/01	2.5
Zambia 2001/02	2.1
Zimbabwe 1999	6.7
North Africa/West Asia/Europe	
Armenia 2000	6.6
Egypt 2000	10.3
Turkey 199	13.9
Central Asia	
Kazakhstan 1999	9.6
Turkmenistan 2000	3.1
South & Southeast Asia	
Bangladesh 1999/2000	2.4
Cambodia 2000	0.8
Nepal 2001	0.8
Philippines 1998	5.7
Latin America & Caribbean	
Colombia 2000	23.6
Dominican Republic 1999	27.9
Guatemala 1998/99	10.8
Haiti 2000	1.6
Peru 2000	12.7

Source: Demographic and Health Surveys

increasing rates of vacuum delivery. However, among women with operative deliveries, the distribution of method varied by age, with women aged 30 years and older more likely to have cesarean section delivery and less likely to have forceps or vacuum delivery than younger women. In the USA during the 1990s, total and primary cesarean section delivery rates were lowest for women aged <25 years and increased with advancing maternal age thereafter (141). Throughout the decade and within most age groups, the total and primary cesarean section delivery rates among non-Hispanic whites were modestly lower than those for non-Hispanic blacks (141). Total cesarean section delivery rates were modestly higher for first births than for second or third births, even though these higher-order births included primary and repeat cesarean deliveries. Women with <12 years of education had lower cesarean rates than those with more education (141).

Attributes of Women with Cesarean Deliveries: The 28-state dataset of NIS shows that, in 2000 in the USA, among women with primary cesarean section delivery, 29.9% were aged 18–24 years, 52.7% were 25–34 years, and 17.4% were ≥34 years. The comparable percentages for those with repeat cesarean deliveries were 18–24 – 18.6%, 25–34 – 57.3%, and >34 – 24.1%. Among women with vaginal deliveries, excluding those with a history of cesarean section delivery, 35.6% were aged 18–24 years, 51.7% were 25–34 years, and 12.7% were >34 years (Care of Women in US Hospitals, 2000. HCUP Fact Book No. 3. AHRQ Publication No. 02-0044, October 2002. Agency for Health-care Research and Quality, Rockville, MD. http://www.ahrq.gov/data/hcup/factbk3/factbk3.htm).

Factors Influencing Occurrence: A diverse range of maternal, fetal, and prac-tice-related factors influence the occurrence of operative deliveries (Table 3.9). Results regarding the risks for cesarean section delivery associated with induction of labor and epidural anesthesia are inconsistent, with some studies showing an increased risk and others showing no association (159, 165, 182–184). If an association with induction is substantiated, the on-going increases in induction rates (which more than doubled from 9.5% in 1990 to 19.4% in 1998) may contribute to future increases in cesarean section delivery rates (185).

Clinical and public health efforts to reduce cesarean section delivery rates have focused on hospital- and practitioner-related practice patterns, because many other risk factors, such as fetal presentation, are immutable. Variations in cesarean section delivery rates among practitioners, hospitals, and countries are consistent with the possibility that practice patterns are a strong determinant of cesarean rates. A study of cesarean section delivery rates in Latin American showed strong, direct ecologic associations between the national cesarean rate and gross national product

Illness caused by obstetrical care:

A recent study used NIS hospital discharge data from 28 states during 2000 to examine medical injuries resulting from care for a wide range of conditions (185). The investigators estimated a rate of obstetrically induced trauma of 7.0% for cesarean deliveries, 8.7% for vaginal births without instrumentation, and a strikingly high rate of 22.4% for vaginal births with instrumentation. Although Patient Safety Indicators (164, 186) have been developed for obstetrical care, virtually no systematic investigations have explored the causes of and remedies for injury due to failed obstetrical care. Such study is especially warranted for operative vaginal deliveries.

Table 3.9 Factors that increase the risk of operative delivery, by type of delivery

Delivery type	Factor	References
Vaginal	<24-years old	
	Midline episiotomy	(134)
	Regional anesthesia	(134)
Primary cesarean	Diabetes (Types 1 and 2 and gestational)	(251)
	Maternal age <16 years	(252)
	Maternal age ≥30 years	(158, 181, 253)
	Short maternal height	(254)
	Maternal bulimia or anorexia nervosa	(255)
	Congenital uterine malformations	(256)
	Maternal preconception high BMI or excessive weight gain during pregnancy	(257)
	Maternal birthweight <2,500 g or >4,000 g	(258, 259)
	Placenta previa or placental abruption	(260)
	Physical violence during pregnancy	(105)
	Multiple gestation	(176)
	Among nulliparas aged ≥40, infertility treatment	(261)
	Breech presentation	(262)
	Prolonged gestation	(181)
	Hospital type	(176, 262, 263)
	Delivery on a weekday (not a weekend)	(264, 265)
	Delivery by an obstetrician (compared with midwife)	(266)
	Obstetrician's practice patterns for management of labor	(175, 267)
	Induced or augmented labor	(158, 181, 268, 269)
	Decreased use of forceps delivery	(152)

per capita, number of doctors per 10,000, the proportion of urban population, and the proportion of institutional deliveries (166). All of these factors are likely to influence obstetric practices.

3.5   Postpartum Morbidity

Many postpartum morbidities stem from problems associated with delivery, particularly infection, perineal trauma, hypertension-related conditions, and hemorrhage (118, 188, 189). Others, notably mastitis, stem from postpartum changes. Less frequently occurring are thromboembolic conditions and cardiac myopathies. In this section we focus on one of the most prevalent postpartum morbidities, depression.

3.5.1   Depression

Although antepartum and postpartum depression occur frequently, they are commonly unrecognized by the depressed women or her health care providers

(190–192). Not surprisingly, women with antepartum or postpartum depression usually do not receive treatment for it (193), despite the risk for suicide that accompanies severe depression, regardless of pregnancy status (194). Anxiety frequently accompanies pregnancy-related depression (195). Some women who experience pregnancy-related depression may have an underlying propensity for depression, regardless of pregnancy status. The findings that women who experience pregnancy-related depression are more likely to have a personal history of depression as well as a family history of psychiatric illness are consistent with this possibility (196–198).

Whether pregnancy itself increases the risk for depression is uncertain. A longitudinal study of child-bearing and nonchild-bearing women observed that child-bearing women had a higher rate of depression only late in pregnancy and shortly after delivery (199). Another study followed women during 12 months following delivery and compared them with a control group of women who were not pregnant, had not delivered during the same 12 months, and were matched to postpartum women by age, marital status, and number of children (200). At 6-months postpartum, the authors observed a similar point prevalence of depression for postnatal women (9.1%) and controls (8.2%). However, postpartum women had a threefold higher onset of depression during the 5 weeks after delivery than control women.

Although several studies suggest that maternal antepartum depression may increase the risk for adverse pregnancy outcomes, including impaired fetal growth and preterm delivery (201–203), the causal nature of this relationship is unclear. One could expect that women at risk of adverse pregnancy are more psychologically stressed than women without this risk and that the stress predisposes the gravida to depression.

Occurrence: Data on temporal trends are lacking and reported rates of depression depend on ascertainment methods. The Edinburgh Postnatal Depression Scale (EPDS) is a validated, widely-used instrument to detect antenatal as well as postnatal depression that can be administered by interview or by the woman herself (204). Other instruments used to measure depression include the National Institute of Health Diagnostic Interview Scale (205), the Center for Epidemiologic Studies Depression Scale (206), and the Primary Care Evaluation of Mental Disorders (205). In comparing reports of depression prevalence, one must consider not only the instrument used to detect depression, but the cutoff used to declare its presence. For example, scores ≥ 13 on the EPDS are usually considered to indicate depression, but some investigators use lower cutoffs to identify women with depressive symptoms.

Table 3.10 displays the range of prevalence of depression during pregnancy and postpartum. Although rates are grouped by their timing relative to pregnancy, repeated measures over time are presented for some cohorts (207). Most investigators have observed similar antepartum and postpartum rates of depression, but some have observed peaks either before or after delivery. A longitudinal study of more than 9,000 women found that depression peaked at 8.3% at 32-weeks gestation, declining thereafter to 6.4% at 8-weeks postpartum and 5.4% at 32-weeks postpartum (207). This finding contradicts conventional wisdom that depression is more prevalent after delivery than before it. These investigators further observed that, of women depressed

Table 3.10 Prevalence of pregnancy-related depression

Population and method of detecting depression	Time period	Depression prevalence	References
9,316 women, Bristol, England, EPDS, 1991–1992	18-weeks gestation	11.9%	(206)
1,795 women in Northern Sweden, PRIME-MD	Second trimester	3.3%	(125, 192)
391 pregnant Finnish women, EPDS	14–37-weeks gestation	7.7%	(270)
9,316 women, Bristol, England, EPDS, 1991–1992	32-weeks gestation	13.7%	(206)
1558 Swedish women, EDPS	35–36-weeks gestation	17%	(271)
417 women in West Midlands, UK, EPDS	Antepartum	9.8%	(272)
1,558 Swedish women, EDPS	At delivery	18%	(271)
327 Israeli women, EPDS	1–2-days postpartum	10–22%	(273)
959 Chinese women in Hong Kong, structured clinical interview for DSM-III-R	1-month postpartum	5.5%	(274)
222 South Australian women, EPDS	6-weeks postpartum	9%	(275)
909 women in Olmsted County, Minnesota, EPDS, 1997–1998	6-weeks postpartum	11.4%	(276)
1,558 Swedish women, EDPS	6–8-weeks postpartum	13%	(271)
9,316 women, Bristol, England, EPDS, 1991–1992	8-weeks postpartum	8.4%	(206)
327 Israeli women, EPDS	6–12-weeks postpartum	5–12%	(273)
359 women in rural South India	6–12 weeks postpartum	11%	(277)
959 Chinese women in Hong Kong, Structured clinical interview for DSM-III-R	3-months postpartum	6.1%	(274)
417 women in West Midlands, UK, EPDS	3-months postpartum	7.4%	(272)
570 women, EPDS	3-months postpartum	10.2%	(278)
396 Lebanese women, EPDS	3–5-months postpartum	21% (urban – 16%, rural – 26%)	(279)

	Incidence of depression between 1 and 4 months postpartum		
465 women in Wisconsin, DIS or CES-D	between 1 and 4 months postpartum	5.8%	(280)
5,252 women delivering at an academic hospital in Denmark, EPDS, 1994–1995	4-months postpartum	5.5%	(281)
222 South Australian women, EPDS	6-months postpartum	10%	(275)
1,558 Swedish women, EDPS	6-months postpartum	13%	(271)
1,336 Australian women, EDPS, 1993	6–7-months postpartum	16.9%	(125, 145)
1,330 women, Christchurch, New Zealand, EPDS	6–9-months postpartum	13%	(189, 190)
9,316 women, Bristol, England, EPDS, 1991–1992	32-weeks postpartum	9.2%	(206)
403 women in Olmsted County, Minnesota, medical chart review	1-year postpartum	3.7%	(282)

at 32-weeks gestation, 62% remained depressed at 8-weeks postpartum, whereas of women not depressed at 32-weeks gestation, 4% were depressed at 8-weeks postpartum. This suggests that antepartum depression is likely to persist postpartum, but that the postpartum risk of developing depression is low among women who were not depressed during pregnancy. A longitudinal study of 293 women observed a peak prevalence at 10-weeks postpartum of 14% (208).

Factors Influencing Occurrence: Investigators have associated psychological, demographic, and obstetrical factors with the risk for postpartum depression (Table 3.11). Data regarding the relationship between obstetric morbidity and subsequent risk for postpartum depression are inconsistent, with some reports showing increased risk (209) and others showing no association (210). No interventions to prevent antepartum or postpartum depression have been rigorously evaluated. Although the presence of thyroid antibodies has been associated with increased risk for postpartum depression, a randomized clinical trial did not find that postpartum administration of thyroxine reduced the risk of postpartum depression (211).

Table 3.11 Risk factors associated with postpartum depression

Psychological factors	References
Previous affective disorder, including depression	(189, 196, 197, 281–283)
Antenatal depression	(272, 279)
Self-perceived antepartum isolation	(281)
Lack of social support postpartum	(279)
Difficulties in relationship with partner or spouse	(189, 190)
Marital disharmony	(272, 284)
Family history of psychiatric illness	(197)
Low level of religious belief	(196)
Demographic factors	
Low maternal education	(189, 190)
Low maternal income	(189, 190, 284)
Single marital status	(282)
Maternal postpartum unemployment	(285)
Paternal postpartum unemployment	(285)
Obstetric and medical factors	
Maternal chronic health problem	(279)
High parity	(281)
Unplanned pregnancy	(285)
Infant gender (usually associated with female when male desired)	(284)
Presence of thyroid peroxidase antibodies at 12-weeks gestation	(286)
Severe antepartum obstetric complications	(208)
High body mass index at 4-months postpartum	(287)
Not breastfeeding	(285)
Low level of docosahexanenoic acid in maternal milk and low fish consumption	(288)
High use of emergency services	(282)

3.6   Public Health Interventions: Their Availability and Use

In this section, we discuss public health interventions that reduce maternal morbidity and consequently often reduce maternal mortality. Additional public health interventions to reduce maternal mortality are discussed at the end of Chap. 4.

Ensuring access to prenatal care is likely to reduce morbidity and mortality from anemia, pyleonephritis, preeclampsia, eclampsia, hemorrhage, operative delivery, and infection. Among the prenatal interventions and their related impacts on maternal morbidity and mortality are the following:

- Providing iron and folate supplements and screening for and treating anemia, which reduces anemia and shows promise for reducing the need for postpartum blood transfusion (212).
- Among women with either high risk of developing hypertension or low baseline dietary calcium intake, providing calcium supplements, which reduces the risk of preeclampsia (212).
- Screening for proteinuria and increases in blood pressure can detect preeclampsia, enabling treatment, including magnesium sulfate to reduce mortality and induced delivery for severe disease. Treatment lowers the risk for hemorrhage that is associated with gestational hypertension (213).
- Screening for asymptomatic bacteriuria and treating appropriately, which prevents pyelonephritis from ascending infections (213).
- Providing tetanus immunization prevents maternal and neonatal tetanus
- Among women with rupture of membranes at or near term, inducing labor, which prevents maternal infection (213).
- Among women with breech presentation at term, external cephalic version, which reduces the risk of cesarean section delivery (213).

In populations with vitamin A deficiency, β-carotene supplementation holds promise for reducing maternal mortality (212, 214). However, vitamin A deficiency is uncommon in the USA (215, 216). Although supplementation with iron and folate may reduce pregnancy-associated morbidity, its impact on reducing maternal mortality is uncertain (217, 218).

Optimizing nutrition during childhood to maximize adult stature (212, 213) and achieving a preconception weight that is appropriate for height are likely to reduce operative delivery due to obstructed labor (Table 3.12).

Notably absent from this list of prenatal clinical interventions are risk-scoring systems. These systems categorize women based on obstetric history and other attributes. Women with higher risk scores receive more intensive and/or specialized obstetrical care. The effectiveness of these approaches for reducing perinatal morbidity has not been established through randomized controlled trials (213).

Secondary Prevention: In developed countries, access to hygienic delivery facilities and availability of tertiary-level care and emergency transport to it are much less of a problem than in developing countries. The FIGO (International

Table 3.12 Public health interventions aimed at decreasing maternal morbidity and mortality

Maternal problem(s)	Public health intervention	Rationale
Ectopic pregnancy	Reducing the prevalence of chlamydia infections through screening and treatment	Chlamydia infections can damage the fallopian tubes
Morbidity or mortality related to induced abortion	Reducing cigarette smoking among women	Smoking increases the risk for ectopic pregnancy
	Ensuring easy access to abortion	Easy access enables women to obtain abortions at earlier gestations, when risks are lowest
Anemia	Removing barriers to prenatal care	Prenatal care reduces the risk of adverse outcomes (see text)
Pyelonephritis		
Preeclampsia		
Eclampsia		
Hemorrhage		
Cesarean delivery		
Endometritis		
Tetanus		
Operative delivery or death secondary to cephalopelvic disproportion (CPD)	Ensuring adequate nutrition during childhood	Short maternal stature increases the risk of CPD. Providing adequate nutrition during pregnancy helps to maximize adult stature
	Reducing preconception overweight/obesity	Maternal overweight/obesity is associated with increased risk for operative delivery.
Death from obstructed labor, hemorrhage, preeclampsia, or eclampsia	Maintaining a rapid transport system to a hospital capable of cesarean section deliveries (in developing countries, usually a referral hospital)	Treatment of hemorrhage, severe preeclampsia, or eclampsia requires prompt care at tertiary facility
Puerpural infection	Providing trained birth attendant and hygienic delivery facilities	Trained attendants and adequate facilities minimize the risk of ascending infection and endometritis
Maternal postpartum tetanus infection	Providing population-based immunization programs	Immunization prevents tetanus

Federation of Obstetrics and Gynecology) initiative (213, 219), which aims to reduce maternal mortality in developing countries, includes four components:

- Skilled attendants at all births
- Basic emergency care in primary-level health facilities
- Comprehensive obstetrical care in referral hospitals
- Rapid transport of women in need of special care

Training a workforce of skilled birth attendants, establishing a network of primary and referral health care facilities, and maintaining a rapid transport system all fall within the realm of public health interventions.

Discussion Topics

1. How could pharmacy or laboratory records be used to categorize the severity of maternal morbidity?
2. For a state or country, what is likely to be the most cost-effective way to reduce maternal morbidity and mortality? How could you test the effectiveness of an intervention to reduce maternal morbidity and mortality? What ethical issues would you need to consider?
3. Define a cohort of women as women born in the same time period, for example, 1974–1979 or 1980–1984. What could you learn from monitoring a cohort's cumulative rate of cesarean section over time (i.e., the percentage of women with ≥ 1 cesarean delivery)? What factors would likely influence the cumulative rate?
4. Cephalopelvic disproportion often necessitates operative delivery. How can obstetric trauma resulting from the cephalopelvic disproportion itself be distinguished from trauma resulting from the operative methods used during delivery?

Promising Areas for Future Research

1. What methods can be developed to use administrative data to monitor severe maternal morbidity?
2. How can the comparability of rates of severe maternal morbidity among developed countries be assessed?
3. What are the best methods to evaluate the impact of interventions to reduce maternal morbidity?

Abbreviations

BMI   Body Mass Index
CPD   Cephalopelvic disproportion

CPT   Current procedural terminology
EPDS   Edinburgh Postnatal Depression Scale
HELLP   Hemolysis, elevated liver enzymes
ICD   International Classification of Diseases
NCHS   National Center for Health Statistics
NHDS   National Hospital Discharge Survey
PMSS   Pregnancy Mortality Surveillance System
SID   State inpatient databases
UTI   Urinary tract infection
WHO   World Health Organization

References

1. Last JM, Spasoff RA, Harris SS (eds.). A Dictionary of Epidemiology, 4th edn. New York City: Oxford University Press, 2001.
2. Savitz DA, Hertz-Picciotto I, Poole C, Olshan AF. Epidemiologic measures of the course and outcome of pregnancy. Epidemiol Rev 2002; 24(2):91–101.
3. Baskett TF, Sternadel J. Maternal intensive care and near-miss mortality in obstetrics. Br J Obstet Gynaecol 1998; 105(9):981–984.
4. Geller SE, Rosenberg D, Cox SM, Kilpatrick S. Defining a conceptual framework for near-miss maternal morbidity. J Am Med Womens Assoc 2002; 57(3):135–139.
5. Mantel GD, Buchmann E, Rees H, Pattinson RC. Severe acute maternal morbidity: a pilot study of a definition for a near-miss. Br J Obstet Gynaecol 1998; 105(9):985–990.
6. Nasrat HA, Youssef MH, Marzoogi A, Talab F. "Near miss" obstetric morbidity in an inner city hospital in Saudi Arabia. East Mediterr Health J 1999; 5(4):717–726.
7. Penny J. Severe acute maternal morbidity: a pilot study of a definition of a near-miss. Br J Obstet Gynaecol 1999; 106(4):397.
8. Geller SE, Rosenberg D, Cox S, Brown M, Simonson L, Kilpatrick S. A scoring system identified near-miss maternal morbidity during pregnancy. J Clin Epidemiol 2004; 57(7): 716–720.
9. Geller SE, Cox SM, Kilpatrick SJ. A descriptive model of preventability in maternal morbidity and mortality. J Perinatol 2006; 26(2):79–84.
10. Geller SE, Cox SM, Callaghan WM, Berg CJ. Morbidity and mortality in pregnancy: laying the groundwork for safe motherhood. Womens Health Issues 2006; 16(4):176–188.
11. Sanderson M, Placek PJ, Keppel KG. The 1988 National Maternal and Infant Health Survey: design, content, and data availability. Birth 1991; 18(1):26–32.
12. Sanderson M, Gonzalez JF. 1988 National Maternal and Infant Health Survey: methods and response characteristics. Vital Health Stat 2 1998; (125):1–39.
13. Lydon-Rochelle MT, Holt VL, Cardenas V, Nelson JC, Easterling TR, Gardella C et al. The reporting of pre-existing maternal medical conditions and complications of pregnancy on birth certificates and in hospital discharge data. Am J Obstet Gynecol 2005; 193(1):125–134.
14. Zane SB, Kieke BA Jr, Kendrick JS, Bruce C. Surveillance in a time of changing health care practices: estimating ectopic pregnancy incidence in the United States. Matern Child Health J 2002; 6(4):227–236.
15. U.S. Department of Health and Human Services. *Healthy People 2010*. 2nd ed. With Understanding and Improving Health and Objectives for Improving Health. 2 vols. Washington, DC: U.S. Government Printing Office, November 2000.

16. Gazmararian JA, Petersen R, Jamieson DJ, Schild L, Adams MM, Deshpande AD et al. Hospitalizations during pregnancy among managed care enrollees. Obstet Gynecol 2002; 100(1):94–100.

17. Bacak SJ, Callaghan WM, Dietz PM, Crouse C. Pregnancy-associated hospitalizations in the United States, 1999–2000. Am J Obstet Gynecol 2005; 192(2):592–597.

18. Liu S, Heaman M, Sauve R, Liston R, Reyes F, Bartholomew S et al. An analysis of antenatal hospitalization in Canada, 1991–2003. Matern Child Health J 2007; 11(2):181–187.

19. Centers for Disease Control and Prevention. Ectopic pregnancy–United States, 1990–1992. MMWR Morb Mortal Wkly Rep 1995; 44(3):46–48.

20. Van Den Eeden SK, Shan J, Bruce C, Glasser M. Ectopic pregnancy rate and treatment utilization in a large managed care organization. Obstet Gynecol 2005; 105(5, Part 1):1052–1057.

21. Irvine LM, Setchell ME. Declining incidence of ectopic pregnancy in a UK city health district between 1990 and 1999. Hum Reprod 2001; 16(10):2230–2234.

22. Coste J, Bouyer J, Germain E, Ughetto S, Pouly JL, Job-Spira N. Recent declining trend in ectopic pregnancy in France: evidence of two clinicoepidemiologic entities. Fertil Steril 2000; 74(5):881–886.

23. Boufous S, Quartararo M, Mohsin M, Parker J. Trends in the incidence of ectopic pregnancy in New South Wales between 1990–1998. Aust N Z J Obstet Gynaecol 2001; 41(4):436–438.

24. Egger M, Low N, Smith GD, Lindblom B, Herrmann B. Screening for chlamydial infections and the risk of ectopic pregnancy in a county in Sweden: ecological analysis. BMJ 1998; 316 (7147):1776–1780.

25. Coste J, Bouyer J, Ughetto S, Gerbaud L, Fernandez H, Pouly JL et al. Ectopic pregnancy is again on the increase. Recent trends in the incidence of ectopic pregnancies in France (1992–2002). Hum Reprod 2004; 19(9):2014–2018.

26. Peterson HB, Xia Z, Hughes JM, Wilcox LS, Tylor LR, Trussell J. The risk of ectopic pregnancy after tubal sterilization. U.S. Collaborative Review of Sterilization Working Group. N Engl J Med 1997; 336(11):762–767.

27. Bouyer J, Coste J, Shojaei T, Pouly JL, Fernandez H, Gerbaud L et al. Risk factors for ectopic pregnancy: a comprehensive analysis based on a large case-control, population-based study in France. Am J Epidemiol 2003; 157(3):185–194.

28. Coste J, Bouyer J, Job-Spira N. [Epidemiology of ectopic pregnancy: incidence and risk factors]. Contracept Fertil Sex 1996; 24(2):135–139.

29. Goldberg JM, Falcone T. Effect of diethylstilbestrol on reproductive function. Fertil Steril 1999; 72(1):1–7.

30. Pisarska MD, Carson SA. Incidence and risk factors for ectopic pregnancy. Clin Obstet Gynecol 1999; 42(1):2–8.

31. Zhang J, Thomas AG, Leybovich E. Vaginal douching and adverse health effects: a meta-analysis. Am J Public Health 1997; 87(7):1207–1211.

32. Kendrick JS, Atrash HK, Strauss LT, Gargiullo PM, Ahn YW. Vaginal douching and the risk of ectopic pregnancy among black women. Am J Obstet Gynecol 1997; 176(5):991–997.

33. Centers for Disease Control and Prevention. Strategies for reducing exposure to environmental tobacco smoke, increase tobacco-use cessation, and reducing initiation in communities and health care systems: a report on recommendations of the Task Force on Community Preventive Services. MMWR Recomm Rep 2000; 49(RR-12):1–12.

34. Bauer JE, Hyland A, Li Q, Steger C, Cummings KM. A longitudinal assessment of the impact of smoke-free worksite policies on tobacco use. Am J Public Health 2005; 95(6): 1024–1029.

35. Preemptive state smoke-free indoor air laws – United States, 1999–2004. MMWR Morb Mortal Wkly Rep 2005; 54(10):250–253.

36. Lacroix R, Eason E, Melzack R. Nausea and vomiting during pregnancy: a prospective study of its frequency, intensity, and patterns of change. Am J Obstet Gynecol 2000; 182(4): 931–937.

37. Quinlan JD. HDA. Nausea and vomiting during pregnancy. Am Fam Physician 2003; 98(1):121–128.
38. Kallen B, Lundberg G, Aberg A. Relationship between vitamin use, smoking, and nausea and vomiting of pregnancy. Acta Obstet Gynecol Scand 2003; 82(10):916–920.
39. Fell DB, Dodds L, Joseph KS, Allen VM, Butler B. Risk factors for hyperemesis gravidarum requiring hospital admission during pregnancy. Obstet Gynecol 2006; 107(2, Part 1): 277–284.
40. Mar Melero-Montes M, Jick H. Hyperemesis gravidarum and the sex of the offspring. Epidemiology 2001; 12(1):123–124.
41. Vilming B, Nesheim BI. Hyperemesis gravidarum in a contemporary population in Oslo. Acta Obstet Gynecol Scand 2000; 79(8):640–643.
42. Anderson BL, Simhan HN, Simons KM, Wiesenfeld HC. Untreated asymptomatic group B streptococcal bacteriuria early in pregnancy and chorioamnionitis at delivery. Am J Obstet Gynecol 2007; 196(6):524–525.
43. Pastore LM, Savitz DA, Thorp JM Jr. Predictors of urinary tract infection at the first prenatal visit. Epidemiology 1999; 10(3):282–287.
44. McIsaac W, Carroll JC, Biringer A, Bernstein P, Lyons E, Low DE et al. Screening for asymptomatic bacteriuria in pregnancy. J Obstet Gynaecol Can 2005; 27(1):20–24.
45. Dempsey C, Harrison RF, Moloney A, Darling M, Walshe J. Characteristics of bacteriuria in a homogeneous maternity hospital population. Eur J Obstet Gynecol Reprod Biol 1992; 44(3):189–193.
46. Pastore LM, Savitz DA, Thorp JM Jr, Koch GG, Hertz-Picciotto I, Irwin DE. Predictors of symptomatic urinary tract infection after 20 weeks' gestation. J Perinatol 1999; 19(7):488–493.
47. Hsu CD, Witter FR. Urogenital infection in preeclampsia. Int J Gynaecol Obstet 1995; 49(3):271–275.
48. Ochoa-Brust GJ, Fernandez AR, Villanueva-Ruiz GJ, Velasco R, Trujillo-Hernandez B, Vasquez C. Daily intake of 100 mg ascorbic acid as urinary tract infection prophylactic agent during pregnancy. Acta Obstet Gynecol Scand 2007; 86(7):783–787.
49. Englund JA. Maternal immunization with inactivated influenza vaccine: rationale and experience. Vaccine 2003; 21(24):3460–3464.
50. Neuzil KM, Reed GW, Mitchel EF, Simonsen L, Griffin MR. Impact of influenza on acute cardiopulmonary hospitalizations in pregnant women. Am J Epidemiol 1998; 148(11): 1094–1102.
51. Fiore AE, Shay DK, Haber P, Iskander JK, Uyeki TM, Mootrey G et al. Prevention and control of influenza. Recommendations of the Advisory Committee on Immunization Practices (ACIP), 2007. MMWR Recomm Rep 2007; 56(RR-6):1–54.
52. American Diabetes Association. Gestational diabetes mellitus. Diabetes Care 2004; 27 Suppl 1:S88–S90.
53. Vidaeff AC, Yeomans ER, Ramin SM. Gestational diabetes: a field of controversy. Obstet Gynecol Surv 2003; 58(11):759–769.
54. Screening for gestational diabetes mellitus: recommendation and rationale. Am Fam Physician 2003; 68(2):331–335.
55. Screening for gestational diabetes mellitus: recommendations and rationale. Obstet Gynecol 2003; 101(2):393–395.
56. Brody SC, Harris R, Lohr K. Screening for gestational diabetes: a summary of the evidence for the U.S. Preventive Services Task Force. Obstet Gynecol 2003; 101(2):380–392.
57. Gestational diabetes mellitus. Diabetes Care 2000; 23 Suppl 1:S77–S79.
58. Ferrara A, Hedderson MM, Quesenberry CP, Selby JV. Prevalence of gestational diabetes mellitus detected by the national diabetes data group or the carpenter and coustan plasma glucose thresholds. Diabetes Care 2002; 25(9):1625–1630.
59. Xiong X, Saunders LD, Wang FL, Demianczuk NN. Gestational diabetes mellitus: prevalence, risk factors, maternal and infant outcomes. Int J Gynaecol Obstet 2001; 75(3):221–228.

60. Cundy T, Gamble G, Townend K, Henley PG, MacPherson P, Roberts AB. Perinatal mortality in Type 2 diabetes mellitus. Diabetes Med 2000; 17(1):33–39.
61. Kim C, Newton KM, Knopp RH. Gestational diabetes and the incidence of type 2 diabetes: a systematic review. Diabetes Care 2002; 25(10):1862–1868.
62. Ferrara A, Kahn HS, Quesenberry CP, Riley C, Hedderson MM. An increase in the incidence of gestational diabetes mellitus: Northern California, 1991–2000. Obstet Gynecol 2004; 103 (3):526–533.
63. Dabelea D, Snell-Bergeon JK, Hartsfield CL, Bischoff KJ, Hamman RF, McDuffie RS. Increasing prevalence of gestational diabetes mellitus (GDM) over time and by birth cohort: Kaiser Permanente of Colorado GDM Screening Program. Diabetes Care 2005; 28(3): 579–584.
64. Gregory KD, Korst LM. Age and racial/ethnic differences in maternal, fetal, and placental conditions in laboring patients. Am J Obstet Gynecol 2003; 188(6):1602–1606.
65. Berkowitz GS, Roman SH, Lapinski RH, Alvarez M. Maternal characteristics, neonatal outcome, and the time of diagnosis of gestational diabetes. Am J Obstet Gynecol 1992; 167 (4, Part 1):976–982.
66. Dornhorst A, Paterson CM, Nicholls JS, Wadsworth J, Chiu DC, Elkeles RS et al. High prevalence of gestational diabetes in women from ethnic minority groups. Diabet Med 1992; 9 (9):820–825.
67. Engelgau MM, Herman WH, Smith PJ, German RR, Aubert RE. The epidemiology of diabetes and pregnancy in the U.S., 1988. Diabetes Care 1995; 18(7):1029–1033.
68. Benjamin E, Winters D, Mayfield J, Gohdes D. Diabetes in pregnancy in Zuni Indian women. Prevalence and subsequent development of clinical diabetes after gestational diabetes. Diabetes Care 1993; 16(9):1231–1235.
69. Rodrigues S, Robinson EJ, Ghezzo H, Gray-Donald K. Interaction of body weight and ethnicity on risk of gestational diabetes mellitus. Am J Clin Nutr 1999; 70(6):1083–1089.
70. Dyck R, Klomp H, Tan LK, Turnell RW, Boctor MA. A comparison of rates, risk factors, and outcomes of gestational diabetes between aboriginal and non-aboriginal women in the Saskatoon health district. Diabetes Care 2002; 25(3):487–493.
71. MacNeill S, Dodds L, Hamilton DC, Armson BA, VandenHof M. Rates and risk factors for recurrence of gestational diabetes. Diabetes Care 2001; 24(4):659–662.
72. MacNeill S, Dodds L, Hamilton DC, Armson BA, VandenHof M. Rate and risk factors for recurrence of gestational diabetes. Diabetes Care 2001; 24(4):663–665.
73. Michlin R, Oettinger M, Odeh M, Khoury S, Ophir E, Barak M et al. Maternal obesity and pregnancy outcome. Isr Med Assoc J 2000; 2(1):10–13.
74. Myles TD, Gooch J, Santolaya J. Obesity as an independent risk factor for infectious morbidity in patients who undergo cesarean delivery. Obstet Gynecol 2002; 100(5, Part 1): 959–964.
75. Carroll CS Sr, Magann EF, Chauhan SP, Klauser CK, Morrison JC. Vaginal birth after cesarean section versus elective repeat cesarean delivery: weight-based outcomes. Am J Obstet Gynecol 2003; 188(6):1516–1520.
76. Rosenberg TJ, Garbers S, Chavkin W, Chiasson MA. Prepregnancy weight and adverse perinatal outcomes in an ethnically diverse population. Obstet Gynecol 2003; 102(5, Part 1): 1022–1027.
77. Jensen DM, Damm P, Sorensen B, Molsted-Pedersen L, Westergaard JG, Ovesen P et al. Pregnancy outcome and prepregnancy body mass index in 2459 glucose-tolerant Danish women. Am J Obstet Gynecol 2003; 189(1):239–244.
78. Nager CW, Helliwell JP. Episiotomy increases perineal laceration length in primiparous women. Am J Obstet Gynecol 2001; 185(2):444–450.
79. Freedman DS, Khan LK, Serdula MK, Galuska DA, Dietz WH. Trends and correlates of class 3 obesity in the United States from 1990 through 2000. JAMA 2002; 288(14):1758–1761.
80. Ogden CL, Flegal KM, Carroll MD, Johnson CL. Prevalence and trends in overweight among US children and adolescents, 1999–2000. JAMA 2002; 288(14):1728–1732.

81. Flegal KM, Carroll MD, Ogden CL, Johnson CL. Prevalence and trends in obesity among US adults, 1999–2000. JAMA 2002; 288(14):1723–1727.

82. von Dadelszen P, Magee LA, Roberts JM. Subclassification of preeclampsia. Hypertens Pregnancy 2003; 22(2):143–148.

83. Rasmussen S, Irgens LM. Fetal growth and body proportion in preeclampsia. Obstet Gynecol 2003; 101(3):575–583.

84. Zhang J, Meikle S, Trumble A. Severe maternal morbidity associated with hypertensive disorders in pregnancy in the United States. Hypertens Pregnancy 2003; 22(2):203–212.

85. Hauth JC, Ewell MG, Levine RJ, Esterlitz JR, Sibai B, Curet LB et al. Pregnancy outcomes in healthy nulliparas who developed hypertension. Calcium for Preeclampsia Prevention Study Group. Obstet Gynecol 2000; 95(1):24–28.

86. van Walraven C, Mamdani M, Cohn A, Katib Y, Walker M, Rodger MA. Risk of subsequent thromboembolism for patients with pre-eclampsia. BMJ 2003; 326(7393):791–792.

87. Wilson ML, Goodwin TM, Pan VL, Ingles SA. Molecular epidemiology of preeclampsia. Obstet Gynecol Surv 2003; 58(1):39–66.

88. Samuels-Kalow ME, Funai EF, Buhimschi C, Norwitz E, Perrin M, Calderon-Margalit R et al. Prepregnancy body mass index, hypertensive disorders of pregnancy, and long-term maternal mortality. Am J Obstet Gynecol 2007; 197(5):490–496.

89. Bellamy L, Casas JP, Hingorani AD, Williams DJ. Pre-eclampsia and risk of cardiovascular disease and cancer in later life: systematic review and meta-analysis. BMJ 2007; 335 (7627):974.

90. Levine RJ, Esterlitz JR, Raymond EG, DerSimonian R, Hauth JC, Ben Curet L et al. Trial of calcium for preeclampsia prevention (CPEP): rationale, design, and methods. Control Clin Trials 1996; 17(5):442–469.

91. Skjaerven R, Wilcox AJ, Lie RT. The interval between pregnancies and the risk of preeclampsia. N Engl J Med 2002; 346(1):33–38.

92. Kullberg G, Lindeberg S, Hanson U. Eclampsia in Sweden. Hypertens Pregnancy 2002; 21(1):13–21.

93. Waterstone M, Bewley S, Wolfe C. Incidence and predictors of severe obstetric morbidity: case-control study. BMJ 2001; 322(7294):1089–1093.

94. Knight M. Eclampsia in the United Kingdom 2005. BJOG 2007; 114(9):1072–1078.

95. Mostello D, Catlin TK, Roman L, Holcomb WL Jr, Leet T. Preeclampsia in the parous woman: who is at risk? Am J Obstet Gynecol 2002; 187(2):425–429.

96. Pridjian G, Puschett JB. Preeclampsia, Part 2: experimental and genetic considerations. Obstet Gynecol Surv 2002; 57(9):619–640.

97. Roberts JM, Lain KY. Recent Insights into the pathogenesis of pre-eclampsia. Placenta 2002; 23(5):359–372.

98. Hibbard JU. Hypertensive disease and pregnancy. J Hypertens 2002; 20 Suppl 2:S29–S33.

99. Wong CA, Scavone BM, Dugan S, Smith JC, Prather H, Ganchiff JN et al. Incidence of postpartum lumbosacral spine and lower extremity nerve injuries. Obstet Gynecol 2003; 101(2):279–288.

100. Lanska DJ, Kryscio RJ. Risk factors for peripartum and postpartum stroke and intracranial venous thrombosis. Stroke 2000; 31(6):1274–1282.

101. Wen SW, Huang L, Liston R, Heaman M, Baskett T, Rusen ID et al. Severe maternal morbidity in Canada, 1991–2001. CMAJ 2005; 173(7):759–764.

102. Gazmararian JA, Petersen R, Jamieson DJ, Schild L, Adams MM, Deshpande AD et al. Hospitalizations during pregnancy among managed care enrollees. Obstet Gynecol 2002; 100(1):94–100.

103. Babinszki A, Kerenyi T, Torok O, Grazi V, Lapinski RH, Berkowitz RL. Perinatal outcome in grand and great-grand multiparity: effects of parity on obstetric risk factors. Am J Obstet Gynecol 1999; 181(3):669–674.

104. Ananth CV, Savitz DA, Luther ER. Maternal cigarette smoking as a risk factor for placental abruption, placenta previa, and uterine bleeding in pregnancy. Am J Epidemiol 1996; 144 (9):881–889.

105. Hauth JC, Ewell MG, Levine RJ, Esterlitz JR, Sibai B, Curet LB et al. Pregnancy outcomes in healthy nulliparas who developed hypertension. Calcium for Preeclampsia Prevention Study Group. Obstet Gynecol 2000; 95(1):24–28.

106. Rachana C, Suraiya K, Hisham AS, Abdulaziz AM, Hai A. Prevalence and complications of physical violence during pregnancy. Eur J Obstet Gynecol Reprod Biol 2002; 103(1):26–29.

107. Sheiner E, Shoham-Vardi I, Hallak M, Hadar A, Gortzak-Uzan L, Katz M et al. Placental abruption in term pregnancies: clinical significance and obstetric risk factors. J Matern Fetal Neonatal Med 2003; 13(1):45–49.

108. Sibai BM, Ramadan MK, Usta I, Salama M, Mercer BM, Friedman SA. Maternal morbidity and mortality in 442 pregnancies with hemolysis, elevated liver enzymes, and low platelets (HELLP syndrome). Am J Obstet Gynecol 1993; 169(4):1000–1006.

109. Schiff MA, Holt VL. The injury severity score in pregnant trauma patients: predicting placental abruption and fetal death. J Trauma 2002; 53(5):946–949.

110. Chen LH, Tan KH, Yeo GS. A ten-year review of uterine rupture in modern obstetric practice. Ann Acad Med Singapore 1995; 24(6):830–835.

111. Delaney T, Young DC. Spontaneous versus induced labor after a previous cesarean delivery. Obstet Gynecol 2003; 102(1):39–44.

112. Stamilio DM, DeFranco E, Pare E, Odibo AO, Peipert JF, Allsworth JE et al. Short interpregnancy interval: risk of uterine rupture and complications of vaginal birth after cesarean delivery. Obstet Gynecol 2007; 110(5):1075–1082.

113. Sebire NJ, Jolly M, Harris JP, Wadsworth J, Joffe M, Beard RW et al. Maternal obesity and pregnancy outcome: a study of 287,213 pregnancies in London. Int J Obes Relat Metab Disord 2001; 25(8):1175–1182.

114. Myles TD, Santolaya J. Maternal and neonatal outcomes in patients with a prolonged second stage of labor. Obstet Gynecol 2003; 102(1):52–58.

115. Ohkuchi A, Onagawa T, Usui R, Koike T, Hiratsuka M, Izumi A et al. Effect of maternal age on blood loss during parturition: a retrospective multivariate analysis of 10,053 cases. J Perinat Med 2003; 31(3):209–215.

116. Olesen AW, Westergaard JG, Olsen J. Perinatal and maternal complications related to postterm delivery: a national register-based study, 1978–1993. Am J Obstet Gynecol 2003; 189(1):222–227.

117. Dunne F, Brydon P, Smith K, Gee H. Pregnancy in women with Type 2 diabetes: 12 years outcome data 1990–2002. Diabetes Med 2003; 20(9):734–738.

118. Lydon-Rochelle M, Holt VL, Martin DP, Easterling TR. Association between method of delivery and maternal rehospitalization. JAMA 2000; 283(18):2411–2416.

119. Martin JA, Hamilton BE, Sutton PD, Ventura SJ, Menacker F, Munson ML. Births: final data for 2002. Natl Vital Stat Rep 2003; 52(10):1–113.

120. Martin JA, Hamilton BE, Ventura SJ, Menacker F, Park MM. Births: final data for 2000. Natl Vital Stat Rep 2002; 50(5):1–101.

121. Martin JA, Hamilton BE, Ventura SJ, Menacker F, Park MM, Sutton PD. Births: final data for 2001. Natl Vital Stat Rep 2002; 51(2):1–102.

122. Martin JA, Hamilton BE, Sutton PD, Ventura SJ, Menacker F, Kirmeyer S. Births: final data for 2004. Natl Vital Stat Rep 2006; 55(1):1–101.

123. Hall W, McCracken K, Osterweil P, Guise JM. Frequency and predictors for postpartum fecal incontinence. Am J Obstet Gynecol 2003; 188(5):1205–1207.

124. Eason E, Labrecque M, Marcoux S, Mondor M. Anal incontinence after childbirth. CMAJ 2002; 166(3):326–330.

125. Elkadry E, Kenton K, White P, Creech S, Brubaker L. Do mothers remember key events during labor? Am J Obstet Gynecol 2003; 189(1):195–200.

126. Weeks JD, Kozak LJ. Trends in the use of episiotomy in the United States: 1980–1998. Birth 2001; 28(3):152–160.
127. Angioli R, Gomez-Marin O, Cantuaria G, O'sullivan MJ. Severe perineal lacerations during vaginal delivery: the University of Miami experience. Am J Obstet Gynecol 2000; 182 (5):1083–1085.
128. Howard D, Davies PS, DeLancey JO, Small Y. Differences in perineal lacerations in black and white primiparas. Obstet Gynecol 2000; 96(4):622–624.
129. Carroll TG, Engelken M, Mosier MC, Nazir N. Epidural analgesia and severe perineal laceration in a community-based obstetric practice. J Am Board Fam Pract 2003; 16(1):1–6.
130. Webb DA, Culhane J. Hospital variation in episiotomy use and the risk of perineal trauma during childbirth. Birth 2002; 29(2):132–136.
131. McLeod NL, Gilmour DT, Joseph KS, Farrell SA, Luther ER. Trends in major risk factors for anal sphincter lacerations: a 10-year study. J Obstet Gynaecol Can 2003; 25(7):586–593.
132. Peleg D, Kennedy CM, Merrill D, Zlatnik FJ. Risk of repetition of a severe perineal laceration. Obstet Gynecol 1999; 93(6):1021–1024.
133. Payne TN, Carey JC, Rayburn WF. Prior third- or fourth-degree perineal tears and recurrence risks. Int J Gynaecol Obstet 1999; 64(1):55–57.
134. Oakley D, Murray ME, Murtland T, Hayashi R, Andersen HF, Mayes F et al. Comparisons of outcomes of maternity care by obstetricians and certified nurse-midwives. Obstet Gynecol 1996; 88(5):823–829.
135. Kabiru WN, Jamieson D, Graves W, Lindsay M. Trends in operative vaginal delivery rates and associated maternal complication rates in an inner-city hospital. Am J Obstet Gynecol 2001; 184(6):1112–1114.
136. Larsen U, Okonofua FE. Female circumcision and obstetric complications. Int J Gynaecol Obstet 2002; 77(3):255–265.
137. Williams A. Third-degree perineal tears: risk factors and outcome after primary repair. J Obstet Gynaecol 2003; 23(6):611–614.
138. Richter HE, Brumfield CG, Cliver SP, Burgio KL, Neely CL, Varner RE. Risk factors associated with anal sphincter tear: a comparison of primiparous patients, vaginal births after cesarean deliveries, and patients with previous vaginal delivery. Am J Obstet Gynecol 2002; 187(5):1194–1198.
139. Handa VL, Danielsen BH, Gilbert WM. Obstetric anal sphincter lacerations. Obstet Gynecol 2001; 98(2):225–230.
140. Sheiner E, Shoham-Vardi I, Silberstein T, Hallak M, Katz M, Mazor M. Failed vacuum extraction. Maternal risk factors and pregnancy outcome. J Reprod Med 2001; 46(9): 819–824.
141. Kozak LJ, Weeks JD. U.S. trends in obstetric procedures, 1990–2000. Birth 2002; 29 (3):157–161.
142. Weber AM, Meyn L. Episiotomy use in the United States, 1979–1997. Obstet Gynecol 2002; 100(6):1177–1182.
143. Jackson N, Paterson-Brown S. Physical sequelae of caesarean section. Best Pract Res Clin Obstet Gynaecol 2001; 15(1):49–61.
144. Lydon-Rochelle M, Holt VL, Easterling TR, Martin DP. Cesarean delivery and postpartum mortality among primiparas in Washington State, 1987–1996(1). Obstet Gynecol 2001; 97 (2):169–174.
145. Schuitemaker N, van Roosmalen J, Dekker G, van Dongen P, van Geijn H, Gravenhorst JB. Maternal mortality after cesarean section in The Netherlands. Acta Obstet Gynecol Scand 1997; 76(4):332–334.
146. Brown S, Lumley J. Maternal health after childbirth: results of an Australian population based survey. Br J Obstet Gynaecol 1998; 105(2):156–161.
147. Lydon-Rochelle MT, Holt VL, Martin DP. Delivery method and self-reported postpartum general health status among primiparous women. Paediatr Perinat Epidemiol 2001; 15(3): 232–240.

148. MacArthur C, Bick DE, Keighley MR. Faecal incontinence after childbirth. Br J Obstet Gynaecol 1997; 104(1):46–50.
149. Johanson RB, Menon BK. Vacuum extraction versus forceps for assisted vaginal delivery. Cochrane Database Syst Rev 2000; 2:CD000224.
150. Allen VM, O'Connell CM, Liston RM, Baskett TF. Maternal morbidity associated with cesarean delivery without labor compared with spontaneous onset of labor at term. Obstet Gynecol 2003; 102(3):477–482.
151. Couto RC, Pedrosa TM, Nogueira JM, Gomes DL, Neto MF, Rezende NA. Post-discharge surveillance and infection rates in obstetric patients. Int J Gynaecol Obstet 1998; 61(3): 227–231.
152. Edwards DR, Porter SA, Stein GS. A pilot study of postnatal depression following caesarean section using two retrospective self-rating instruments. J Psychosom Res 1994; 38(2):111–117.
153. Joseph KS, Young DC, Dodds L, O'Connell CM, Allen VM, Chandra S et al. Changes in maternal characteristics and obstetric practice and recent increases in primary cesarean delivery. Obstet Gynecol 2003; 102(4):791–800.
154. Lydon-Rochelle M, Holt VL, Easterling TR, Martin DP. Risk of uterine rupture during labor among women with a prior cesarean delivery. N Engl J Med 2001; 345(1):3–8.
155. Hibbard JU, Ismail MA, Wang Y, Te C, Karrison T, Ismail MA. Failed vaginal birth after a cesarean section: how risky is it? I. Maternal morbidity. Am J Obstet Gynecol 2001; 184 (7):1365–1371.
156. Gregory KD, Korst LM, Cane P, Platt LD, Kahn K. Vaginal birth after cesarean and uterine rupture rates in California. Obstet Gynecol 1999; 94(6):985–989.
157. Green DC, Moore JM, Adams MM, Berg CJ, Wilcox LS, McCarthy BJ. Are we under-estimating rates of vaginal birth after previous cesarean birth? The validity of delivery methods from birth certificates. Am J Epidemiol 1998; 147(6):581–586.
158. Learman LA. Regional differences in operative obstetrics: a look to the South. Obstet Gynecol 1998; 92(4, Part 1):514–519.
159. Roberts CL, Algert CS, Carnegie M, Peat B. Operative delivery during labour: trends and predictive factors. Paediatr Perinat Epidemiol 2002; 16(2):115–123.
160. O'Connell MP, Lindow W. Caesarean section controversy. Further research is needed on why rates of caesarean section are increasing. BMJ 2000; 320(7241):1074.
161. Rasmussen OB, Pedersen BL, Wilken-Jensen C, Vejerslev LO. Stratified rates of cesarean sections and spontaneous vaginal deliveries. Data from five labor wards in Denmark – 1996. Acta Obstet Gynecol Scand 2000; 79(3):227–231.
162. Odlind V, Haglund B, Pakkanen M, Otterblad OP. Deliveries, mothers and newborn infants in Sweden, 1973–2000. Trends in obstetrics as reported to the Swedish Medical Birth Register. Acta Obstet Gynecol Scand 2003; 82(6):516–528.
163. Zanetta G, Tampieri A, Currado I, Regalia A, Nespoli A, Midwife T et al. Changes in cesarean delivery in an Italian university hospital, 1982–1996: a comparison with the national trend. Birth 1999; 26(3):144–148.
164. Lin HC, Xirasagar S. Institutional factors in cesarean delivery rates: policy and research implications. Obstet Gynecol 2004; 103(1):128–136.
165. Roberts CL, Tracy S, Peat B. Rates for obstetric intervention among private and public patients in Australia: population based descriptive study. BMJ 2000; 321(7254):137–141.
166. Belizan JM, Althabe F, Barros FC, Alexander S, Showalter E, Griffin A et al. Rates and implications of caesarean sections in Latin America: ecological study ò Commentary: all women should have a choice ò Commentary: increase in caesarean sections may reflect medical control not women's choice ò Commentary: "health has become secondary to a sexually attractive body". BMJ 1999; 319(7222):1397–1402.
167. Baskett TF. Cesarean section: what is an acceptable rate? Can Med Assoc J 1978; 118 (9):1019–1020.

168. Ash AK, Okoh D. What is the right number of caesarean sections? Lancet 1997; 349 (9064):1557.
169. Li T, Rhoads GG, Smulian J, Demissie K, Wartenberg D, Kruse L. Physician cesarean delivery rates and risk-adjusted perinatal outcomes. Obstet Gynecol 2003; 101(6):1204–1212.
170. Hofmeyr GJ, Hannah ME. Planned caesarean section for term breech delivery. Cochrane Database Syst Rev 2003; 3:CD000166.
171. Brocklehurst P. Interventions for reducing the risk of mother-to-child transmission of HIV infection. Cochrane Database Syst Rev 2002; 1:CD000102.
172. Grant A, Glazener CM. Elective caesarean section versus expectant management for delivery of the small baby. Cochrane Database Syst Rev 2001; 2:CD000078.
173. Boulvain M, Stan C, Irion O. Elective delivery in diabetic pregnant women. Cochrane Database Syst Rev 2000; 2:CD001997.
174. Hofmeyr GJ, Kulier R. Operative versus conservative management for 'fetal distress' in labour. Cochrane Database Syst Rev 2000; 2:CD001065.
175. Crowther CA. Caesarean delivery for the second twin. Cochrane Database Syst Rev 2000; 2:CD000047.
176. Lagrew DC Jr, Adashek JA. Lowering the cesarean section rate in a private hospital: comparison of individual physicians' rates, risk factors, and outcomes. Am J Obstet Gynecol 1998; 178(6):1207–1214.
177. Gregory KD, Korst LM, Platt LD. Variation in elective primary cesarean delivery by patient and hospital factors. Am J Obstet Gynecol 2001; 184(7):1521–1532.
178. Walker R, Turnbull D, Wilkinson C. Strategies to address global cesarean section rates: a review of the evidence. Birth 2002; 29(1):28–39.
179. Flamm BL, Berwick DM, Kabcenell A. Reducing cesarean section rates safely: lessons from a "breakthrough series" collaborative. Birth 1998; 25(2):117–124.
180. Mehta A, Apers L, Verstraelen H, Temmerman M. Trends in caesarean section rates at a maternity hospital in Mumbai, India. J Health Popul Nutr 2001; 19(4):306–312.
181. Naiden J, Deshpande P. Using active management of labor and vaginal birth after previous cesarean delivery to lower cesarean delivery rates: a 10-year experience. Am J Obstet Gynecol 2001; 184(7):1535–1541.
182. Heffner LJ, Elkin E, Fretts RC. Impact of labor induction, gestational age, and maternal age on cesarean delivery rates. Obstet Gynecol 2003; 102(2):287–293.
183. Heinberg EM, Wood RA, Chambers RB. Elective induction of labor in multiparous women. Does it increase the risk of cesarean section? J Reprod Med 2002; 47(5):399–403.
184. Leighton BL, Halpern SH. Epidural analgesia: effects on labor progress and maternal and neonatal outcome. Semin Perinatol 2002; 26(2):122–135.
185. Zhang J, Yancey MK, Henderson CE. U.S. national trends in labor induction, 1989–1998. J Reprod Med 2002; 47(2):120–124.
186. Zhan C, Miller MR. Excess length of stay, charges, and mortality attributable to medical injuries during hospitalization. JAMA 2003; 290(14):1868–1874.
187. Johantgen M, Elixhauser A, Bali JK, Goldfarb M, Harris DR. Quality indicators using hospital discharge data: state and national applications. Jt Comm J Qual Improv 1998; 24 (2):88–105.
188. Hebert PR, Reed G, Entman SS, Mitchel EF Jr, Berg C, Griffin MR. Serious maternal morbidity after childbirth: prolonged hospital stays and readmissions. Obstet Gynecol 1999; 94(6):942–947.
189. Liu S, Heaman M, Kramer MS, Demissie K, Wen SW, Marcoux S. Length of hospital stay, obstetric conditions at childbirth, and maternal readmission: a population-based cohort study. Am J Obstet Gynecol 2002; 187(3):681–687.
190. Lee DT, Yip AS, Leung TY, Chung TK. Identifying women at risk of postnatal depression: prospective longitudinal study. Hong Kong Med J 2000; 6(4):349–354.

191. McGill H, Burrows VL, Holland LA, Langer HJ, Sweet MA. Postnatal depression: a Christchurch study. N Z Med J 1995; 108(999):162–165.

192. Johanson R, Chapman G, Murray D, Johnson I, Cox J. The North Staffordshire Maternity Hospital prospective study of pregnancy-associated depression. J Psychosom Obstet Gynaecol 2000; 21(2):93–97.

193. Andersson L, Sundstrom-Poromaa I, Bixo M, Wulff M, Bondestam K, aStrom M. Point prevalence of psychiatric disorders during the second trimester of pregnancy: a population-based study. Am J Obstet Gynecol 2003; 189(1):148–154.

194. Parsons LH, Harper MA. Violent maternal deaths in North Carolina. Obstet Gynecol 1999; 94(6):990–993.

195. Ross LE, Gilbert Evans SE, Sellers EM, Romach MK. Measurement issues in postpartum depression, Part 1: anxiety as a feature of postpartum depression. Arch Women Ment Health 2003; 6(1):51–57.

196. Bryan TL, Georgiopoulos AM, Harms RW, Huxsahl JE, Larson DR, Yawn BP. Incidence of postpartum depression in Olmsted County, Minnesota. A population-based, retrospective study. J Reprod Med 1999; 44(4):351–358.

197. Dankner R, Goldberg RP, Fisch RZ, Crum RM. Cultural elements of postpartum depression. A study of 327 Jewish Jerusalem women. J Reprod Med 2000; 45(2):97–104.

198. Johnstone SJ, Boyce PM, Hickey AR, Morris-Yatees AD, Harris MG. Obstetric risk factors for postnatal depression in urban and rural community samples. Aust N Z J Psychiatry 2001; 35(1):69–74.

199. O'Hara MW, Zekoski EM, Philipps LH, Wright EJ. Controlled prospective study of postpartum mood disorders: comparison of childbearing and nonchildbearing women. J Abnorm Psychol 1990; 99(1):3–15.

200. Cox JL, Murray D, Chapman G. A controlled study of the onset, duration and prevalence of postnatal depression. Br J Psychiatry 1993; 163:27–31.

201. Orr ST, James SA, Blackmore PC. Maternal prenatal depressive symptoms and spontaneous preterm births among African-American women in Baltimore, Maryland. Am J Epidemiol 2002; 156(9):797–802.

202. Hoffman S, Hatch MC. Depressive symptomatology during pregnancy: evidence for an association with decreased fetal growth in pregnancies of lower social class women. Health Psychol 2000; 19(6):535–543.

203. Orr ST, Miller CA. Maternal depressive symptoms and the risk of poor pregnancy outcome. Review of the literature and preliminary findings. Epidemiol Rev 1995; 17(1):165–171.

204. Cox JL, Holden JM, Sagovsky R. Detection of postnatal depression. Development of the 10-item Edinburgh Postnatal Depression Scale. Br J Psychiatry 1987; 150:782–786.

205. Gilbody SM, House AO, Sheldon TA. Routinely administered questionnaires for depression and anxiety: systematic review. BMJ 2001; 322(7283):406–409.

206. Roberts RE, Vernon SW. The Center for Epidemiologic Studies Depression Scale: its use in a community sample. Am J Psychiatry 1983; 140(1):41–46.

207. Fergusson DM, Horwood LJ, Thorpe K. Changes in depression during and following pregnancy. ALSPAC Study Team. Study of pregnancy and children. Paediatr Perinat Epidemiol 1996; 10(3):279–293.

208. Pop VJ, Essed GG, de Geus CA, van Son MM, Komproe IH. Prevalence of post partum depression – or is it post-puerperium depression? Acta Obstet Gynecol Scand 1993; 72 (5):354–358.

209. Verdoux H, Sutter AL, Glatigny-Dallay E, Minisini A. Obstetrical complications and the development of postpartum depressive symptoms: a prospective survey of the MATQUID cohort. Acta Psychiatr Scand 2002; 106(3):212–219.

210. Waterstone M, Wolfe C, Hooper R, Bewley S. Postnatal morbidity after childbirth and severe obstetric morbidity. BJOG 2003; 110(2):128–133.

211. Harris B, Oretti R, Lazarus J, Parkes A, John R, Richards C et al. Randomised trial of thyroxine to prevent postnatal depression in thyroid-antibody-positive women. Br J Psychiatry 2002; 180:327–330.
212. Villar J, Merialdi M, Gulmezoglu AM, Abalos E, Carroli G, Kulier R et al. Nutritional interventions during pregnancy for the prevention or treatment of maternal morbidity and preterm delivery: an overview of randomized controlled trials. J Nutr 2003; 133(5) Suppl 2): 1606S–1625S.
213. Carroli G, Rooney C, Villar J. How effective is antenatal care in preventing maternal mortality and serious morbidity? An overview of the evidence. Paediatr Perinat Epidemiol 2001; 15 Suppl 1:1–42.
214. Tomkins A. Nutrition and maternal morbidity and mortality. Br J Nutr 2001; 85 Suppl 2: S93–S99.
215. Baker H, DeAngelis B, Holland B, Gittens-Williams L, Barrett T Jr. Vitamin profile of 563 gravidas during trimesters of pregnancy. J Am Coll Nutr 2002; 21(1):33–37.
216. Ballew C, Bowman BA, Sowell AL, Gillespie C. Serum retinol distributions in residents of the United States: third National Health and Nutrition Examination Survey, 1988–1994. Am J Clin Nutr 2001; 73(3):586–593.
217. Brabin BJ, Hakimi M, Pelletier D. An analysis of anemia and pregnancy-related maternal mortality. J Nutr 2001; 131(2S-2):604S–614S.
218. Rush D. Nutrition and maternal mortality in the developing world. Am J Clin Nutr 2000; 72 (1 Suppl):212S–240S.
219. Benagiano G, Thomas B. Saving mothers' lives: the FIGO Save the Mothers Initiative. Int J Gynaecol Obstet 2003; 80(2):198–203.
220. Jones KD. Incidence and risk factors for third degree perineal tears. Int J Gynaecol Obstet 2000; 71(3):227–229.
221. Samuelsson E, Ladfors L, Lindblom BG, Hagberg H. A prospective observational study on tears during vaginal delivery: occurrences and risk factors. Acta Obstet Gynecol Scand 2002; 81(1):44–49.
222. Bodner K, Bodner-Adler B, Wagenbichler P, Kaider A, Leodolter S, Husslein P et al. Perineal lacerations during spontaneous vaginal delivery. Wien Klin Wochenschr 2001; 113(19):743–746.
223. O'Brien TE, Ray JG, Chan WS. Maternal body mass index and the risk of preeclampsia: a systematic overview. Epidemiology 2003; 14(3):368–374.
224. Lockshin MD, Sammaritano LR. Lupus pregnancy. Autoimmunity 2003; 36(1):33–40.
225. Basso O, Olsen J. Sex ratio and twinning in women with hyperemesis or pre-eclampsia. Epidemiology 2001; 12(6):747–749.
226. Coomarasamy A, Honest H, Papaioannou S, Gee H, Khan KS. Aspirin for prevention of preeclampsia in women with historical risk factors: a systematic review. Obstet Gynecol 2003; 101(6):1319–1332.
227. Dawson LM, Parfrey PS, Hefferton D, Dicks EL, Cooper MJ, Young D et al. Familial risk of preeclampsia in Newfoundland: a population-based study. J Am Soc Nephrol 2002; 13 (7):1901–1906.
228. Skjaerven R, Vatten LJ, Wilcox AJ, Ronning T, Irgens LM, Lie RT. Recurrence of pre-eclampsia across generations: exploring fetal and maternal genetic components in a population based cohort. BMJ 2005; 331(7521):877.
229. Harlap S, Paltiel O, Deutsch L, Knaanie A, Masalha S, Tiram E et al. Paternal age and preeclampsia. Epidemiology 2002; 13(6):660–667.
230. Zhang C, Williams MA, King IB, Dashow EE, Sorensen TK, Frederick IO et al. Vitamin C and the risk of preeclampsia – results from dietary questionnaire and plasma assay. Epidemiology 2002; 13(4):409–416.
231. Heine RP, Ness RB, Roberts JM. Seroprevalence of antibodies to Chlamydia pneumoniae in women with preeclampsia. Obstet Gynecol 2003; 101(2):221–226.

232. Hernandez-Diaz S, Werler MM, Louik C, Mitchell AA. Risk of gestational hypertension in relation to folic acid supplementation during pregnancy. Am J Epidemiol 2002; 156 (9):806–812.

233. Qiu C, Williams MA, Leisenring WM, Sorensen TK, Frederick IO, Dempsey JC et al. Family history of hypertension and type 2 diabetes in relation to preeclampsia risk. Hypertension 2003; 41(3):408–413.

234. Qiu C, Williams MA, Leisenring WM, Sorensen TK, Frederick IO, Dempsey JC et al. Family history of hypertension and type 2 diabetes in relation to preeclampsia risk. Hypertension 2003; 41(3):408–413.

235. Boggess KA, Lieff S, Murtha AP, Moss K, Beck J, Offenbacher S. Maternal periodontal disease is associated with an increased risk for preeclampsia. Obstet Gynecol 2003; 101 (2):227–231.

236. Basso O, Christensen K, Olsen J. Higher risk of pre-eclampsia after change of partner. An effect of longer interpregnancy intervals? Epidemiology 2001; 12(6):624–629.

237. Said J, Dekker G. Pre-eclampsia and thrombophilia. Best Pract Res Clin Obstet Gynaecol 2003; 17(3):441–458.

238. Morrison ER, Miedzybrodzka ZH, Campbell DM, Haites NE, Wilson BJ, Watson MS et al. Prothrombotic genotypes are not associated with pre-eclampsia and gestational hypertension: results from a large population-based study and systematic review. Thromb Haemost 2002; 87(5):779–785.

239. Walker ID. Prothrombotic genotypes and pre-eclampsia. Thromb Haemost 2002; 87(5):777–778.

240. D'Elia AV, Driul L, Giacomello R, Colaone R, Fabbro D, Di Leonardo C et al. Frequency of factor V, prothrombin and methylenetetrahydrofolate reductase gene variants in preeclampsia. Gynecol Obstet Invest 2002; 53(2):84–87.

241. Saftlas AF, Levine RJ, Klebanoff MA, Martz KL, Ewell MG, Morris CD et al. Abortion, changed paternity, and risk of preeclampsia in nulliparous women. Am J Epidemiol 2003; 157(12):1108–1114.

242. Verwoerd GR, Hall DR, Grove D, Maritz JS, Odendaal HJ. Primipaternity and duration of exposure to sperm antigens as risk factors for pre-eclampsia. Int J Gynaecol Obstet 2002; 78 (2):121–126.

243. Einarsson JI, Sangi-Haghpeykar H, Gardner MO. Sperm exposure and development of preeclampsia. Am J Obstet Gynecol 2003; 188(5):1241–1243.

244. Eras JL, Saftlas AF, Triche E, Hsu CD, Risch HA, Bracken MB. Abortion and its effect on risk of preeclampsia and transient hypertension. Epidemiology 2000; 11(1):36–43.

245. Ioka A, Tsukuma H, Nakamuro K. Lifestyles and pre-eclampsia with special attention to cigarette smoking. J Epidemiol 2003; 13(2):90–95.

246. Kobashi G, Ohta K, Hata A, Shido K, Yamada H, Fujimoto S et al. An association between maternal smoking and preeclampsia in Japanese women. Semin Thromb Hemost 2002; 28 (6):507–510.

247. Cnattingius S, Lambe M. Trends in smoking and overweight during pregnancy: prevalence, risks of pregnancy complications, and adverse pregnancy outcomes. Semin Perinatol 2002; 26(4):286–295.

248. England LJ, Levine RJ, Qian C, Morris CD, Sibai BM, Catalano PM et al. Smoking before pregnancy and risk of gestational hypertension and preeclampsia. Am J Obstet Gynecol 2002; 186(5):1035–1040.

249. Sibai BM, Ewell M, Levine RJ, Klebanoff MA, Esterlitz J, Catalano PM et al. Risk factors associated with preeclampsia in healthy nulliparous women. The Calcium for Preeclampsia Prevention (CPEP) Study Group. Am J Obstet Gynecol 1997; 177(5):1003–1010.

250. Sibai BM, Caritis S, Hauth J. What we have learned about preeclampsia. Semin Perinatol 2003; 27(3):239–246.

251. Villar J, Merialdi M, Gulmezoglu AM, Abalos E, Carroli G, Kulier R et al. Nutritional interventions during pregnancy for the prevention or treatment of maternal morbidity and preterm delivery: an overview of randomized controlled trials. J Nutr 2003; 133(5) Suppl 2): 1606S–1625S.
252. Multicenter survey of diabetic pregnancy in France. Gestation and Diabetes in France Study Group. Diabetes Care 1991; 14(11):994–1000.
253. Amini SB, Catalano PM, Dierker LJ, Mann LI. Births to teenagers: trends and obstetric outcomes. Obstet Gynecol 1996; 87(5, Part 1):668–674.
254. Bell JS, Campbell DM, Graham WJ, Penney GC, Ryan M, Hall MH. Can obstetric complications explain the high levels of obstetric interventions and maternity service use among older women? A retrospective analysis of routinely collected data. BJOG 2001; 108(9):910–918.
255. Read AW, Prendiville WJ, Dawes VP, Stanley FJ. Cesarean section and operative vaginal delivery in low-risk primiparous women, Western Australia. Am J Public Health 1994; 84 (1):37–42.
256. Franko DL, Blais MA, Becker AE, Delinsky SS, Greenwood DN, Flores AT et al. Pregnancy complications and neonatal outcomes in women with eating disorders. Am J Psychiatry 2001; 158(9):1461–1466.
257. Golan A, Langer R, Neuman M, Wexler S, Segev E, David MP. Obstetric outcome in women with congenital uterine malformations. J Reprod Med 1992; 37(3):233–236.
258. Johnson JW, Longmate JA, Frentzen B. Excessive maternal weight and pregnancy outcome. Am J Obstet Gynecol 1992; 167(2):353–370.
259. McCord C, Premkumar R, Arole S, Arole R. Efficient and effective emergency obstetric care in a rural Indian community where most deliveries are at home. Int J Gynaecol Obstet 2001; 75(3):297–307.
260. Shy K, Kimpo C, Emanuel I, Leisenring W, Williams MA. Maternal birth weight and cesarean delivery in four race-ethnic groups. Am J Obstet Gynecol 2000; 182(6):1363–1370.
261. Iyasu S, Saftlas AK, Rowley DL, Koonin LM, Lawson HW, Atrash HK. The epidemiology of placenta previa in the United States, 1979 through 1987. Am J Obstet Gynecol 1993; 168 (5):1424–1429.
262. Sheiner E, Shoham-Vardi I, Hershkovitz R, Katz M, Mazor M. Infertility treatment is an independent risk factor for cesarean section among nulliparous women aged 40 and above. Am J Obstet Gynecol 2001; 185(4):888–892.
263. Gregory KD, Korst LM, Krychman M, Cane P, Platt LD. Variation in vaginal breech delivery rates by hospital type. Obstet Gynecol 2001; 97(3):385–390.
264. Garcia FA, Miller HB, Huggins GR, Gordon TA. Effect of academic affiliation and obstetric volume on clinical outcome and cost of childbirth. Obstet Gynecol 2001; 97(4):567–576.
265. Gould JB, Qin C, Marks AR, Chavez G. Neonatal mortality in weekend vs weekday births. JAMA 2003; 289(22):2958–2962.
266. Curtin SC, Park MM. Trends in the attendant, place, and timing of births, and in the use of obstetric interventions: United States, 1989–97. Natl Vital Stat Rep 1999; 47(27):1–12.
267. Janssen PA, Lee SK, Ryan EM, Etches DJ, Farquharson DF, Peacock D et al. Outcomes of planned home births versus planned hospital births after regulation of midwifery in British Columbia. CMAJ 2002; 166(3):315–323.
268. Sandmire HF, DeMott RK. The Green Bay cesarean section study. IV. The physician factor as a determinant of cesarean birth rates for the large fetus. Am J Obstet Gynecol 1996; 174 (5):1557–1564.
269. Seyb ST, Berka RJ, Socol ML, Dooley SL. Risk of cesarean delivery with elective induction of labor at term in nulliparous women. Obstet Gynecol 1999; 94(4):600–607.
270. Maslow AS, Sweeny AL. Elective induction of labor as a risk factor for cesarean delivery among low-risk women at term. Obstet Gynecol 2000; 95(6, Part 1):917–922.
271. Pajulo M, Savonlahti E, Sourander A, Helenius H, Piha J. Antenatal depression, substance dependency and social support. J Affect Disord 2001; 65(1):9–17.

272. Josefsson A, Berg G, Nordin C, Sydsjo G. Prevalence of depressive symptoms in late pregnancy and postpartum. Acta Obstet Gynecol Scand 2001; 80(3):251–255.
273. Johanson R, Chapman G, Murray D, Johnson I, Cox J. The North Staffordshire Maternity Hospital prospective study of pregnancy-associated depression. J Psychosom Obstet Gynaecol 2000; 21(2):93–97.
274. Fisch RZ, Tadmor OP, Dankner R, Diamant YZ. Postnatal depression: a prospective study of its prevalence, incidence and psychosocial determinants in an Israeli sample. J Obstet Gynaecol Res 1997; 23(6):547–554.
275. Lee D, Yip A, Chiu H, Leung T, Chung T. A psychiatric epidemiological study of postpartum Chinese women. Am J Psychiatry 2001; 158(2):220–226.
276. Stamp GE, Crowther CA. Postnatal depression: a South Australian prospective survey. Aust N Z J Obstet Gynaecol 1994; 34(2):164–167.
277. Georgiopoulos AM, Bryan TL, Yawn BP, Houston MS, Rummans TA, Therneau TM. Population-based screening for postpartum depression. Obstet Gynecol 1999; 93(5, Part 1):653–657.
278. Chandran M, Tharyan P, Muliyil J, Abraham S. Post-partum depression in a cohort of women from a rural area of Tamil Nadu, India. Incidence and risk factors. Br J Psychiatry 2002; 181:499–504.
279. Righetti-Veltema M, Conne-Perreard E, Bousquet A, Manzano J. Postpartum depression and mother-infant relationship at 3 months old. J Affect Disord 2002; 70(3):291–306.
280. Chaaya M, Campbell OM, El Kak F, Shaar D, Harb H, Kaddour A. Postpartum depression: prevalence and determinants in Lebanon. Arch Women Ment Health 2002; 5(2):65–72.
281. Chaudron LH, Klein MH, Remington P, Palta M, Allen C, Essex MJ. Predictors, prodromes and incidence of postpartum depression. J Psychosom Obstet Gynaecol 2001; 22(2):103–112.
282. Nielsen FD, Videbech P, Hedegaard M, Dalby SJ, Secher NJ. Postpartum depression: identification of women at risk. BJOG 2000; 107(10):1210–1217.
283. Bryan TL, Georgiopoulos AM, Harms RW, Huxsahl JE, Larson DR, Yawn BP. Incidence of postpartum depression in Olmsted County, Minnesota. A population-based, retrospective study. J Reprod Med 1999; 44(4):351–358.
284. Morris-Rush JK, Freda MC, Bernstein PS. Screening for postpartum depression in an inner-city population. Am J Obstet Gynecol 2003; 188(5):1217–1219.
285. Patel V, Rodrigues M, DeSouza N. Gender, poverty, and postnatal depression: a study of mothers in Goa, India. Am J Psychiatry 2002; 159(1):43–47.
286. Warner R, Appleby L, Whitton A, Faragher B. Demographic and obstetric risk factors for postnatal psychiatric morbidity. Br J Psychiatry 1996; 168(5):607–611.
287. Kuijpens JL, Vader HL, Drexhage HA, Wiersinga WM, van Son MJ, Pop VJ. Thyroid peroxidase antibodies during gestation are a marker for subsequent depression postpartum. Eur J Endocrinol 2001; 145(5):579–584.
288. Carter AS, Baker CW, Brownell KD. Body mass index, eating attitudes, and symptoms of depression and anxiety in pregnancy and the postpartum period. Psychosom Med 2000; 62(2):264–270.

Chapter 4
Maternal Mortality

4.1 Definitions, Measures, and Measurement Issues

Definition: The definition of maternal death has evolved along with progress in understanding the role of pregnancy in causing death. Differences in the definition of maternal death persist, as demonstrated in Table 4.1 (1, 2).

The most recent definitions reflect the understanding that deaths that are caused by pregnancy may occur well beyond 6 weeks after pregnancy termination. The length of time after pregnancy termination when pregnancy-related deaths do *not* occur has not been assessed empirically. For convenience, more recent definitions of maternal death use 365 days. We use *pregnancy termination* to encompass all pregnancy outcomes: ectopic pregnancies, induced and spontaneous abortions, fetal deaths, live births, and on-going pregnancies. The World Health Organization (WHO) definition does not account for potential advances in our understanding of the role of pregnancy in causing death. In contrast, the ACOG/CDC definition allows for this possibility by including pregnancy-associated deaths. These deaths are temporally associated with pregnancy, but pregnancy's role in causing them cannot be determined. As our understanding of the role of pregnancy in causing death evolves in the future, these deaths may be definitively reclassified as pregnancy-related or not pregnancy-related.

Direct maternal deaths are those that result directly from the pregnancy itself. *Indirect* maternal deaths are those that occur because pregnancy exacerbates an illness that existed before conception.

An important rationale for monitoring maternal mortality is its use as a sentinel for maternal morbidity. Experts judge that higher levels of maternal mortality correspond to higher levels of maternal morbidity. Empirical evidence supporting this assumption is sparse, especially when the maternal mortality ratio (MMR) is at the low level currently observed in developed countries. One study of maternal mortality in Europe – an area with low overall maternal mortality – reports that cause-of-death patterns are consistent with this assumption (3). Other investigators have found that analysis of maternal mortality and severe acute maternal morbidity

M.M. Adams et al., *Perinatal Epidemiology for Public Health Practice.*
doi: 10.1007/978-0-387-09439-7_4; © Springer Science + Business Media, LLC 2009

Table 4.1 Definitions of death in relation to pregnancy (*Source*: (72))

Relationship between pregnancy and cause of death	Source of definition		
	ACOG/CDC[a]	ICD-9[b]	ICD-10[c]
When death and pregnancy are causally related:			
Death during pregnancy or within 42 days postpartum	Pregnancy-related death	Maternal death	Maternal death
Death 43–365 days postpartum	Pregnancy-related death	Not defined	Late maternal death
When death and pregnancy are not causally related:			
Death during pregnancy or within 365 days postpartum	Not pregnancy-related death	Not defined	Not defined
When death and pregnancy may or may not be causally related:			
Death during pregnancy or within 42 days postpartum	Pregnancy-associated death	Not defined	Pregnancy-related death
Death 43–365 days postpartum	Pregnancy-associated death	Not defined	Not defined

[a] American College of Obstetricians and Gynecologists/Centers for Disease Control and Prevention Maternal Mortality Study Group
[b] WHO 1977

(akin to "near-miss" morbidity) provide more useful information for monitoring trends and targeting interventions than mortality alone (4).

Measures: Table 4.2 lists the most frequently used measures of maternal mortality.

Data sources – developed countries: Maternal deaths are difficult to completely ascertain, because the pregnancy-related etiology of a death is not always apparent. Typically, maternal deaths are ascertained from review of the causes of death on the death certificate, which are assigned International Classification of Diseases (ICD) codes. Although the ICD includes specific codes for pregnancy-related conditions (ICD-9: 630–676; ICD-10: O10-O99 ["O" is a letter]), certifiers of death may neglect to note that the cause of death was related to pregnancy or nosologists may use ICD codes that do not convey the condition's pregnancy-related nature.

Identifying maternal deaths solely from pregnancy-related codes on death certificates will miss many pregnancy-related deaths (10, 11). Thus, many states use additional strategies to identify maternal deaths. By 1997, 12 states and New York City had modified their death certificates to include a pregnancy-related check box on the certificate. Certifiers were requested to mark in it if the death occurred either while the decedent was pregnant or within a specified interval after a pregnancy termination. The interval ranged among states from 42 days to 18 months.

Table 4.2 Common measures of maternal mortality

Measure	Interpretation	Computation
Pregnancy related mortality ratio; maternal mortality ratio (MMR)	Likelihood of death per pregnancy; case fatality rate for pregnancy.	$\dfrac{\text{Number of pregnancy–related deaths in a year}}{\text{Number of live births in a year}} \times 100,000$
Pregnancy-related mortality rate	Frequency of maternal death among reproductive-age women	$\dfrac{\text{Number of pregnancy–related deaths in a year}}{\text{Number of women of reproductive age}} \times 100,000$
Proportional mortality ratio	Contribution of pregnancy-related death to all deaths among reproductive-age women	$\dfrac{\text{Number of pregnancy–related deaths in an interval}}{\text{Number of deaths to women of reproductive age in an interval}}$
Cause-specific mortality ratio	Proportion of all pregnancy-related deaths due to a specific cause	$\dfrac{\text{Number of pregnancy–related deaths due to a specific cause in an interval}}{\text{Number of pregnancy–related deaths due to all causes in an interval}}$

Many states routinely attempt to match the names on death certificates of reproductive-age women to mothers' names on certificates for fetal deaths and live births that occurred in the preceding 12 months. Matches are then further investigated to determine if the woman's death was due to her pregnancy or another cause. This matching approach is also used in Finland (12). In view of the difficulties of distinguishing deaths that are pregnancy-related from those that are not, most surveillance experts recommend identifying all deaths that are temporally associated with pregnancy. Using additional data collected for each death, surveillance personnel can then determine whether pregnancy contributed to or caused death. If the death becomes the subject of malpractice litigation, additional information may be severely restricted or unavailable. Less frequently used supplemental sources for pregnancy-related deaths are hospital discharge data, autopsy, and medical examiner data. Often these sources are not available in an electronic format or are not available for an entire population, limiting their utility.

Data sources – developing countries: In areas without reliable on-going vital record systems, deaths are ascertained by survey interviews. In the "sisterhood" method, analysts estimate the maternal mortality rate by using the proportion of deaths due to pregnancy for all deaths among respondents' reproductive-age sisters (13). Estimates take into account the age of the decedent relative to the respondent. The primary measure is lifetime risk of pregnancy-related death.

A modification of the sisterhood approach that avoids the need for a population-based survey is the clinic-based approach (14). In this method, individuals attending clinics are queried about pregnancy-related deaths.

Case–case control studies can be used to estimate the population proportional attributable risk, which is the proportion of deaths among reproductive-age women attributable to pregnancy. Cases are deaths among reproductive-age women that occurred during a defined interval and controls are reproductive-age women alive at the end of the interval. Pregnancy history is compared for cases and controls (15).

Measurement issues: The biggest measurement problem is underascertainment of pregnancy-related deaths (16–18). Despite the use of multiple methods to ascertain pregnancy-related deaths, researchers estimate that approximately half of pregnancy-related deaths in the United States are not ascertained (17, 19). In a study of maternal deaths from 1988 through 1992 in Canada, investigators found that one-third of total direct maternal deaths were not identified as such (18). The greatest underreporting was for deaths from cerebrovascular disorders, pulmonary embolism, and causes indirectly related to pregnancy. These investigators extended their study to compare identification of maternal deaths using ICD-9 and ICD-10. They found that the maximum number of direct maternal deaths was 20% *less* using ICD-10. Contributing to this difference is that deaths from cerebrovascular disorders during pregnancy or within 42 days after its termination are classified as direct maternal deaths in ICD-9, but not in ICD-10.

A study of pregnancy-associated deaths in 13 European countries showed substantial variability among countries in the completeness and accuracy of ascertainment of maternal deaths from vital records (20). Official statistics correctly identified 215 (83%) of 260 deaths from obstetrical causes. They also incorrectly identified 14 (14%) of 99 nonobstetric deaths as having obstetric causes. The percentage of correctly identified obstetric deaths ranged from 59% in Hungary and 60% in Austria to 100% in Belgium and France.

Problems in accurately counting the appropriate denominator also impede accurate assessment of MMRs. Ideally, the denominator for the pregnancy-related mortality rate should be the number of pregnancies, rather than the number of women. Counting the number of pregnancies in a population is difficult, but not impossible (21, 22). Alternative measures for the denominator are the number of women of reproductive age and the number of live births. Because nearly all countries have a system for registering live births, live births are a surrogate for the number of pregnancies. Because live births do not include all pregnancies (i.e., the denominator), we calculate the MMR rather than the maternal mortality rate. In countries where a relatively high proportion of pregnancies end in spontaneous or induced abortion, the number of live births may substantially underestimate the number of pregnancies. As a result, the MMR may appear higher than in a country with a comparable mortality experience, but where more of the pregnancies end in live birth. Similarly, changes over time within a country in the percentage of pregnancies that end in live births will confound temporal trends in the MMR.

The sisterhood method has several disadvantages. Because it typically ascertains deaths during the past 5 or 10 years, it provides historical, rather than current information about maternal deaths. Furthermore, the sisterhood requires the expense and effort of a survey (15, 23). It is limited by the accuracy of the respondent's understanding of the decedent's cause of death. Investigators have noted underacertainment of maternal deaths due to respondents' failure to recognize the pregnancy-related nature of a death (23). At least one analyst has voiced concern that, as used for international comparisons of maternal mortality rates, the sisterhood method underestimates variability (24).

In view of the difficulties of accurately measuring maternal mortality, the WHO and United Nations' Children's Fund (UNICEF) recently recommended using obstetric process indicators in place of the MMR (25, 26). Such measures include the availability of essential obstetric care, proportion of births by Cesarean section, and the proportion of deliveries assisted by skilled attendants. Analysts recommend process indicators because they may increase the validity of international comparisons and may be more immediately useful for needs assessment and program evaluation.

Maternal Mortality Review

Case-by-case review of detailed information for each maternal death continues to be at the heart of maternal mortality surveillance domestically and internationally (5–9). Typically, review committees include local clinicians (obstetricians, midwives, and nurses), as well as public health and hospital staff. In reviewing deaths, committee members aim to identify potentially preventable factors that contributed to death (8). Using this knowledge, they propose approaches to avert future deaths. Often these approaches involve improving the quality of clinical care. They may also involve public health interventions, such as improving access to prenatal or assuring the availability of emergency transport to referral facilities.

4.2   Overall Maternal Mortality

Occurrence and trends. Maternal mortality declined markedly during the twentieth century from ~600–900 deaths per 100,000 live births in 1900 to 10 per 100,000 live births in 1999 (Fig. 4.1). From 1900 to the mid-1930s, puerperal infections caused by virulent streptococcal and poor obstetric delivery practices, due largely to inadequately trained practitioners or unnecessary obstetric procedures, accounted for most of the deaths (27, 28). From 1938 to 1948, the percentage of deliveries occurring in hospitals shifted from 55% to 90% and maternal mortality declined by 71% (29). Concomitantly, obstetric training improved, technical advances increased treatment options (e.g., antibiotics, safer anesthesia, and trans- fusion), and hospitals restricted delivery privileges to qualified practitioners. Maternal mortality continued to decline during the 1950s and 1960s (89% decline from 1950 through 1973 (30), accompanied by continuing improvements in obstet- ric practice as well as the introduction of oral contraceptives and the legalization of abortion. A mortality study in North Carolina from 1963 through 1992 demon- strates the reduction in maternal mortality that followed the legalization of abortion (31). From 1973–1977, immediately following legalization of abortion in North Carolina, the MMR dropped by 85%. A decrease in abortion-related mortality accounted for about 46% of this total decline.

Since the 1980s, the national trend in the MMR has been essentially flat or slightly increasing (18, 32, 33). States report similar experience (31). The lack of

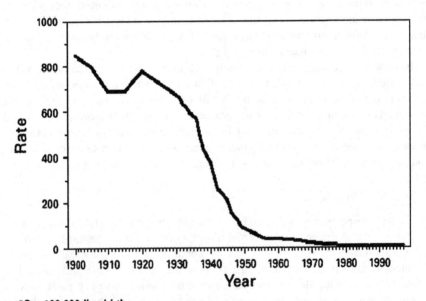

*Per 100,000 live births.

Fig. 4.1 Maternal mortality ratio, by year, United States, 1990–1997

change, however, may conceal a true decrease that has been offset by improved reporting of maternal deaths (34). Analysts have estimated that up to 50% of maternal deaths from 1987 through 1990 were not reported (19).

Using data from death certificates, the National Center for Health Statistics (NCHS) computes the MMR for the United States (34). During the 1990s, the NCHS's MMR ranged from 8.2 per 100,000 live births in 1990 to 7.1 in 1995 and 1998, ending the decade at 9.9. Before 1999, data for the MMR included only deaths occurring within 42 days after pregnancy termination. Reflecting the 1999 transition to ICD-10, since 1999, the MMR has included pregnancy-related deaths that occurred up to 1 year following pregnancy termination. The annual number of pregnancy-related deaths ranged from a low of 294 in 1996 to a high of 391 in 1999. During the 1990s, data from death certificates showed that direct obstetric causes (such as hemorrhage, embolism, or pregnancy-induced hypertension) accounted for the majority of deaths (overall 81%), followed by deaths related to pregnancies ending in abortive outcomes (11%) and indirect obstetric causes (8%).

Healthy People 2010 Objective for Maternal Mortality (1)

- Reduce maternal deaths to 3.3 per 100,000 live births (objective unchanged from 2000)

The Healthy People 2010 Objectives comprise more than 400 health-related objectives for the United States. They were developed and are monitored by federal agencies with broad public consultation.

The Pregnancy Mortality Surveillance System (PMSS) reports a higher MMR for the 1990s than the NCHS. The PMSS uses multiple sources to ascertain maternal deaths and includes deaths that occur within 1 year after pregnancy termination (32). From 1991 through 1999, 4,200 deaths were identified, yielding an overall 9-year MMR of 11.8. The MMR increased from 10.3 in 1991 to 13.2 in 1999, probably due to improved ascertainment. Overall, 60% of deaths followed a live birth, 7% a stillbirth, 6% an ectopic pregnancy, 4% an abortion, and 10% of decedents had not delivered when they died. Pregnancy outcome was unknown for 13% of decedents.

In the United States from 1991 to 1999, risk of pregnancy-related death varied by pregnancy outcome (35). It was lowest following legal abortion (0.6 per 100,000 legal abortions) or spontaneous abortion (1.2 per 100,000 spontaneous abortions), followed by live birth (7.1 per 100,000 pregnancies ending in live birth) and ectopic pregnancy (31.9 per 100,000 ectopic pregnancies). It was highest after pregnancies ending in fetal death (96.3 per 100,000 pregnancies ending in fetal death). The risk also varied by method of delivery. Some authors reported a risk of maternal mortality that was 3.6 times higher for Cesarean deliveries compared with vaginal deliveries (36). Other authors, however, did not detect this increase (37).

Table 4.3 Percentage distribution and pregnancy-related mortality ratio for causes of pregnancy-related death, United States, 1991–1999 (*Source*: (32))

Cause	Percent distribution (n = 4,200)	Deaths per 100,000 live births
Embolism	19.6	2.3
Hemorrhage	17.2	2.0
Pregnancy-induced hypertension	15.7	1.8
Infection	12.6	1.5
Cardiomyopathy	8.3	1.0
Cerebrovascular accidents	5.0	0.6
Anesthesia	1.6	0.6
Others	9.2	2.3
Unknown	0.7	0.1
Total	*100.0*	*11.8*

In the United States during the 1990s, the most frequent causes of maternal death were hemorrhage and embolism, followed by hypertensive disorders, infection, and cardiomyopathy (Table 4.3) (32).

Cause of death varied by pregnancy outcome (32). Among pregnancies that ended in live birth, embolism accounted for 21% of deaths, pregnancy-induced hypertension for 19.3%, infection for 11.7%, and cardiomyopathy for 10.1%. Deaths following pregnancies that ended in stillbirth showed a similar overall pattern, except hemorrhage accounted for a notable portion of deaths (21.1%) and cardiomyopathy accounted for a smaller portion of deaths (5.1%). Nearly all deaths (93.3%) associated with ectopic pregnancy were caused by hemorrhage. Compared with deaths following all other pregnancy outcomes, deaths following spontaneous or induced abortions had the highest portion attributed to infection (33.9%). Embolism and hemorrhage accounted for 13.9% and 21.8% of deaths following abortion, respectively.

Describing specific causes of death may conceal factors that contribute to their underlying etiologies. Such factors include the trends toward delayed childbearing and increased use of reproductive technology (38). The latter often results in multifetal pregnancies, which themselves are related to a higher risk of maternal mortality (39).

PMSS data concerning the length of time from pregnancy termination to maternal death were available for 3,400 decedents (32). Overall, relative to pregnancy termination, 34% died within 24 h, 55% during 1–42 days afterwards, and 11% during 43–365 days afterwards. The length of time between pregnancy termination and maternal death varied by cause of death and pregnancy outcome. More than half of the deaths from hemorrhage and embolism occurred within 48 h after pregnancy termination. In contrast, more than half of the deaths from infection and pregnancy-induced hypertension occurred from 3 through 42 days after delivery. Deaths from cardiomyopathy occurred at the longest interval after pregnancy termination: 45% occurred from 43 through 365 days after pregnancy termination.

International findings: The WHO and UNICEF estimated maternal mortality in 188 countries for 1995 (26). Because of changes in estimation methods, assessment of trends is difficult. Nonetheless, 1995 data show large variation in MMRs among regions and countries. An estimated 515,000 deaths occurred worldwide, with more than half (273,000) occurring in Africa. Although the global MMR was estimated as 397 per 100,000 live births (95% confidence interval, 234, 635), the estimated MMR in Africa exceeded 1,000 (i.e., one maternal death occurred for every 100 live births). The estimated MMRs for developed countries with 500,000 or more live births annually ranged from 84 in Argentina, to 74 in the Russian Federation, 45 in Ukraine, 20 in France, 12 in Germany, Japan, and the United States, 11 in Italy, and 10 in the United Kingdom. The estimated MMRs were high in several of the most populated countries: China – 62, India – 437, Indonesia – 472, Brazil – 262, and Mexico – 67.

Analyses performed by WHO, UNICEF, and UNFPA estimate that, in 2000, 529,000 maternal deaths occurred globally (http://www.childinfo.org/maternal_mortality_in_2000.pdf). In developed countries, an estimated one out of 2,800 women died from a pregnancy-related cause. The highest lifetime risks occurred in sub-Saharan Africa, where an estimated one out of 16 women died from a pregnancy-related cause.

A report of the Maternal Mortality Working Group, which calculated the MMR using improved methods, estimated that, in 2005, 535,900 maternal deaths occurred worldwide, of which 533,100 were in developing regions (40). This Group also reported that MMRs in sub-Saharan Africa remained very high in 2005.

Demographic variability. During the 1990s in the United States, the MMR varied by:

- Maternal race (lowest for Whites),
- Marital status (lowest for married women),
- Age (lowest for women ≤19 years),
- Education (lowest for women with ≥12 years education, after accounting for age),
- Use of prenatal care initiation (lowest for any care compared with no care), and
- Live-birth order (highest for fifth and higher-order births) (32).

Of these characteristics, disparities are the largest and most consistent for race and maternal age. In general, African-American women have a three-to-four-fold higher risk of pregnancy-related death than White women, depending on the cause of death (32). Exceptions are deaths from ectopic pregnancy and cardiomyopathy, for which African-Americans have a six-fold higher risk of death than Whites (32, 41, 42). Analyses of state-specific MMRs also reveal a higher risk for African-American women during 1987–1996 (43), 1992–1998 (44), and 1994–1998 (45). For maternal deaths following pregnancies that ended in live birth, the excess mortality among African-Americans is not explained by racial differences in maternal age, marital status, education, use of prenatal care, urban or rural residence, infant weight, gestation, or live birth order (46). One author has attributed the excess risk of maternal mortality for African-American women to infection and microvascular dysfunction (47). Other authors attribute the excess risk of African-American women to their more severe comorbidities and differentials in pregnancy-related care (44).

Advanced maternal age ($\geq$35 years for Whites; $\geq$30 years for Blacks) also increases the risk of maternal death due to medical causes (48–51). For Black women aged 30 and above, the risk of pregnancy-related death is especially elevated compared with either younger Black women or White women of any age.

Apart from deaths due to pregnancy-related conditions, studies in Georgia and Finland found that, during the year after delivery, women who have recently given birth generally have a lower risk of death than women who have not been pregnant or given birth (52, 53). An exception occurred for women aged 15–19, who have 2.6 times the risk of postpartum death due to homicide than women who have not been pregnant (52). Researchers examining data from Massachusetts, the United States, and Mozambique also have reported elevated numbers of homicides among young women who have recently delivered (5, 54, 55).

4.3   Cause-Specific Mortality

4.3.1.   Abortion

Occurrence: In the United States, the number of deaths related to legal abortion was 10 in 1998 and 4 in 1999 (56). The legal abortion-related case fatality rate during the 1990s ranged from 8 deaths per 1,000,000 abortions to 3 deaths per 1,000,000 abortions. No deaths related to illegal abortions occurred from 1995 through 1999. The number of maternal deaths related to spontaneous abortion was 11 in 1998 and 10 in 1999 (56). From 1991 through 1999 in the United States, deaths related to induced or spontaneous abortion accounted for 4% of all pregnancy-related deaths and occurred at a rate of 0.5 per 100,000 births (32). Of abortion-related deaths, 34% were caused by infection and 22% by hemorrhage.

Abortion-related mortality is a much bigger problem in developing countries than in developed countries. This is particularly true in Africa, where access to legal abortion is limited. For example, in Nigeria, 20,000 deaths annually are attributed to unsafe induced abortion (57). In a study of maternal deaths in Benin, Ivory Coast, and Senegal during 1999, induced abortion-related deaths accounted for just under half of all pregnancy-related deaths and were 37 times more frequent than deaths associated with spontaneous abortion (58).

Factors influencing occurrence: The most important cause of death from induced abortion is the safety of the procedure itself. The rates of unsafe abortion vary by location: Latin America and the Caribbean – one unsafe abortion per three live births; Asia (excluding east Asia) – one per five live births; Africa – one per seven live births; and developed countries – one per 25 live births (59).

4.4   Public Health Interventions, their Availability, and Use

Here, we focus on interventions to reduce maternal morbidity and mortality that are implemented immediately before or during pregnancy. Interventions range in when they need to occur from preconception (e.g., family planning), to during pregnancy as well as to during and after delivery (60). Many interventions involve clinical practice, rather than public health practice. Furthermore, many public health interventions have their impact by directly or indirectly supporting clinical care. Few public health interventions have been rigorously evaluated through randomized clinical trials, although many hold the potential for positive benefits.

Primary prevention: Although the effectiveness of preconception care has not been evaluated in randomized controlled trials, helping women to have pregnancies when they want to have them and are in good health likely would have substantial impact on reducing maternal as well as neonatal morbidity. As discussed in Chap. 2, we are far from achieving this goal. Broadly based public health interventions, such as eliminating barriers to family planning services, encouraging pregnancy planning, and ensuring universal access to health, are needed to achieve it. Compared with other developed countries, the United States has achieved only moderate success in applying these interventions.

Reducing cigarette smoking and the prevalence of chlamydia infections are likely to reduce ectopic pregnancy (Table 4.4). Methods to reduce smoking that have strong evidence of their effectiveness include smoking bans and restrictions; increasing the unit price for tobacco; media campaigns with interventions; and quitter telephone support with interventions (61). An ecologic study in Sweden found a correlation between temporal trends of lower rates of chlamydial infection detected on screening and lower rates of ectopic pregnancy (62). Community rates of chlamydia infection can be lowered by screening and treatment of infected individuals and their partners.

The risks for complications from abortion are lowest early in gestation. Ensuring women's easy access to safe, legal abortion is associated with shorter lengths of gestation when abortions are performed (63). Although death from induced abortion is rare in developed countries, it accounts for a substantial number of deaths in developing countries. In contrast with an estimated death rate from abortions of 0.2–1.2 per 100,000 abortions in the developed world, the rate is 680 deaths per 100,000 abortions in Africa, 283 in South and Southeast Asia, and 119 in Latin America (63). At least five public health actions improve access to abortions:

- Making abortion available at an affordable price;
- Providing abortion facilities in geographically accessible locations,
- Insuring adequate capacity to perform abortions, so that waiting time is minimized;
- Eliminating legally prescribed waiting periods before the procedure as well as psychological harassment of women seeking abortions; and
- Training an adequate number of clinicians skilled in abortion procedures.

Table 4.4 Public health interventions aimed at decreasing maternal morbidity and mortality

Maternal problem(s)	Public health intervention	Rationale
Ectopic pregnancy	Reducing the prevalence of chlamydia infections through screening and treatment	Chlamydia infections can damage the fallopian tubes
	Reducing cigarette smoking among women	Smoking increases the risk for ectopic pregnancy
Morbidity or mortality related to induced abortion	Ensuring easy access to abortion	Easy access enables women to obtain abortions at earlier gestations, when risks are lowest
Anemia; pyelonephritis; preeclampsia; eclampsia; hemorrhage; Cesarean delivery; endometritis; tetanus	Removing barriers to prenatal care	Prenatal care reduces the risk of adverse outcomes (see text)
Operative delivery or death secondary to cephalopelvic disproportion (CPD)	Ensuring adequate nutrition during childhood	Short maternal stature increases the risk of CPD. Providing adequate nutrition during pregnancy helps to maximize adult stature
	Reducing preconception overweight/obesity	Maternal overweight/obesity is associated with increased risk for operative delivery
Death from obstructed labor, hemorrhage, preeclampsia, or eclampsia	Maintaining a rapid transport system to a hospital capable of Cesarean section deliveries (in developing countries, usually a referral hospital)	Treatment of hemorrhage, severe preeclampsia, or eclampsia requires prompt care at tertiary facility
Puerpural infection	Providing trained birth attendant and hygienic delivery facilities	Trained attendants and adequate facilities minimize the risk of ascending infection and endometritis
Maternal postpartum tetanus infection	Providing population-based immunization programs	Immunization prevents tetanus

Ensuring access to prenatal care is likely to reduce morbidity and mortality from anemia, pyleonephritis, preeclampsia, eclampsia, hemorrhage, operative delivery, and infection. Among the prenatal interventions and their related impacts on maternal morbidity and mortality are:

- Providing iron and folate supplements and screening for and treating anemia, which reduces anemia and shows promise for reducing the need for postpartum blood transfusion (64);
- Among women with either high risk of developing hypertension or low baseline dietary calcium intake, providing calcium supplements reduces the risk of preeclampsia (64);

- Screening for proteinuria and increases in blood pressure can detect preeclampsia, enabling treatment, including magnesium sulfate to reduce mortality and induced delivery for severe disease. Treatment lowers the risk for hemorrhage that is associated with gestational hypertension (65);
- Screening for asymptomatic bacteriuria and treating appropriately, which prevents pyelonephritis from ascending infections (65);
- Providing tetanus immunization prevents maternal and neonatal tetanus;
- Among women with rupture of membranes at or near term, inducing labor, which prevents maternal infection (65); and
- Among women with breech presentation at term, external cephalic version, which reduces the risk of Cesarean section delivery (65).

In populations with vitamin A deficiency, β-carotene supplementation holds promise for reducing maternal mortality (64, 66). However, vitamin A deficiency is uncommon in the United States (67, 68). Although supplementation with iron and folate may reduce pregnancy-associated morbidity, its impact on reducing maternal mortality is uncertain (69, 70).

Optimizing nutrition during childhood to maximize adult stature (64, 65) and achieving a preconception weight that is appropriate for height are likely to reduce operative delivery due to obstructed labor (Table 4.4).

Notably absent from this list of prenatal clinical interventions is risk-scoring systems. These systems categorize women based on obstetric history and other attributes. Women with higher risk scores receive more intensive and/or specialized obstetrical care. The effectiveness of this approach for reducing perinatal morbidity has not been established through randomized controlled trials (65).

Secondary prevention: In developed countries, access to hygienic delivery facilities and availability of tertiary-level care and emergency transport to it are much less of a problem than in developing countries. The FIGO (International Federation of Obstetrics and Gynecology) initiative (65, 71), which aims to reduce maternal mortality in developing countries, includes four components:

- Skilled attendants at all births;
- Basic emergency care in primary-level health facilities;
- Comprehensive obstetrical care in referral hospitals; and
- Rapid transport of women in need of special care.

Training a workforce of skilled birth attendants, establishing a network of primary and referral health care facilities, and maintaining a rapid transport system all fall within the realm of public health interventions.

Discussion Topics

1. What is the best balance between spending funds to prevent maternal mortality and funds to conduct surveillance of maternal mortality? What factors could change this balance?

2. Would one expect that the rate of "near-miss" maternal morbidity will increase as the rate of maternal mortality decreases? Are the two outcomes directly related to each other?
3. How can persistent racial disparities in maternal mortality be reduced in the United States? What impact are these disparities likely to have on other pregnancy outcomes?

Promising Areas for Future Research

1. How can changes in the rates of maternal mortality in developing countries be assessed when accounting for improvements in ascertainment of maternal deaths?
2. What are the best methods for assessing the comparability of rates of maternal mortality among developed countries with differing methods of ascertainment and differing health-care systems?
3. What are the best methods to evaluate the impact of interventions to reduce maternal mortality?

Abbreviations

ICD	International Classification of Diseases
MMR	Maternal mortality ratio
NCHS	National Center for Health Statistics
PMSS	Pregnancy Mortality Surveillance System
UNICEF	United Nations' Children's Fund
WHO	World Health Organization

References

1. U.S. Department of Health and Human Services. Healthy People 2010: Understanding and Improving Health, 2nd ed. Washington, DC: U.S. Government Printing Office, 2000.
2. Strategies to reduce pregnancy-related deaths: from identification and review to action. Berg C. Diahzsble, editor. Atlanta: Centers for Disease Control and Prevention, 2001.
3. Wildman K, Bouvier-Colle MH. Maternal mortality as an indicator of obstetric care in Europe. BJOG 2004; 111(2):164–169.
4. Cochet L, Pattinson RC, Macdonald AP. Severe acute maternal morbidity and maternal death audit – a rapid diagnostic tool for evaluating maternal care. S Afr Med J 2003; 93(9):700–702.
5. Thomas TA, Cooper GM. Maternal deaths from anaesthesia. An extract from Why mothers die 1997–1999, the Confidential Enquiries into Maternal Deaths in the United Kingdom. Br J Anaesth 2002; 89(3):499–508.

6. Nannini A, Weiss J, Goldstein R, Fogerty S. Pregnancy-associated mortality at the end of the twentieth century: Massachusetts, 1990–1999. J Am Med Womens Assoc 2002; 57 (3):140–143.

7. Chichakli LO, Atrash HK, Musani AS, Mahaini R, Arnaoute S. Maternal mortality surveillance and maternal death reviews in countries of the Eastern Mediterranean Region. East Mediterr Health J 2000; 6(4):625–635.

8. Mantel GD, Moodley J. Can a developed country's maternal mortality review be used as the 'gold standard' for a developing country? Eur J Obstet Gynecol Reprod Biol 2002; 100 (2):189–195.

9. A review of maternal deaths in South Africa during 1998. National Committee on Confidential Enquiries into Maternal Deaths. S Afr Med J 2000; 90(4):367–373.

10. MacKay AP, Rochat R, Smith JC, Berg CJ. The check box: determining pregnancy status to improve maternal mortality surveillance. Am J Prev Med 2000; 19(1 Suppl):35–39.

11. Starzyk P, Frost F, Kobayashi J. Misclassification of maternal deaths – Washington State. MMWR 2003; 35(39):621–623.

12. Gissler M, Kauppila R, Merilainen J, Toukomaa H, Hemminki E. Pregnancy-associated deaths in Finland 1987–1994 – definition problems and benefits of record linkage. Acta Obstet Gynecol Scand 1997; 76(7):651–657.

13. Graham W, Brass W, Snow RW. Estimating maternal mortality: the sisterhood method. Stud Fam Plann 1989; 20(3):125–135.

14. Danel I, Graham W, Stupp P, Castillo P. Applying the sisterhood method for estimating maternal mortality to a health facility-based sample: a comparison with results from a household-based sample. Int J Epidemiol 1996; 25(5):1017–1022.

15. Berhane Y, Andersson T, Wall S, Byass P, Hogberg U. Aims, options and outcomes in measuring maternal mortality in developing societies. Acta Obstet Gynecol Scand 2000; 79(11):968–972.

16. Atrash HK, Alexander S, Berg CJ. Maternal mortality in developed countries: not just a concern of the past. Obstet Gynecol 1995; 86(4 Pt 2):700–705.

17. Callaghan WM, Berg CJ. Maternal mortality surveillance in the United States: moving into the twenty-first century. J Am Med Womens Assoc 2002; 57(3):131–134, 139.

18. Turner LA, Kramer MS, Liu S. Cause-specific mortality during and after pregnancy and the definition of maternal death. Chronic Dis Can 2002; 23(1):31–36.

19. Berg CJ, Atrash HK, Koonin LM, Tucker M. Pregnancy-related mortality in the United States, 1987–1990. Obstet Gynecol 1996; 88(2):161–167.

20. Salanave B, Bouvier-Colle MH, Varnoux N, Alexander S, Macfarlane A. Classification differences and maternal mortality: a European study. MOMS Group. Mothers' Mortality and Severe morbidity. Int J Epidemiol 1999; 28(1):64–69.

21. Saraiya M, Berg CJ, Shulman H, Green CA, Atrash HK. Estimates of the annual number of clinically recognized pregnancies in the United States, 1981–1991. Am J Epidemiol 1999; 149 (11):1025–1029.

22. Goldhaber MK, Fireman BH. Re: "Estimates of the annual number of clinically recognized pregnancies in the United States, 1981–1991". Am J Epidemiol 2000; 152(3):287–289.

23. Shahidullah M. The sisterhood method of estimating maternal mortality: the Matlab experience. Stud Fam Plann 1995; 26(2):101–106.

24. Hakkert R. Country estimates of maternal mortality: an alternative model. Stat Med 2001; 20 (23):3505–3524.

25. UNICEF/WHO/UNFPA. Guidelines for monitoring the availability and use of obstetric services. New York: UNICEF, 1997.

26. Hill K, AbouZahr C, Wardlaw T. Estimates of maternal mortality for 1995. Bulletin of the World Health Orgaization 2001; 79(3):182–193.

27. Achievements in public health, 1900–1999: healthier mothers and babies. MMWR 1999; 48 (38):849–858.

28. Loudon I. Maternal mortality in the past and its relevance to developing countries today. Am J Clin Nutr 2000; 72(1 Suppl):241S–246S.
29. Children's Bureau. Changes in infant, childhood, and maternal mortality over the decade of 1939–1948: a graphic analysis. 1950. Washington, DC: Children's Bureau, Social Security Administration.
30. National Center for Health Statistics. Vital statistics of the United States, 1973. Vol II, mortality, part A. Rockville, Maryland: US Department of Health, Education, and Welfare, 1977.
31. Meyer RE, Buescher PA. Maternal mortality related to induced abortion in North Carolina: a historical study. Fam Plann Perspect 1994; 26(4):179–180, 191.
32. Chang J, Elam-Evans L, Berg C, Herndon J, Flowers L, Seed K, et al. Pregnancy-related mortality surveillance – United States, 1991–1999. MMWR Surveill Summ 2003; 52(SS-2):1–8.
33. Berg CJ, Chang J, Callaghan WM, Whitehead SJ. Pregnancy-related mortality in the United States, 1991–1997. Obstet Gynecol 2003; 101(2):289–296.
34. Hoyert DL. Maternal mortality and related concepts. Vital Health Stat 3 2007; 33:1–13.
35. Grimes DA. Estimation of pregnancy-related mortality risk by pregnancy outcome, United States, 1991 to 1999. Am J Obstet Gynecol 2006; 194(1):92–94.
36. Deneux-Tharaux C, Carmona E, Bouvier-Colle MH, Breart G. Postpartum maternal mortality and cesarean delivery. Obstet Gynecol 2006; 108(3 Pt 1):541–548.
37. Vadnais M, Sachs B. Maternal mortality with cesarean delivery: a literature review. Semin Perinatol 2006; 30(5):242–246.
38. Lang CT, King JC. Maternal mortality in the United States. Best Pract Res Clin Obstet Gynaecol 2008; 22(3):517–531.
39. MacKay AP, Berg CJ, King JC, Duran C, Chang J. Pregnancy-related mortality among women with multifetal pregnancies. Obstet Gynecol 2006; 107(3):563–568.
40. Hill K, Thomas K, AbouZahr C, Walker N, Say L, Inoue M, et al. Estimates of maternal mortality worldwide between 1990 and 2005: an assessment of available data. Lancet 2007; 370(9595):1311–1319.
41. Fang J, Madhavan S, Alderman MH. Maternal mortality in New York City: excess mortality of Black women. J Urban Health 2000; 77(4):735–744.
42. Whitehead SJ, Berg CJ, Chang J. Pregnancy-related mortality due to cardiomyopathy: United States, 1991–1997. Obstet Gynecol 2003; 102(6):1326–1331.
43. State-specific maternal mortality among Black and White women – United States, 1987–1996. MMWR 1999; 48(23):492–495.
44. Harper M, Dugan E, Espeland M, Martinez-Borges A, Mcquellon C. Why African-American women are at greater risk for pregnancy-related death. Ann Epidemiol 2007; 17(3):180–185.
45. Rosenberg D, Geller SE, Studee L, Cox SM. Disparities in mortality among high risk pregnant women in Illinois: A population based study. Ann Epidemiol 2006; 16(1):26–32.
46. Saftlas AF, Koonin LM, Atrash HK. Racial disparity in pregnancy-related mortality associated with livebirth: can established risk factors explain it? Am J Epidemiol 2000; 152 (5):413–419.
47. Fiscella K. Racial disparity in infant and maternal mortality: confluence of infection, and microvascular dysfunction. Matern Child Health J 2004; 8(2):45–54.
48. Chichakli LO, Atrash HK, MacKay AP, Musani AS, Berg CJ. Pregnancy-related mortality in the United States due to hemorrhage: 1979–1992. Obstet Gynecol 1999; 94(5 Pt 1):721–725.
49. MacKay AP, Berg CJ, Atrash HK. Pregnancy-related mortality from preeclampsia and eclampsia. Obstet Gynecol 2001; 97(4):533–538.
50. Saraiya M, Green CA, Berg CJ, Hopkins FW, Koonin LM, Atrash HK. Spontaneous abortion-related deaths among women in the United States – 1981–1991. Obstet Gynecol 1999; 94 (2):172–176.
51. Callaghan WM, Berg CJ. Pregnancy-related mortality among women aged 35 years and older, United States, 1991–1997. Obstet Gynecol 2003; 102(5 Pt 1):1015–1021.

52. Dietz PM, Rochat RW, Thompson BL, Berg CJ, Griffin GW. Differences in the risk of homicide and other fatal injuries between postpartum women and other women of childbearing age: implications for prevention. Am J Public Health 1998; 88(4):641–643.

53. Gissler M, Berg C, Bouvier-Colle MH, Buekens P. Pregnancy-associated mortality after birth, spontaneous abortion, or induced abortion in Finland, 1987–2000. Am J Obstet Gynecol 2004; 190(2):422–427.

54. Granja AC, Zacarias E, Bergstrom S. Violent deaths: the hidden face of maternal mortality. BJOG 2002; 109(1):5–8.

55. Chang J, Berg CJ, Saltzman LE, Herndon J. Homicide: a leading cause of injury deaths among pregnant and postpartum women in the United States, 1991–1999. Am J Public Health 2005; 95(3):471–477.

56. Elam-Evans LD, Strauss LT, Herndon J, Parker WY, Bowens SV, Zane S, et al. Abortion surveillance – United States, 2000. MMWR Surveill Summ 2003; 52(12):1–32.

57. Raufu A. Unsafe abortions cause 20 000 deaths a year in Nigeria. BMJ 2002; 325(7371):988d.

58. Thonneau P, Goyaux N, Goufodji S, Sundby J. Abortion and maternal mortality in Africa. N Engl J Med 2002; 347(24):1984–1985.

59. Ahman E, Shah I. Unsafe abortion: worldwide estimates for 2000. Reprod Health Matters 2002; 10(19):13–17.

60. Campbell OM, Graham WJ. Strategies for reducing maternal mortality: getting on with what works. Lancet 2006; 368(9543):1284–1299.

61. Strategies for reducing exposure to environmental tobacco smoke, increase tobacco-use cessation, and reducing initiation in communities and health care systems: A report on recommendations of the Task Force on Community Preventive Services. MMWR Recomm Rep 2000; 49(RR-12):1–12.

62. Egger M, Low N, Smith GD, Lindblom B, Herrmann B. Screening for chlamydial infections and the risk of ectopic pregnancy in a county in Sweden: ecological analysis. BMJ 1998; 316 (7147):1776–1780.

63. The Alan Guttmacher Institute. Sharing responsibility: women, society, and abortion worldwide. 1999. The Alan Guttmacher Institute, New York.

64. Villar J, Merialdi M, Gulmezoglu AM, Abalos E, Carroli G, Kulier R, et al. Nutritional interventions during pregnancy for the prevention or treatment of maternal morbidity and preterm delivery: an overview of randomized controlled trials. J Nutr 2003; 133(5 Suppl 2):1606S–1625S.

65. Carroli G, Rooney C, Villar J. How effective is antenatal care in preventing maternal mortality and serious morbidity? An overview of the evidence. Paediatr Perinat Epidemiol 2001; 15 (Suppl 1):1–42.

66. Tomkins A. Nutrition and maternal morbidity and mortality. Br J Nutr 2001; 85 (Suppl 2): S93–S99.

67. Baker H, DeAngelis B, Holland B, Gittens-Williams L, Barrett T, Jr. Vitamin profile of 563 gravidas during trimesters of pregnancy. J Am Coll Nutr 2002; 21(1):33–37.

68. Ballew C, Bowman BA, Sowell AL, Gillespie C. Serum retinol distributions in residents of the United States: third National Health and Nutrition Examination Survey, 1988–1994. Am J Clin Nutr 2001; 73(3):586–593.

69. Brabin BJ, Hakimi M, Pelletier D. An analysis of anemia and pregnancy-related maternal mortality. J Nutr 2001; 131(2S-2):604S–614S.

70. Rush D. Nutrition and maternal mortality in the developing world. Am J Clin Nutr 2000; 72 (1 Suppl):212S–240S.

71. Benagiano G, Thomas B. Saving mothers' lives: the FIGO Save the Mothers Initiative. Int J Gynaecol Obstet 2003; 80(2):198–203.

72. Atrash HK, Lawson HW, Ellerbrock RV, Rowley DL, Koonin LM. Pregnancy-related mortality. In: Wilcox LS, Marks JS, eds. From Data to Action: CDC's Public Health Surveillance for Women, Infants, and Children. Washington, DC: U.S. Department of Health and Human Services/CDC, 1995:141–154.

Chapter 5
Infant Morbidity

While epidemiologic research occasionally results in identification of novel associations between exposures and disease, more often it is the astute clinician who makes the initial observations that begin the process. Such was the case in the late 1950s, when a German pediatrician, Dr. Widikund Lenz, began to observe a very unusual pattern of birth defects involving phocomelia. Fetuses affected by this extremely rare condition have limb reduction defects including the absence of hands and/or feet, together with other abnormalities. Dr. Lenz queried colleagues, and compiled a case series with more than 50 cases by late 1961. The common exposure was the use of a new anti-nausea medication, thalidomide. Additional studies demonstrated the power teratogenic effect of this drug, and the timing of fetal development during which its effects were most pronounced. Thalidomide was removed for the market for several decades, but is now prescribed for patients suffering terminal illness.

Rajkumar (1)

Most babies are born healthy and experience growth and development within typical limits. However, normative growth and development differs for very small infants with underlying disease and those who are not provided sufficient nutrition and developmental stimulation. In the United States, standards exist for routine infant care and immunization, under the rubric of *Bright Futures* (2).

From an epidemiologic perspective, opportunities exist to assess the association between adverse perinatal outcomes or infant health problems and use of health care services by race and ethnicity, socioeconomic status, and insurance or membership in specific health programs or plans. Sources of infant morbidity may originate in the perinatal period, or arise from insults or infections postnatally acquired in the family or community.

This chapter begins by defining infant morbidity, and then it describes general measures, data sources, and measurement issues. Subsequent sections examine specific types of morbidity, focusing on epidemiology, risk factors, and protective factors, as well as public health interventions.

M.M. Adams et al., *Perinatal Epidemiology for Public Health Practice.*
doi: 10.1007/978-0-387-09439-7_5; © Springer Science + Business Media, LLC 2009

5.1   General Issues of Infant Morbidity

5.1.1   Definitions, Measures, Data Sources, and Measurement Issues

5.1.1.1   Definitions

Infant morbidity is defined as any physiologic or structural departure from a state of well-being that is manifest during the infant's first year of life. This broad definition covers conditions with a broad range of etiologies, including those that are determined genetically (e.g., phenylketonuria – PKU), those that arise from adverse exposures while in utero (e.g., birth defects), those that are consequences of shortened gestation and/or abnormal fetal growth, those related to infections, and those stemming from injuries. We have not included most developmental disorders, largely because they typically do not manifest until after the first year of life nor have we included psychological disorders, because of the difficulty of diagnosing them during infancy.

5.1.1.2   Measures

The frequency of infant morbidity may be assessed by prevalence at birth, proportion of affected infants, or proportion of infants experiencing a first episode of a morbidity (Table 5.1). Typically, birth defects are measured by prevalence at birth (3). Birth defects occur early in gestation and many affected fetuses do not survive. Thus, the number of infants with birth defects at delivery is only a portion of all

Table 5.1 Measures of infant morbidity

Measure	Computation	Comment and example
Prevalence rate at birth	$\dfrac{\text{Number of live born infants with the morbidity}}{\text{Total number of live births}}$	Suitable for conditions that arise during gestation
		Example: Rate of spina bifida
Incidence rate during infancy	$\dfrac{\text{Number of infants with the morbidity}}{\text{Total Number of live births}}$	Suitable for conditions that can occur only once
		Example: Retinopathy of prematurity
Incidence rate of first occurrence during infancy	$\dfrac{\text{Infants with first occurrence of the morbidity}}{\text{Total number of live births}}$	Suitable for conditions that can occur more than once
		Example: Rate of motor vehicle-associated injuries

occurrences of birth defects. These affected infants represent prevalent (i.e., existing), rather than incident (i.e., newly occurring) cases.

Some morbidities, including some viral illnesses, can occur only once, because affected individuals develop immunity. In this case, occurrence can be measured accurately by counting the number of infants who have the illness, regardless of when during infancy it occurs. In contrast, other morbidities, notably injuries, may recur. In computing the *rates* of morbidities that can recur, one must count the first occurrences of the illness, not the total number of episodes of illness. (Using the total number of occurrences of illness is fine, however, for computing the *ratio* of morbidity occurrences to the number of infants.) To further refine the available information, one can compute the rate of first occurrences of the morbidity, the rate of second occurrences, and so on. Along with the total number of times that the morbidity occurs, these computations help to show whether the morbidity occurs repeatedly in a small group of infants or usually just once among the overall population of infants.

5.1.1.3 Data Sources

Sources for the study of infant morbidity are similar to those enumerated for maternal morbidity in Chap. 3, and range from vital statistics to service utilization records – including hospital discharge data, emergency room, outpatient care visits, and claims databases such as Medicaid, to data from public health programs. The latter include results from newborn screening for metabolic disorders and inborn errors of metabolism, newborn hearing screening, birth defects surveillance, and communicable disease surveillance. Additional programs that may collect clinical data of relevance to infant morbidity include early intervention, children with special health care needs, blood lead screening, WIC, and child protective services.

Figure 5.1 provides a conceptual framework for data integration to investigate the epidemiology of infant morbidity from a population-based perspective. At the center is the population reference base, typically the database of birth certificates (this database may be enhanced by adding records for infants entering the population after birth but during the first year of life). Although birth certificates contain some information concerning infant health status, these observations relate only to infant characteristics at birth or during the first few days of life at best. However, birth certificates serve as the population reference base and can enable record linkages between administrative, surveillance, or public health services databases.

All of the data sources surrounding the certificates of live birth in Fig. 5.1 contain sufficient personal identifiers to link individual records from health services programs to their birth certificates, if not directly to records on the same infant in the other data sources shown. The examples shown in this diagram include the most commonly analyzed databases as well as several that have been utilized less infrequently by perinatal epidemiologists.

Databases specific to infancy include newborn metabolic screening, newborn hearing screening, neonatal intensive care unit (NICU) discharge data, and to a

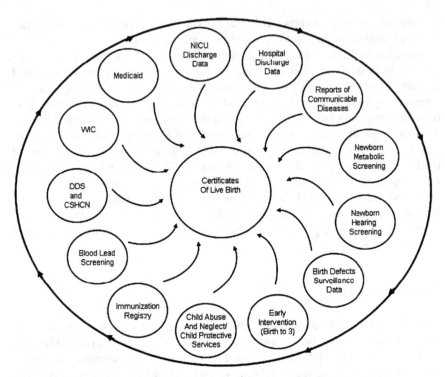

Fig. 5.1 Schematic diagram of population-based and public health data sources useful for study of infant morbidity. *WIC* women, infants and children, *NICU* neonatal intensive care unit, *DDS* developmental disability services, *CSHCN* children with special health care needs

greater extent birth defects surveillance data. Public health programs in all states have been designed to screen all newborns, shortly after birth, for a growing list of disorders (PKU, congenital hypothyroidism, galactosemia, biotinidase deficiency, medium chain acyl CoA dehydrogenase (MCAD) disorder and sickle cell disease, among others) (4–6).

Screening for conditions such as cystic fibrosis has recently been added to state newborn screening panels in most U.S. (7). Most states have implemented mandatory or voluntary programs for early hearing detection and screening to ensure that infants born with congenital hearing loss receive treatment and follow-up to minimize the developmental sequelae of moderate to severe hearing loss (8, 9). Several regions have maintained databases that collect systematic information at discharge from the NICU, which can be linked to birth certificates for risk factor epidemiologic studies and to examine the efficiency of the perinatal health care system (10, 11). Unfortunately these data systems have been difficult to sustain (12); in their place, newer programs such as the Vermont-Oxford Network and the National Institutes of Child Health and Human Development (NICHD) Neonatal Network collect standardized data on NICU diagnoses, treatments, and outcomes from participating hospitals. These data have the limitation of not being population-based (13–15). In contrast many European nations have collaborated in the development of regional measures of the quality of perinatal care services (e.g., 16). Population-based birth defects surveillance programs have been implemented in most states; these data must be linked to birth certificates to provide unduplicated counts of individuals and the resultant linked files can be used for a variety of epidemiologic analyses and health services research studies (17).

Several databases (early intervention – birth to three, immunization, blood lead screening, developmental disabilities services and children with special health care needs, and child abuse and neglect/child protective services) collect information concerning issues affecting infant and child health that have become foci of public health attention, but are not limited to events during the first year of life. Research using these databases often provides information specific to infant morbidity, but the data must be used with caution and attention to detail (e.g., 18–20).

Three databases included in Fig. 5.1 cover the entire age span, but include records of special interest for perinatal epidemiology. Reports of communicable disease must be filed with state epidemiologists whenever physicians diagnose reportable conditions. Many of these conditions (syphilis, pertussis) can have devastating consequences for the infant. However, communicable disease reporting is imperfect, and many perinatal infections are not reportable or are highly under-reported. Hospital discharge databases potentially can identify these cases as well as other infant morbidities requiring hospitalization. This source is described in more detail in Chap. 3. Here we note not only that all infants should have a newborn hospital discharge, but also that when properly designed and implemented subsequent discharges also can be linked for the same infant, and these records can be linked to the infant's birth certificate. Two projects that demonstrate the potential value of these data are the Birth Event Record Database (BERD) maintained by the state of Washington and the Pregnancy and Early Life Longitudinal Study (PELL), at Boston University. Methods for linking vital statistics with hospital discharge records should include scientific analysis of data quality and validation (21, 22).

Medicaid data are another potential source for perinatal epidemiologists. These data can provide information on eligibility for Medicaid services, as well as diagnoses, procedures, and source of care. When linked with birth certificates and other population-based infant health data sources, many aspects of infant morbidity can be studied, both within the Medicaid service population and comparing Medicaid recipients with other infants.

5.1.1.4 Measurement Issues

For most of the data sources described in Fig. 5.1 and discussed in the previous section, programs are maintained at the state level, and obtaining national data is difficult, even for programs that exist in most or all states, such as newborn metabolic screening, newborn hearing screening, and birth defects surveillance. Vital statistics are an exception, most useful as a reference data set for the study of infant morbidities. Other data sources are administrative program databases, which often are not maintained and frequently not designed for use in epidemiologic or evaluation research. While the databases may be population-based, records are frequently duplicated, may or may not match the population of resident live births in the jurisdiction, and can have clerical or coding errors that may prove impossible to correct (23).

Hospital discharge data, when linked to vital statistics and unduplicated or linked across subsequent hospital stays, are a potential source, but only for conditions requiring hospitalization (e.g., intussusception, certain birth defects, or respiratory infections among neonates with lung disease). These data have been underutilized in perinatal epidemiology in the past, but have received considerable attention since the development of the Agency for Healthcare Research and Quality (AHRQ) databases and the creation of linked vital statistics-hospital discharge databases in several states, including California, Massachusetts, Michigan, Missouri, New Jersey, New York, and Washington, among others.

Researchers utilizing Medicaid databases should recognize that these data are not population-based. Medicaid data are often used for health services research, in particular, to measure perinatal outcomes before and after the implementation of policy changes (i.e., presumptive eligibility, Temporary Assistance to Needy Families (TANF), changes in eligibility based on the federal poverty level in specific states). Particularly when linked with birth certificates and other public health program administrative databases, Medicaid data can be a rich source of information concerning infant morbidity and health services utilization (e.g., 24, 25).

Race/ethnicity data have tended to be unreliable when reported in hospital sources, and there is the additional problem of *whose* race to use in classifying and analyzing the data: mother or child. Recent work summarizing these issues and their implications for research in public health include (26) and (27).

Although the fields of public and population health informatics (28–31) are in their infancy, developments in computational methods, data storage and retrieval capacity, and system integration will facilitate the rapid development of child health information systems (32, 33), building on earlier concepts of child health profiles (34) in the coming years. While limited opportunities for systematic population-based study of infant morbidity currently exist, we anticipate rapid advances in both epidemiologic research and application to public health practice.

5.2 Morbidity Associated with Shortened Gestation, Near-Term Intrauterine Growth Restriction, and Sequelae of Prematurity

In this section we focus on infant morbidity associated with preterm birth and intrauterine growth restriction (IUGR) among neonates born moderately preterm or very preterm. While these outcomes are often referred to as *sequelae of prematurity*, some infant diseases and health conditions in the sequelae of prematurity are acquired postnatally rather than perinatally and could be considered a developmental burden in preterm infants compared with their term peers.

5.2.1 Definitions, Measures, Data Sources, and Measurement Issues

5.2.1.1 Definitions

Preterm birth is discussed in considerable detail in Chap. 7. The generally accepted definition is birth at less than 37-weeks gestation, but variants on this definition occasionally occur in the research literature. IUGR (see Chap. 7) is also subject to varying definitions, with the most commonly accepted being birth weight at less than the 10th percentile for gestational age at delivery. The term *small-for-gestational age* is often used synonymously with IUGR. We focus on neurodevelopmental outcomes in infants born preterm and/or IUGR.

5.2.1.2 Measures

While some analyses study patterns of morbidity among preterm and IUGR infants overall, gestational age-specific or birth weight-specific analyses are much more common. Most perinatal sequelae show strong inverse associations with gestational age prior to term. IUGR, on the other hand, is more commonly analyzed as a category, typically comparing small-for-gestational age (SGA, less than 10th percentile of birth weight for given gestational age) with appropriate-for-gestational age (AGA, 10th–90th percentile) and large-for-gestational age (LGA, greater than 90th percentile). Measures utilized are more commonly rate-based rather than incidence-density measures, although the latter are sometimes used in hospital-based research.

5.2.1.3 Data Sources

Many preterm and virtually all very low birth weight or very preterm infants surviving the first 24 h of life receive care in NICUs. Most studies examining the characteristics of infants with NICU stays draw from the experiences of single hospitals or research networks, with limited research examining morbidity during NICU stays or postdischarge from a population-based perspective. Few studies provide a comprehensive overview, focusing instead on specific birth weight or gestational age subgroups, or clinical treatments and outcomes. While population-based studies in US samples are infrequent, numerous studies in the international literature are available. Although birth certificates are limited as a source for data on infant morbidity in general and outcomes for high-risk neonates in particular, these data are essential to population-based research. Hospital discharge summaries also provide information concerning diagnoses and procedures during initial and subsequent inpatient hospitalizations, but these data often fail to provide sufficient clinical details, and long-term outcomes beyond the index hospital stay are not reported.

5.2.1.4   Measurement Issues

The most serious challenge in population-based epidemiologic analysis of sequelae of preterm birth and/or IUGR stems from the difficulty involved in identifying the birth cohort and following all cases systematically through infancy or into early childhood. By no means are all high-risk infants enrolled in infant follow-up programs, and even when they do receive these services, clinical practices and diagnostic criteria differ considerably from program to program. Perinatal sequelae that occur early in infancy, during NICU stays or rehospitalizations, may be more readily identified. However, conditions such as retinopathy of prematurity (ROP) and intraventricular hemorrhage (IVH) vary in severity and ICD-9-CM codes lack the specificity to classify these cases appropriately. Additionally, unless records for preterm or IUGR infants are linked to vital statistics, demographic information concerning the infant's race/ethnicity and maternal characteristics may be incomplete or subject to reporting bias.

International and state-to-state comparisons in incidence of sequelae of prematurity may be hampered by variations in NICU care resulting in greater or lesser rates of mortality. Since many assessments of these morbidities are conducted only on infants surviving the neonatal period, or the NICU stay, regional variations in mortality rates can materially affect these comparisons.

5.2.2   Descriptive Epidemiology

5.2.2.1   Temporal Trends

Since their inception in the 1960s, NICUs have been the focal point for improvements in high-risk infant treatment and management, resulting in dramatic improvements in survival and gradual downward shifts to earlier gestational ages in the limits of neonatal viability. Carter and Stahlman recently reviewed this history from the perspective of clinical ethics (2001).

One recent study examined in-hospital morbidity among less than 25-week gestation infants surviving at least 12 h, comparing those born between 1991 and 1994 with those born between 1995 and 1998, using NICHD neonatal research network data (35). Controlling for use of antenatal steroids, antibiotics, and neonatal surfactant, mortality decreased in the more recent cohort. This decrease occurred concomitantly with increased major morbidity (defined for this study as necrotizing enterocolitis (NEC), IVH grade 3 or 4, periventricular leukomalacia (PVL), or bronchopulmonary dysplasia (BPD)).

Infant morbidity varies with gestational age. Acute and chronic morbidities present in well over half of all extremely preterm neonatal survivors (23–26 weeks) include respiratory distress syndrome (RDS), BPD, and ROP. Less prevalent although very frequently present are neonatal sepsis (early or late) and IVH (grades III or IV), while PVL occurs in approximately 10% of cases and NEC in approximately 5% (36). The prevalence of these conditions, all of which generally manifest during the early stages of extended NICU stays, declines with increasing gestational age. Neurological and developmental sequelae of preterm birth – such as cerebral palsy, cognitive deficits, neurosensory, and gross/fine motor impairment – also are modified to some extent by external factors. These factors include parenting, home environment, early intervention, and community-acquired infections, among others.

Although survival of infants at the lowest birth weights and earliest gestational ages has improved throughout the 1980s and 1990s, rates of cerebral palsy, blindness, deafness, and neurosensory disability have not decreased. For example, a recent study of survivors to age 2 found similar rates among those born in 1991–1992 and 1997 (37). Several meta-analyses examining studies over longer time intervals have made similar observations (38, 39, 40). In general, although mortality has decreased dramatically, especially at shorter gestations, and rates of intact central nervous system (CNS) have increased, the shift of the birth distribution to shorter gestations increases the burden on the perinatal health care system and society.

At the other end of the spectrum of low birth weight infants are those born moderately low birth weight (1,500–2,499 g). While there are at least four times as many of these infants as there are VLBW infants, they receive considerably less public health attention (41, 42). These infants are much less likely to experience NICU stays, yet they account for perhaps 25% of all cases of cerebral palsy as well as a disproportionate share of neonatal deaths and mental retardation.

Infants born preterm are significantly more likely than term infants to require rehospitalization, at higher cost, as are multiple births, which are frequently delivered preterm (43, 44).

5.2.2.2 Geographic Variability

While there are definite differences in patterns of perinatal sequelae in cross-national comparisons, differences observed in the United States are based primarily on analyses using hospital NICUs as the units of analysis, especially with data from the Vermont-Oxford Neonatal Network. Extreme variations have been observed in patterns of ROP, grade III–IV IVH, and related outcomes. These variations have led to implementation of quality improvement and quality monitoring programs (45) that have reduced the hospital variability. Infants born at facilities with NICUs tend to have better outcomes than those born elsewhere and transferred after delivery; access to care and availability of tertiary perinatal services clearly plays some role (46–48). Available data do not support comprehensive regional or state level comparisons within the United States.

5.2.3 Factors That Influence Occurrence and the Availability and Effectiveness of Related Public Health Interventions

5.2.3.1 Interventions

Prevention of infant morbidity among high-risk infants requires the joining of hands between health care delivery systems and public health programs. Although public health agencies no longer have sufficient funds to support long-term multidisciplinary follow-up clinics for high-risk infants, these babies need developmental assessments at regular intervals during the first 2 years of life. These assessments include neurological, intellectual, speech/language, growth and developmental, and psychosocial aspects of the child and the family/home environment. Many of these infants are *at-risk* for or have identified developmental delays. Referrals from NICUs and follow-up programs to publicly funded Birth–to-Three programs and programs for CSHCN can implement care arrangements. Public health agencies can support the development of family-centered NICU services, and aid in the transition from hospital to caregiving in the family home. Developmentally sensitive approaches to nursing care for high-risk infants may play an important role in supporting the abilities of parents to act as primary caregivers. Insufficient evidence presently supports the assertion that individualized developmental care programs such as the Newborn Individualized Developmental Care and Assessment Program (NIDCAP) are effective in improving short-term medical and neurodevelopmental or long-term neurodevelopmental outcomes in preterm or low birth weight infants (49, 50).

Determining which infants are at highest risk for adverse neurodevelopmental outcomes remains elusive. While a number of indices and measures have been developed over the years, beginning with Dr. Virginia Apgar's eponymously named score (51), measures of acuity of the condition of the ill neonate such as the CRIB (clinical risk index for babies) and SNAP (score for neonatal acute physiology) have been generally more effective at predicting mortality or severe central nervous system deficits than for predicting short- or long-term developmental outcomes (52–54). These and other proposed neonatal disease severity scores are summarized in (55).

Infants born preterm, with SGA, or adverse perinatal outcomes are especially vulnerable, and at greatest need for linkages to pediatric health care services through the medical home (56, 57). Special attention can also be paid to preventive health measures, including immunizations, and hearing and vision screening, as well as early intervention and prompt treatment of infections such as otitis media.

Developmental Delay/Disabilities

Pediatricians recognize that infant development is a *moving target* within which developmental and behavioral abilities develop over time. *Normal* development is generally defined by achievement of developmental milestones within specified age ranges (58). Developmental disabilities include neurosensory deficits or impairments (especially vision and hearing), neurological disorders including gross and fine motor development, and physical disabilities that limit intellectual development.

The term *developmental delay* is used in a variety of settings, with different definitions and intentions. In infancy, some use it to refer to neurodevelopmental disabilities, while others use it to identify at-risk infants who test lower on developmental assessments than established norms or control groups (59). Developmental disorders are somewhat less likely to be diagnosed in infancy. Pediatricians prefer not to diagnose mental retardation or cognitive or neurological deficits at young ages, choosing less specific terms wherever possible (e.g., *delayed milestones*). However, routine developmental assessments recommended for all infants at well-child visits, utilizing validated screening instruments and with referral to specialists for more careful assessment would uncover many of these (2). Although developmental disabilities can occur among any group of infants, those born preterm or requiring extended stays in the NICU are at increased risk.

Public health interventions include screening at well-child visits with referrals, the Early Periodic Screening Diagnosis and Treatment (EPSDT) in the Medicaid program, Birth-to-Three early intervention services, CSHCN, developmental disabilities services, and high-risk infant follow-up services. Ideally these services are provided within the context of a pediatric medical home, focused on family-centered, community-based, culturally appropriate care.

5.3   Infection

Infectious diseases were the principal cause of infant morbidity and mortality at the beginning of the twentieth century (60). While their role has been greatly reduced, especially in developed countries, babies continue to die from infectious diseases, and infections may result in permanent disability or impairment. Some infections affect the fetus in utero, particularly when the mother contracts a primary infection at critical stages of fetal growth and development. Fetuses exposed to rubella early in the pregnancy (before the 16th week) may have serious birth defects or result in spontaneous abortion, while those affected later in pregnancy develop ear malformations or hearing impairments – this spectrum of perinatal morbidity has been termed the congenital rubella syndrome (CRS). In many ways this disease process and its sequelae are a paradigm for a clinical and public health approach to primary prevention. Prior to the 1930s, the association of rubella with congenital hearing loss and birth defects was not known. Once it was identified, researchers developed vaccines to immunize children against this formerly common childhood disease, and today women are routinely tested for antibodies to rubella early in their pregnancies, and some health services quality experts regard the occurrence of CRS as a sentinel event indicating vaccine failure, failure of health care access, or poor quality prenatal care (61).

5.3.1 Definitions, Measures, Data Sources, and Measurement Issues

5.3.1.1 Definitions

Infectious diseases affecting infants can be classified in several ways. For example, some have advocated the categorization of infections among infants into endogenous (those arising congenitally or during the perinatal period) and exogenous (those occurring after the first month of life), paralleling the classification of infant deaths into neonatal and postneonatal categories (62). Here we chose to differentiate among congenital infections, acquired in utero or during the perinatal course, other typical infections of infants. This classification is helpful for focusing on the public health implications of infectious disease during infancy.

5.3.1.2 Measures

Measures useful for assessing infections in infancy include incidence and prevalence, as well as co-occurrence with other infant morbidities and specific measures stratified by birth characteristics and other factors. While mortality is not the subject of the present chapter, case fatality rates are also commonly used measures, as well as developmental sequelae secondary to the infectious disease process.

5.3.1.3 Data Sources

While infants are susceptible to a variety of common infections, most of these have a short duration, are managed at home, and have limited effects on growth and development. Thus, most are not reportable, do not require hospitalization, and do not require health services utilization. Many are not captured by our data systems. Here we focus on infections with developmental sequelae, including otitis media, retrosynctial virus (RSV) and related respiratory infections that require health care utilization, and group B streptococcus (GBS), congenital (acquired in utero/ perinatally): e.g., rubella, syphilis, HIV. While some infectious diseases affecting infants are reportable communicable diseases (e.g., congenital syphilis), despite their potentially serious effects and sequelae most are not directly under public health surveillance. Data on specific organisms affecting infants hospitalized in the NICU can be obtained from the Vermont-Oxford Network, and some data on infections occurring in hospitals can be obtained from the National Nosocomial Infection Surveillance System maintained by the Centers for Disease Control and Prevention (http://www.cdc.gov/ncidod/dhqp/nnis.html). Data on infections occurring during infant hospitalizations that warrant diagnosis and treatment can be obtained from hospital discharge databases as well. Data on infant infectious disease diagnosed and treated outside hospital settings are much more difficult to obtain.

5.3.1.4 Measurement Issues

Because most of these infections are not carefully monitored on a population basis, available data may be subject to significant reporting bias and incomplete or selective ascertainment, rendering comparisons across geographic areas or over time difficult to interpret.

5.3.2 Descriptive Epidemiology

Pathogens capable of infecting the placenta and damaging the development of the fetus have traditionally been classed as toxoplasmosis, other pathogens (including varicella and parvovirus), rubella, cytomegalovirus (CMV), and herpes simplex under the mnemonic TORCH infections. These infections, particularly CMV, are important causes of sensorineural impairment in infants and children worldwide, and continue to play a role in infant morbidity in the United States (63).

Acquired CMV infections typically produce no recognizable symptoms in healthy infants. Even among CMV-infected neonates, most show no symptoms at birth. Some 10% of affected newborns do show systemic signs, ranging from jaundice, hepato- or splenomegaly, petechiae, IUGR, or RDS to microcephaly, seizures, sensorineural hearing loss, and abnormal tone. Approximately 5% of infants who are symptomatic may die (64). Neonates with silent CMV infections have no neurodevelopmental sequelae, but some may later develop sensorineural hearing loss. According to one estimate, annually approximately 9,000 infants in the United States have either audiologic or neurologic deficits as a result of congenital CMV infection (65, 66).

There are two primary opportunities for prevention of congenital CMV exposure. CMV vaccines are progressing through clinical trials, and may reduce exposure to some extent; however, it is possible for seropositive women to become reinfected with new CMV strains, suggesting that vaccines may be of limited efficacy for prevention of transmission from mother via placenta to the developing fetus. Avoidance of direct contact with urine and saliva of young children during pregnancy, with immediate hand washing with soap and water in the event of exposure, is an important precautionary measure.

Toxoplasma gondii infection, caused by a protozoan, can cause central nervous system damage with primary exposure during pregnancy. Infected cats are the primary host, although *T. gondii* can be found in undercooked meats and in some fruits and vegetables contaminated with the oocyst form of the *T. gondii* organism. In the US, perhaps 15% of women of reproductive age show evidence of prior infection. Estimates of rates of congenital infection in the US are in the range of 0.8–10/10,000 live births. This suggests that perhaps 400–4,000 infants are born with congenital toxoplasmosis in this country each year (63). Infants with congenital toxoplasmosis may present with neonatal clinical features similar to congenital CMV, including microcephaly, IUGR, hydrocephaly, jaundice, and chorioretinitis toxoplasmosis or with no clinical symptoms at birth. The best clinical practice is to establish the seropositivity of the mother early in pregnancy, and treat with antibiotics those who seroconvert within 4 weeks of the diagnosis of intrauterine exposure (63). Infants with proven congenital toxoplasmosis treated have lower risk for epilepsy, cerebral palsy, visual impairment, and mental retardation.

While as many as 2% of pregnant women become infected with herpes simplex virus (HSV) during pregnancy, most infections do not result in disease in the fetus or newborn. Fetuses exposed to genital infections near the time of delivery are more likely to have neonatal disease. Cesarean sections have been advocated to avoid neonatal exposure to herpes in the birth canal.

CRS is caused by maternal rubella (German measles) infection. Severity of outcomes is associated with timing of infection – exposures in the first 8 weeks of gestation can result in congenital heart defects and cataracts, and hearing loss. CRS can also cause stillbirth or spontaneous abortion. Maternal infections after 16 weeks of gestation may result in sensorineural hearing loss (63). Since 1969 and the introduction of the rubella vaccine, incidence of CRS in the United States has declined dramatically to rates of less than 0.1 per 100,000 live births. Most cases today occur among infants of immigrants from countries that have not implemented compulsory immunization; however, epidemiologists should carefully monitor the incidence of CRS as a sentinel event for vaccine-preventable neurodevelopmental sequelae.

Similarly, congenital syphilis is caused by untreated maternal syphilis infections during pregnancy. Perhaps as many as one million infants worldwide are born with congenital syphilis each year (67). Although the incidence of congenital syphilis was much higher in the late 1980s and early 1990s, in recent years fewer than 600 cases have been reported annually in the United States (CDC 2004). Laws concerning the testing and reporting of prenatal syphilis infection vary by state (68). Most reported cases are untreated or have inadequate or undocumented treatment, and occur much more commonly among Black non-Hispanic and Hispanic women. From 1992 to 1998, the case-fatality rate for congenital syphilis was 6.4%, with approximately 60% of cases reported as stillbirths (69).

Group B streptococci (GBS) emerged as a leading cause of neonatal infection in the United States since 1970. Perhaps 20–30% of all pregnant women are carriers of

GBS, and GBS colonization rates are higher among African-American than among White or Asian women (70). Maternal GBS infection can manifest as urinary tract infection, chorioamnionitis, bacteremia, and postpartum endometritis. In the neonate, early-onset disease is defined as onset in the first week of life, and most typically is seen within 72 h of birth. Early onset GBS infections, typically transmitted from mother to infant can cause sepsis, meningitis, and pneumonia, among others. Late-onset disease first manifests after 7 days of life, and can result in similar symptoms but may have different sources. Improved screening of mothers and clinical management techniques have dramatically reduced the incidence of early-onset neonatal GBS (71). Overall incidence of early-onset disease was 0.4 cases per 1,000 live births during 2002 (71). Case fatality rates have fallen below 5%, but mortality increases with decreasing gestational age (72).

Neonatal nosocomial infections also fall under the rubric of perinatally acquired infections. Bloodstream infections are the most common site recognized among NICU patients, with higher incidence with decreasing birth weight (73, 74). These infections were most commonly associated with umbilical or central intravenous catheters. Most bloodstream infections were acquired after birth, as were the large majority of nosocomial pneumonias and reflect the length of time in intensive care. NEC affects preterm infants (75). Some nosocomial outbreaks have occurred (76), pathogens vary, and in several outbreaks no significant pathogen could be identified.

Respiratory infections are extremely common in infants. Most are of little consequence in otherwise healthy infants. Approximately one in five infants may have RSV-associated wheezing during the first year of life (77). An analysis of National Hospital Discharge Survey (NHDS) data for 1997–2000 identified bronchiolitis due to RSV, unspecified bronchiolitis, and unspecified pneumonia as the top three primary diagnoses among hospitalized infants under the age of 1 in the United States. When both primary and secondary diagnoses of RSV are included, 24.3 hospitalizations for RSV per 1,000 infants occurred (78). Most infants hospitalized for bronchiolitis or RSV pneumonia have complications, with serious complications in 24% of cases in one multicenter study (79). Available data thus suggest that RSV leads to hospitalization of 2–3% of otherwise healthy infants hospitalized per year. Incidence of RSV is higher in the first 6 months of life (4.4 per 100 child-years compared with 1.5 in the second 6 months). Severity of RSV infection is much higher among preterm infants and those with congenital heart disease or BPD (77, 80).

Pertussis is a respiratory illness caused by *Bordetella pertussis*, with a paroxysmal cough that may last several weeks. Prior to the 1940s when a pertussis vaccine became commonly available, later combined with vaccines for diphtheria and tetanus into the diptheria–tetanus–pertussis (DTP) vaccine, pertussis was a major cause of morbidity and mortality in infants and young children in the United States. Reported cases of pertussis among infants still occur and the incidence appears to be rising (81). Infants with fewer than recommended doses of DTP vaccine were at greater risk of pertussis-associated hospitalization. Newer vaccine strategies may target infant caretakers.

Otitis media is a very common infection that may accompany respiratory infection. An analysis of National Health and Nutrition Examination Survey (NHANES) data for 1988–1994 estimated the prevalence of otitis media among infants in the United States at 34.1%, with 8.2% of infants having recurrence of otitis media (110). The prevalence among children under age 6 was higher among White children (also confirmed by Vernacchio et al. (83) in a study focusing on infants), increased with increasing education level of the head of household, among children attending child care, and with family income above the federal poverty level.

Diarrheal illnesses of infancy were once a leading cause of mortality in developed countries and remain an important cause of morbidity. Diarrhea is influenced by feeding practices, almost unknown in breastfed infants without supplementary feedings. Among infants, incidence of diarrheal illness rises with supplemental feeds, particularly where sanitary conditions are not good. Common reported pathogens causing infectious diarrhea include rotavirus, enteric adenovirus, salmonella, camplyobacter, yersinia, and giardia. Diarrhea in the newborn is more likely the result of a systemic infection or urinary tract infection than infectious diarrhea (84).

Salmonellosis resulted in 120.8 reported cases, and 25.0 hospitalizations per 100,000 person-years among infants in California during the 1990s, with gastroenteritis the most common site of infection (85). Data from the FoodNet study area, comprised of several states and metropolitan areas in the United States, show higher incidence of invasive Salmonella infections among male infants and among Black infants (86). Approximately 25% of infants with Salmonella infections were hospitalized, with a case-fatality rate of 0.1% (87).

A review of the world literature suggests that exclusive breastfeeding provides a protective effect against diarrhea or gastroenteritis, with odds ratios of 3.0 or more compared with infants fed non-breast milk (88). This observation was confirmed in a case-control study of sporadic Salmonellosis derived from the FoodNet surveillance data (89).

Intussusception, the most common cause of intestinal obstruction in infants and young children, gained attention with the introduction of the rotavirus vaccine in 1999 (90). While the etiology is unknown and possibly multifactorial, some children have anatomical predisposition (e.g., everted Meckel's diverticulum) and pathogens such as respiratory adenoviruses may be involved (91). Intussusception-associated hospitalization rates in infancy are 1.2–1.7 times higher among males, but do not appear to differ among white and black infants while infants of other races have higher incidence (91).

5.3.2.1 Temporal Trends and Geographic Variability

While there is evidence for declining patterns of specific infectious diseases in infancy following development and widespread implementation of vaccines (e.g., *Haemophilus influenzae*) available data in the United States are insufficient to enable careful consideration of geographic or temporal variation in the incidence of specific diseases affecting infants.

5.3.3 Factors That Influence Occurrence and the Availability and Effectiveness of Related Public Health Interventions

5.3.3.1 Interventions

Public health interventions to prevent infections in infancy focus on primary prevention with vaccines, good hygiene, breastfeeding, and avoidance of opportunities for exposure. Invasive pneumococcal disease could be dramatically reduced, including many infections causing otitis media, with widespread use of the heptavalent pneumococcal conjugate vaccine. Vaccines have also been developed and are in a testing phase for *Neisseria meningitides* and rotavirus (92). For RSV, while there is hope for an eventual vaccine, avoidance of day care, crowding, and effective hand washing are good precautionary measures. While vaccines for rubella are available, maternal seropositivity for each of the infectious agents in the TORCH mnemonic should be assessed early in pregnancy, and precautionary measures should be taken as indicated. Avoidance of environmental tobacco smoke exposure for infants will reduce the likelihood of respiratory disease as well as acute and chronic otitis media, and environmental tobacco smoke has also been associated with developmental delay.

Oral rehydration therapy has proven especially effective in preventing infant and child mortality associated with diarrheal diseases. While life-threatening cases of severe dehydration are infrequent in the United States, this therapy saves thousands of lives each year in developing nations.

5.4 Birth Defects

Birth defects occur in 3–5% of all live births, with higher frequencies at earlier gestations, among stillbirths, and among spontaneous pregnancy losses (93). Birth defects are a leading cause of infant mortality, and contribute to deaths in early childhood (94, 95). Birth defects also contribute disproportionately to infant morbidity and health services utilization. Next to cancers, birth defects are the most common source of public concerns for community-level environmental exposures. In this section, we will review common definitions, methods for identification of pregnancies and infants affected by birth defects, risk factors and etiology for common birth defects, and opportunities for public health intervention.

5.4.1 Definitions, Measures, Data Sources, and Measurement Issues

5.4.1.1 Definitions

Birth defects include "abnormalities of structure or function, including metabolism, which are present from birth. Serious birth defects are life threatening or have the potential to disability (physical, intellectual, visual or hearing impairment or epilepsy)" (96). Structural or functional anomalies include malformations, deformations, disruptions of normal embryonic/fetal growth, and development.

5.4.1.2 Measures

Identification of fetuses affected by birth defects often occurs antenatally, but the full extent and severity may not be known until after delivery. Improvements in laboratory methods, screening techniques, and imaging technology have increased the range of birth defects that can be diagnosed in utero, including anueploidy (especially Down syndrome – Trisomy 21, Trisomy 18, Trisomy 13), other chromosomal abnormalities, central nervous system defects, ventral wall defects (including gastroschisis and omphalocele), facial clefts, limb reduction defects, and congenital heart defects and other conditions affecting major organ systems. However, many birth defects go undetected until well after birth, with some congenital heart defects diagnosed only in adolescence or even adulthood. Surveillance and measurement of birth defects are complicated by the perception that existing public health data systems (vital statistics, hospital discharge summaries, program data for early intervention services, and children with special health care needs) are sufficient to provide comprehensive population-based data. Studies of the reliability and validity of these sources demonstrate that birth and death certificates have extremely poor sensitivity and unacceptable positive predictive value, with limited diagnostic specificity (97); while hospital discharge data fare somewhat better this source misses significant numbers of cases diagnosed outside the context of inpatient hospital stays (98). In most states, public health program data from programs that provide services to children with special health care needs or for early intervention are incomplete because some families do not utilize these services or because public funding is inadequate to make these services available to all eligible children.

Independent, focused programs for birth defects surveillance are necessary for adequate monitoring, surveillance, and descriptive epidemiologic analysis of trends in the prevalence of specific conditions, syndromes, and their outcomes. In the United States, population-based programs have been established in most states since the creation of the model surveillance program in the metropolitan Atlanta area in the late 1960s (99). Guidelines for the implementation and operation of birth defects surveillance programs in the United States have recently been published (108).

Birth prevalence is the preferred measure for assessing the relative frequency of specific birth defects (3); these measures are typically calculated after including all confirmed cases whether diagnosed prenatally, identified at birth or reported in infancy in the numerator, using the total number of live births as the denominator. Case fatality rates for specific birth defects can be calculated following linkage to infant or child death certificate data (100).

5.4.1.3   Data Sources

Birth defects registries typically utilize multisource data acquisition strategies to identify cases for inclusion in their databases. The preferred methodology involves active case-finding with records reviewed and abstracted at clinical sites by trained staff (see 92 for more detailed discussion of public health surveillance methods; (17, 102) Some programs utilize passive case-finding, requiring health facilities or providers to file case reports when birth defects diagnoses are made. When conducted with diligence, these programs yield prevalence rates that are comparable to those from active case-finding and appear valid for use in descriptive epidemiology and case-control studies. Programs that accept all case reports, while failing to interact with providers to improve reporting compliance or to review the accuracy of reported information, have results that are less than valid for epidemiologic research or to support public health programmatic activities. Some databases are populated through automated record linkage methods, without any birth defects diagnoses reported specifically to the registry; this case-ascertainment methodology has been termed *impassive* case-finding (103).

While most birth defects are not life-threatening, birth defects are a leading cause of infant and child mortality. Most birth defects surveillance programs link their records to birth and infant death certificates, providing the necessary database for analysis of both case fatality rates and the contribution of birth defects to infant mortality. Many birth defects lead to disabilities and limitations of daily activity (104–106); however, population-based surveillance of developmental disabilities in the United States is quite limited.

5.4.1.4   Measurement Issues

In the United States, although birth defects surveillance programs exist in approximately 40 states (107), numerous variations in methodology create complexities for the calculation of national estimates of the prevalence of birth defects. Some researchers prefer to focus on the prevalence of specific birth defects, rather than the overall prevalence, due to the heterogeneity of etiologies involved. Infants with a specific birth defect may have an isolated condition, or several birth defects that may be associated manifestations of a genetic disease, sequence, or syndrome. While there are some notable examples of specific exposures associated with particular syndromes or patterns of birth defects manifestations (e.g., fetal alcohol syndrome, thalidomide embryopathy), most birth defects probably result from complex gene–environment interactions, even among disorders primarily genetic in origin.

5.4.2   Descriptive Epidemiology

5.4.2.1   Temporal Trends

Because population-based birth defects surveillance is largely a late twentieth century phenomenon, limited data on which to base analyses of long-term secular trends are available. Data on secular trends are regularly published by the International Clearinghouse for Birth Defects Surveillance and Research (108), and analyses of data from metropolitan Atlanta demonstrate declining trends for neural tube defects (109), while gastroschisis appears to be increasing in prevalence in the United States and elsewhere (110).

5.4.2.2 Geographic Variability

Because of differences in surveillance methods, comparisons across US states may result in invalid inferences concerning specific defects. A recent study identified 11 states with similar methods, and calculated national prevalence estimates from these data (111). Even within this limited group of states, the range of reported prevalence varied by an order of magnitude or more for some birth defects, suggesting that differences in diagnosis, documentation, or surveillance methods may remain even after carefully selecting states with the most similar case ascertainment methods.

5.4.2.3 Demographic Variability

Racial/Ethnic Variation: Overall rates of birth defects in the United States are similar among White non-Hispanic and Black non-Hispanic infants, and lower among infants born to Asian mothers. Hispanic infants have higher prevalence of selected birth defects, with prevalence similar to that for White non-Hispanics for many others, as demonstrated in two multistate collaborative studies (112, 113).

Maternal/Paternal Age: Although some birth defects increase in prevalence with increasing age of mother, e.g., chromosomal abnormalities, especially Down syndrome (114), others have higher prevalence among younger mothers, e.g., gastroschisis (110, 115, 116). Paternal age effects have been less well studied, but research does suggest that older paternal age influences the risk for chromosomal abnormalities independent of maternal age (117).

Multiple Births: Infants born of multiple gestation pregnancies have higher prevalence of birth defects than do singleton infants (118). Multiple gestations are frequently discordant for specific birth defects. Most population-based data sources do not explicitly measure zygosity, chorionicity, or amnionicity of each set of multiple births. There is a need for perinatally ascertained multiple birth registers (119), through which these important characteristics of multiple gestations would be documented prospectively.

5.4.3 Factors That Influence Occurrence and the Availability and Effectiveness of Related Public Health Interventions

5.4.3.1 Risk and Protective Factors

The epidemiologic research literature on maternal, environmental, and behavioral risk and protective factors for birth defects is voluminous. Readers interested in risk factors for specific birth defects will find numerous condition-specific monographs as well as review papers in the periodical literature. Here we note only a few observations. Increasing birth order is associated with some birth defects, including oral clefts and spina bifida (120, 121). Maternal weight and stature appears to play some role in birth defect causation (122). High pregravid body mass index (BMI) (obesity) has been implicated as a risk factor for neural tube defects, possibly other birth defects (e.g., 123, 124). Hyperthermia, whether caused by fever or thermal exposure (hot tub use) shows an approximately twofold increased risk for neural tube defects in a recent systematic review (125). Many other hypotheses concerning diet, use of over-the-counter medications, electric blankets, proximity of maternal residence to sources of environmental exposure, to name only a few, have been examined. Interested readers should consult textbooks on specific birth defects (i.e., 126, 127), as well as the PubMed database of health research publications.

5.4.3.2 Interventions

Primary prevention of birth defects involves preconception care for women with chronic health conditions that may affect embryologic or fetal development as well as avoidance of risky behaviors and reduction of exposure to known teratogens including prescription drugs. Opportunities for preventive interventions include, but are not limited to, folic acid, maternal PKU, avoidance of alcohol consumption, genetic disorders associated with specific populations (i.e., Tay-Sachs), management of maternal diabetes, epilepsy, heart disease, and autoimmune disorders (i.e., lupus). Women considering pregnancy should reduce exposure to known drug teratogens (e.g., thalidomide, accutane, antiepileptic medications); this topic is comprehensively reviewed in (128).

For secondary prevention, infants with specific birth defects should be referred to comprehensive treatment and follow-up clinics for their condition (e.g., spina bifida, Down syndrome, PKU, craniofacial anomalies), and linked with Birth-to-Three, DD services, CSHCN programs, and educational interventions. Families with previously affected pregnancies should be offered genetics counseling and linked to preconception care services.

For primary prevention, preconceptional care, perinatal risk assessment in subsequent pregnancies, and avoidance of medications and known teratogens during preconception and pregnancy are recommended. For women with a previous history of neural tube defect-affected pregnancy, 4 mg per day of folic acid supplementation periconceptionally is recommended, with follow-up and preconceptional care.

5.5   Infant Morbidity Due to Injuries

5.5.1   Definition, Measures, and Measurement Issues

5.5.1.1   Definition

An injury is defined generally as a wound, hurt, or harm to the structure or function of the body. Injuries are often categorized into two groups by their intentionality: unintentional and intentional. Violence is defined by the CDC as "intentional use of physical force or power against oneself, another person, or against a group or community" (129). Causes differ for fatal and nonfatal infant injuries (130).

5.5.1.2   Measures

The occurrence of nonfatal injuries is measured often by medical visits for an injury during the first year of life per 1,000 or 10,000 infants at risk. Medical visits include visits to a doctor's office or a hospital emergency department. Much less frequently, occurrence is measured by surveying parents and asking them to report information about injuries that occurred to their infants.

Why Should We Care About Nonfatal Injuries in Infants?

Nonfatal injuries are not rare and are much more common than fatal injuries (130). Nonfatal injuries are associated with substantial costs for immediate treatment and for rehabilitative care during childhood (131).

5.5.1.3   Data Sources

Several federal surveys provide information about the occurrence of injuries. Some of these surveys are listed in Table 5.2.

5.5.1.4   Measurement Issues

The rate of medical visits for injuries does not permit one to know the percentage of infants who had one or more injuries during their first year of life. This occurs because an infant can have multiple medical visits for different injuries. Not all injuries result in a visit for medical care.

Table 5.2 Selected systems providing data about the national occurrence of nonfatal injuries in infants

Type of injury	Name of system	Sponsor of system
All	National Health Interview Survey	Federal government
	Injury Control & Risk of Injury Survey	Federal government
	National Ambulatory Medical Care Survey	Federal government
	National Hospital Ambulatory Medical Care Survey	Federal government
	National Hospital Discharge Survey	Federal government
	Medical Expenditure Panel Survey	Federal government
	National EMS Information System	Multiple sponsors
Cause-specific	National Electronic Injury Surveillance System	Federal government
	National Automotive Sampling System – General Estimates System	Federal government
	National Child Abuse and Neglect Data System	Federal government
	National Incidence Study of Child Abuse and Neglect	Federal Government
	National Fire Incident Reporting System	Federal Government
	National Trauma Data Bank	American College of Surgeons
	Toxic Exposure Surveillance System	American Association of Poisoning Control Centers
	United States Eye Injury Registry	American Society of Ocular Trauma

Source: CDC. http://www.cdc.gov/ncipc/osp/InventoryInjuryDataSys.htm (accessed November 10, 2007).

5.5.2 Descriptive Epidemiology

5.5.2.1 Occurrence and Trends

In 2006, infants accounted for 244,444 visits to hospital emergency departments for nonfatal injuries. Nearly all (98%) of these visits were for unintentional injuries. These visits occurred at a rate of 5.9 visits per 100 infants. From 2001 through 2006, the rate of visits to hospital emergency departments for nonfatal injuries ranged from a low of 5.8 per 100 infants (2005) to a high of 6.3 per 100 infants (2002) (http://www.cdc.gov/ncipc/wisqars/nonfatal/datasources.htm. Accessed November 11, 2007). Table 5.3 shows the ten leading causes of nonfatal injuries among infants in the United States in 2006. Falls were the most frequently occurring injury.

5.5.2.2 Geographic Variability

CDC's Web-based Injury Statistics Query and Reporting System provides data on fatal and nonfatal injuries. Mortality data, however, may shed the best light

Table 5.3 Ten leading causes of nonfatal injuries among infants in the United States in 2006

Cause	Visits to hospital emergency departments
Unintentional fall	124,747
Unintentional struck by/against	30,872
Unintentional other bite/sting	12,456
Unintentional foreign body	10.903
Unintentional fire/burn	10,378
Unintentional other specified	7,965
Unintentional overexertion	7,531
Unintentional motor vehicle occupant	6,885
Unintentional poisoning	6.877
Unintentional cut/pierce	6,479

Source: http://www.cdc.gov/ncipc/wisqars/nonfatal/datasources.htm (accessed November 11, 2007).

on regional differences. Examination of race-specific postneonatal mortality rates due to injuries in the United States for 1988 and 1998 showed the highest rates in Midwest for Black postneonates (77.8 per 100,000 in 1988; 86.6 per 100,000 in 1998) and in the South for Whites (27.8; 25.6). The lowest rates occurred in the Northeast for Blacks (39.3; 33.3) and Whites (16.4; 11.8) (132).

5.5.2.3 International Comparisons

The World Health Organization (WHO) reported for children aged 0–4 years, injuries were the twelfth (falls) and thirteenth (drowning) leading causes of the global burden of disease for both sexes in 2000 (133).

5.5.2.4 Demographic Variability

For 2006, the rate of visits by infants to hospital emergency departments for nonfatal injuries was higher overall among males compared with that among females. This pattern was true for non-Hispanic White as well as Hispanic infants, but not for Black infants (http://www.cdc.gov/ncipc/wisqars/nonfatal/datasources. htm. Accessed November 11, 2007). From 2001–2006, the rate of visits to hospital emergency departments for nonfatal injuries was consistently the highest for Black infants. White infants had the next highest rate and Hispanic infants the lowest rate. For example, in 2006 the rate of visits to hospital emergency departments for nonfatal injuries was 5.5 per 100 Black infants, followed by 4.4 for non-Hispanic White infants and 3.4 for Hispanic infants.

Studies from Canada reported an inverse relationship between the risk of nonfatal childhood and socioeconomic status. Children from lower socioeconomic useholds had higher rates of injuries than their peers with higher socioeconomic

Table 5.4 Cause-specific rates of hospitalization or death per 100,000 infants, by age, California, 1996–1998 (*source:* (138))

Cause	Age (months)			
	0–2	3–5	6–8	9–11
Fall	92	80	114	101
Poisoning	35	18	23	64
Transportation	20	23	22	21
Foreign Body	33	15	45	84
Burn/fire	15	14	32	50
Assault and neglect	76	62	36	22
Submersion/drowning	–	4	17	26
All injuries	337	262	333	423

status (134, 135). A similar relationship was observed for Dutch young children (136). This pattern was not found in Sweden, however, where little variation in injury rates by socioeconomic status was observed for children aged 0–4 years (137).

Dutch children living in rural areas as well as those with three or more siblings had a higher risk for injuries (136).

Data for infants in California during 1996, 1997, and 1998 showed the age- and cause-specific rates of hospitalization or death displayed in Table 5.4 (138). Overall, falls account for the highest injury rate. Cause-specific rates vary by age during injury. For example, the highest rates for abuse and neglect occur during the infant's first 0–5 months of life. Another report has shown that the highest risk for homicide before age 17 years occurs during the first 4 months of life (139).

5.5.3 *Factors Influencing Occurrence and the Availability and Use of Public Health Interventions*

Factors influencing occurrence: unintentional injuries. Pickett et al. observed that "infant injuries...all involve unplanned contact between a physical or other force and an unprotected child" (140). Inadequate parental supervision has been often identified as an important contributor to unintentional injuries (141). A recent study from Brazil identified low maternal involvement with or responsiveness as risk factor for unintentional injuries to her infant (142).

Factors influencing occurrence: intentional injuries. Parents who themselves experienced abuse as children have increased risk for abusing their infants (143). Poverty, family disorganization, and parental stress have also been identified as risk factors. One study reported that children living in households with adults who were not biologically related to them had an increased risk for fatal injuries (144).

Public health interventions: unintentional injuries. Pickett et al. state that "...given that it is more difficult to modify circumstances and adult behaviors, prevention efforts should be focused on environmental modifications., [i.e.,] placing limits on infant mobility through the use of passive safety devices, and similarly

limiting contact between physical hazards and children via other forms of environmental vigilance" (140). Child safety seats are an excellent example of a safety
device. Currently, 50 states mandate use of infant safety seats. Parental education
about the proper use of seats and stricter enforcement of state laws are important
public health interventions to prevent infant morbidity and mortality due to motor
vehicle crashes (145). Parental training on the importance of providing adequate
supervision and home visiting aimed at supporting parental supervision offer the
promise of preventing injuries. Neither the efficacy nor cost-effectiveness of these
strategies has been evaluated.

> *Shaken Baby Syndrome*
>
> Shaken Baby Syndrome occurs when a baby is violently shaken by the baby's
> parent or caregiver (146). The abuse may cause intracranial injury, retinal
> hemorrhage, or long bone fractures (146). An effective intervention provided
> education to parents of newborns concerning the dangers of violent shaking
> and alternative strategies for persistent infant crying (147).

Public Health Interventions: *Intentional Injuries*: Few prevention interventions
have been assessed adequately (148). The interventions that investigators currently
are evaluating include parenting programs and home visiting – especially for
parents with substance abuse problems, mental illness, disabilities, or histories of
intimate partner violence (145).

5.6   Conclusion

While infant mortality has been a primary focus for research and prevention
activities in the US and internationally, diseases and health conditions affecting
infants in the first year of life contribute to the population disease burden. Opportunities for primary prevention exist for some birth defects, injuries, and infectious
diseases, and preventive interventions can improve outcomes for many infants
affected by sequelae of prematurity and less than optimal growth and development.
Primary and secondary prevention of infant morbidity will require collaborative
strategies involving both primary care providers and public health agencies working together on the local level to implement best practices identified through
research and developed through state/national public policies.

Abbreviations

BPD	bronchopulmonary dysplasia
CDC	Centers for Disease Control and Prevention
CMV	cytomegalovirus

CRS   congenital rubella syndrome
CSHCN   Children with Special Health Care Needs
DTP   diphtheria-tetanus-pertussis
GBS   Group B Streptococcus
IUGR   intrauterine growth restriction
IVH   intraventricular hemorrhage
NEC   necrotizing enterocolitis
PKU   phenylketonuria
PVL   periventricular leukomalacia
ROP   retinopathy of prematurity
RSV   retrosynctial virus
SGA   small-for-gestational age
NICU   neonatal intensive care unit
WIC   Special Supplemental Food Program for Women, Infants
             and Children

Discussion Topics

1. Why is prevalence the preferred measure for examining the frequency of birth defects among deliveries?
2. From a population perspective, how should *high-risk infant* be defined? What data resources are needed to study high-risk infant health outcomes?
3. How might studies focusing on environmental exposures associated with infant morbidity best be designed?

Promising Areas for Future Research

1. Development of methods for population-based assessment of infectious disease affecting infants, both congenital and community-acquired.
2. Are infants with adverse reproductive outcomes at greater risk for injury during the first year of life?

References

1. Rajkumar SV. Thalidomide: tragic past and promising future *Mayo Clin Proc*. 2004;79:899–903.
2. Hagen HF Jr, Shaw JS, Duncan P, Eds. *Bright Futures: Guidelines for Health Supervision of Infants, Children, and Adolescents* – 3rd Ed. Elk Grove Village, IL: American Academy of Pediatrics, 2007.

3. Mason CA, Kirby RS, Sever LE, Langlois PH. Prevalence is the preferred measure of frequency of birth defects. *Birth Defects Res A Clin Mol Teratol* 2005;73:690–692.
4. Khoury MJ, McCabe LL, McCabe ERB. Population screening in the age of genomic medicine. *N Engl J Med* 2003;348:50–58.
5. McCabe LL, McCabe ERB. Minireview: newborn screening as a model for population screening. *Mol Genet Metab* 2002;75:299–307.
6. Newborn Screening Task Force. Serving the family from birth to the medical home. Newborn screening: a blueprint for the future – a call for a national agenda on newborn screening programs. *Pediatrics* 2000;106S:386–427.
7. Castellani C. Evidence for newborn screening for cystic fibrosis. *Paediatr Resp Rev* 2003;4:278–284.
8. Prince CB, Miyashiro L, Weirather Y, Heu P. Epidemiology of early hearing loss detection in Hawaii. *Pediatrics* 2003;111:1202–1206.
9. White KB. The current status of EHDI programs in the United States. *Ment Retard Dev Disabil Res Rev* 2003;8:79–88.
10. Kirby RS. Perinatal Regionalization in Wisconsin. Unpublished M.S. thesis. Madison, WI: Department of Preventive Medicine, University of Wisconsin-Madison, 1991.
11. Synnes AR, Berry M, Jones H, Pendray M, Stewart S, Lee SK. Infants with congenital anomalies admitted to neonatal intensive care units. *Am J Perinatol* 2004;21:199–207.
12. Kirby RS. From public health to population health: epidemiologic yardsticks for perinatal care. *J Perinatol* 1999;19:S16–S20.
13. Fanaroff AA, Hack M, Walsh MC. The NICHD neonatal research network: changes in practice and outcomes during the first 15 years. *Semin Perinatol* 2003;27:281–287.
14. Horbar JD. The Vermont-Oxford Neonatal Network: integrating research and clinical practice to improve to quality of medical care. *Semin Perinatol* 1995;19:124–131.
15. Wright LL, McNellis D. National Institute of Child Health and Human Development (NICHD)-sponsored perinatal research networks. *Semin Perinatol* 1995;19:112–123.
16. Lindmark G, Langhoff-Roos J. Regional quality assessment in perinatal care. *Semin Neonatol* 2004;9:145–153.
17. National Birth Defects Prevention Network (NBDPN). State Birth Defects Surveillance Program Directory. *Birth Defects Res A Clin Mol Teratol* 2007;79:815–873.
18. Freeman VA, DeFriese GH. The challenge and potential of childhood immunization registries. *Annu Rev Public Health* 2003;24:227–246.
19. Gessner BD, Moore M, Hamilton B, Muth PT. The incidence of infant physical abuse in Alaska. *Child Abuse Neglect* 2004;28:9–13.
20. Papadouka V, Schaeffer P, Metroka A, Borthwick A, Tehranifar P, Leighton J, Aponte A, Liao R, Ternier A, Friedman S, Arzt N. Integrating the New York citywide immunization registry and the childhood blood lead registry. *J Public Health Manage Pract* 2004;10:S72–S80.
21. Herrchen B, Gould JB, Nesbitt TS. Vital statistics linked birth/infant death and hospital discharge record linkage for epidemiological studies. *Comput Biomed Res* 1997;30:290–305.
22. Zingmond DS, Ye Z, Ettner SL, Liu H. Linking hospital discharge and death records – accuracy and sources of bias. *J Clin Epidemiol* 2004;57:21–29.
23. Iezzoni LI. Assessing quality using administrative data. *Ann Intern Med* 1997;127:666–674.
24. Gyllstrom ME, Jensen JL, Vaughan JN, Castellano SE, Oswald JW. Linking birth certificates with Medicaid data to enhance population health assessment: methodological issues addressed. *J Public Health Manage Pract* 2002;8:38–44.
25. Marshall LM, Howard RN, Sullivan A, Hgo DL, Woodward JA, Kohn MA. Public health surveillance approaches in Oregon's Medicaid population. *J Public Health Manage Pract* 2002;8,4:63–69.
26. Mays VM, Ponce NA, Washington DL, Cochran SD. Classification of race and ethnicity: implications for public health. *Annu Rev Public Health* 2003;24:83–110.

27. Chen W, Pettiti DB, Enger S. Limitations of potential uses of Census-based data on ethnicity in a diverse community. *Ann Epidemiol* 2004;14:339–345.
28. Friede A, Blum HL, McDonald M. Public health informatics: how information-age technology can strengthen public health. *Annu Rev Public Health* 1995;16:239–252.
29. Kirby RS. A parable wrapped in an enigma: population-based assessments of outcomes among high-risk neonates are even less achievable in the age of clinical informatics. *Arch Pediatr Adolesc Med* 1999;153:789–792.
30. Yasnoff WA, O'Carroll PW, Koo D, Linkins RW, Kilbourne E, Editors Public health informatics: improving and transforming public health in the information age. *Public Health Management Pract* 2000;6:67–75.
31. O'Carroll PW, Yasnoff WA, Ward ME, Ripp LH, Guegan YN. *Public Health Informatics and Information Systems.* New York: Springer, 2003.
32. Hinman AR, Atkinson D, Diehn TN, Eichwald J, Heberer J, Hoyle T, King P, Kossack RE, Williams DC, Zimmerman A. Principles and core functions for integrated child health information systems. *J Public Health Manage Pract* 2004;10:S52–S56.
33. Shiffman RN. A convocation of wizards: synergies at the intersection of child health care, public health, and information technology. *J Public Health Manage Pract* 2004;10:S87–S90.
34. Linzer DS, Lloyd-Puryear MA, Mann M, Kogan MD. Evolution of a child health profile initiative. *J Public Health Manage Pract* 2004;10:S16–S23.
35. Hintz SR, Poole WK, Wright LL, Fanaroff AA, Kendrick DE, Laptook AR, Goldberg R, Duara S, Stoll BJ, Oh W, for the NICHD Neonatal Research Network. Changes in mortality and morbidities among infants born at less than 25 weeks during the post-surfactant era. *Arch Dis Child Fetal Neonatal Ed* 2005;90:F128–F135.
36. Louis JM, Ehrenberg HM, Collin MF, Mercer BM. Perinatal intervention and neonatal outcomes near the limit of viability. *Am J Obstet Gynecol* 2004;191:1398–1402.
37. Doyle LW and the Victorian Infant Collaborative Study Group. Neonatal intensive care at the borderline of viability – is it worth it? *Early Hum Dev* 2004;80:103–113.
38. Lee K, Kim BI, Khoshnood B, Hsieh H, Chen T-J, Herschel M et al. Outcome of very low birth weight infants in industrialized countries: 1947–1987. *Am J Epidemiol* 1995;141:1188–1193.
39. Lorenz JM, Wooliever DE, Jetton JR, Paneth N. A quantitative review of mortality and developmental disability in extremely premature newborns. *Arch Pediatr Adolesc Med* 1998;152:425–435.
40. Lorenz JM. The outcome of extreme prematurity. *Semin Perinatol* 2001;25:348–359.
41. Amiel-Tison C, Allen MC, Lebrun F, Rogowski J. Macropremies: underprivileged newborns. *Ment Retard Dev Disabil Res Rev* 2002;8:281–292.
42. Wang ML, Dorer DJ, Fleming MP, Catlin EA. Clinical outcomes of near-term infants. *Pediatrics* 2004;114:372–376.
43. Henderson J, Hockley C, Petrou S, Goldacre M, Davidson L. Economic implications of multiple births: inpatient hospital costs in the first 5 years of life. *Arch Dis Child Fetal Neonatal Ed* 2004;89:F542–F545.
44. Petrou S, Mehta Z, Hockley C, Cook-Mozaffari P, Henderson J, Goldacre M. The impact of preterm birth on hospital inpatient admissions and costs during the first 5 years of life. *Pediatrics* 2003;112:1290–1297.
45. Ohlinger J, Brown MS, Laudert S, Swanson S, Fofah O. Development of potentially better practices for the neonatal intensive care unit as a culture of collaboration: communication, accountability, respect, and empowerment. *Pediatrics* 2003;111(4 Pt 2):e471–e481.
46. McCormick MC, Shapiro S, Starfield BH. The regionalization of perinatal services: summary of the evaluation of a national demonstration program. *JAMA* 1985;253:799–804.
47. Paneth N, Kiely JL, Wallenstein S, Susser M. The choice of place of delivery: effect of hospital level on mortality in all singleton births in New York City. *Am J Dis Child* 1987;141:60–64.

48. Kirby RS. Perinatal mortality: the role of hospital of birth. *J Perinatol* 1996;16:43–49.
49. Als H. *Program Guide: Newborn Individualized Developmental Care and Assessment Program (NIDCAP): An Education and Training Program for Health Care Professionals.* Boston, MA: Children's Medical Center Corporation, 1997.
50. Jacobs SE, Sokol J, Ohlsson A. The Newborn Individualized Developmental Care and Assessment Program is not supported by meta-analyses of the data. *J Pediatr* 2002;140:699–706.
51. Baskett TF. Virginia Apgar and the newborn Apgar score. Resuscitation 2000;47:215–217.
52. The International Neonatal Network. The CRIB (clinical risk index for babies) score: a tool for assessing initial neonatal risk and comparing performance of neonatal intensive care units. *Lancet* 1993;342:193–198.
53. Lago P, Freato F, Bettiol T, Chiandetti L, Vianello A, Zaramella P. Is the CRIB Score (Clinical Risk Index for Babies) a valid tool in predicting neurodevelopmental outcome in extremely low birth weight infants? *Biol Neonate* 1999;76:220–227.
54. Richardson DK, Gray JE, McCormick MC, et al. Score for neonatal acute physiology: a physiology severity index for neonatal intensive care. *Pediatrics* 1993;91:617–623.
55. Darling JS, Field DJ, Manktelow B. Neonatal disease severity scoring systems. *Arch Dis Child Fetal Neonatal Ed* 2005;90:F11–F16.
56. Johnson CP, Kastner TA. American Academy of Pediatrics Section on Children with Disabilities. Helping families raise children with special health care needs at home. *Pediatrics* 2005;115:507–511.
57. Sia C, Tonniges TF, Osterhus E, Taba S. History of the medical home concept. *Pediatrics* 2004;133:1473–1478.
58. Glascoe FP. Eary detection of developmental and behavioral problems. *Pediatr Rev* 2000;21:272–280.
59. Petersen MC, Kube DA, Palmer FB. Classification of developmental delays. *Semin Pediatr Neurol* 1998;5:2–14.
60. Meckel RA. *Save the Babies: American Public Health Reform and the Prevention of Infant Mortality, 1850–1929.* Baltimore, MD: *Johns Hopkins University Press,* 1990.
61. Reef S, Frey TK, Abernathy K, Burnett CL, Icenogle J, McCauley MM, Wharton M. The changing epidemiology of rubella in the 1990s: on the verge of elimination and new challenges for control and prevention. *JAMA* 2002;287:464–472.
62. Kirby RS. Neonatal and postneonatal mortality: useful concepts or outdated constructs? *J Perinatol* 1993;13:433–441.
63. Bale JF Jr. Congenital infections. *Neurol Clin* 2002;20:1039–1060.
64. Istas AS, Demmler GJ, Dobbins JG, Stewart JA. Surveillance for congenital cytomegalovirun disease: a report from the National Congenital Cytomegalovirus Disease Registry. *Clin Infect Dis* 1995;20:665–670.
65. Demmler GJ. Summary of a workshop on surveillance of congenital cytomegalovirus disease. *Rev Infect Dis* 1991;13:315–329.
66. Fowler KB, Boppana SB. Congenital cytomegalovirus (CMV) infection and hearing deficit. *J Clin Virol* 2006;35:226–231.
67. Saloojee H, Velaphi S, Goga Y, Afadapa N, Steen R, Lincetto O. The prevention and management of congenital syphilis: an overview and recommendations. *Bull World Health Organization* 2004;82:424–430.
68. Hollier LM, Hill J, Sheffield JS, Wendel GD Jr. State laws regarding prenatal syphilis screening in the United States. *Am J Obstet Gynecol* 2003;189:1178–1183.
69. Gust DA, Levine WC, St. Louis ME, Braxton J, Berman SM. Mortality associated with congenital syphilis in the United States, 1992–1998. *Pediatrics* 2002;109:e79. http:www.pediatrics.org/cgi/content/full/109/5/e79. Accessed September 6, 2008.
70. Regan JA, Klebanoff MA, Nugent RP. The epidemiology of group B streptococcal colonization in pregnancy. Vaginal Infections and Prematurity Study Group. *Obstet Gynecol* 1991;77:604–610.
71. Gibbs RS, Schrag S, Schucha. A. *Perinatal infections due to Group B streptococci. Obstet Gynecol* 2004;104:1062–1076.

72. Schrag SG, Zywicki S, Farley MM, Reingold AL, Harrison LH, Lefkowitz LB, et al. Group B streptococcal disease in the era of intrapartum antibiotic prophylaxsis. *N Engl J Med* 2000;342:15–20.

73. Gaynes RP, Edwards JR, Jarvis WR, Culver DH, Tolson JS, Martone WJ. Nosocomial infections among neonates in high-risk nurseries in the United States. National Nosocomial Infections Surveillance System. *Pediatrics* 1996;98:357–361.

74. National Nosocomial Infections Surveillance System, National Nosocomial Infections Surveillance (NNIS). System Report, data summary from January 1992 through June 2004, issued October 2004. *Am J Infect Control* 2004;32:470–485.

75. Fell JME. Neonatal inflammatory intestinal diseases: necrotising enterocolitis and allergic colitis. *Early Human Dev* 2005;81:117–122.

76. Boccia D, Stolfi I, Lana S, Moro ML. Nosocomial necrotising enterocolitis outbreaks: epidemiology and control measures. *Eur J Pediatr* 2001;160:385–391.

77. Welliver RC. Review of epidemiology and clinical risk factors for severe respiratory synctial virus (RSV) infection. *J Pediatr* 2003;143:S112–S117.

78. Leader S, Kohlhase K. Recent trends in severe respiratory synctial virus (RSV) among US infants, 1997–2000. *J Pediatr* 2003;143:S127–S132.

79. Willson DF, Landrigan CP, Horn SD, Smout RJ. Complications in infants hospitalized for bronchiolitis or respiratory synctial virus pneumonia. *J Pediatr* 2003;143:S142–S149.

80. Boyce TB, Mellen BG, Mitchel EF Jr, Wright PF, Griffin MR. Rates of hospitalization for respiratory synctial virus infection among children in Medicaid. *J Pediatr* 2000;137:865–870.

81. Tanaka M, Vitek CR, Pascual FB, Bisgard KM, Tate JE, Murphy TV. Trends in pertussis among infants in the United States, 1980–1999. *JAMA* 2003;290:2968–2975.

82. Auinger P, Lanphear BP, Kalkwarf HJ, Mansour ME. Trends in otitis media among children in the United States. *Pediatrics* 2003;112:514–520.

83. Vernacchio L, Lesko SM, Vezina RM, Corwin MJ, Hunt CE, Hoffman HJ, Mitchell AA. Racial/ethnic disparities in the diagnosis of otitis media in infancy. *Int J Pediatr Otorhinolaryngol* 2004;68:795–804.

84. Ramaswamy K, Jacobson K. Infectious diarrhea in children. *Gastroenterol Clin N A* 2001;30:611–624.

85. Trevejo RT, Courtney JG, Starr M, Vugia DJ. Epidemiology of salmonellosis in California, 1990–1999: morbidity, mortality, and hospitalization costs. *Am J Epidemiol* 2003;157:48–57.

86. Vugia DJ, Samuel M, Farley MM, Marcus R, Shiferaw B, Shallow S, Smith K, Angulo FJ, for the Emerging Infections Program FoodNet Working Group. Invasive Salmonella infections in the United States, FoodNet, 1996–1999: incidence, serotype distribution, and outcome. *Clin Infect Dis* 2004;38 Suppl 3:S149–S156.

87. Kennedy M, Villar R, Vugia DJ, Rabatsky-Her T, Farley MM, Pass M, Smith K, Smith P, Cieslak PR, Imhoff B, Griffin PM, for the Emerging Infections Program FoodNet Working Group. Hospitalizations and deaths due to Salmonella infections, FoodNet, 1996–1999. *Clin Infect Dis* 2004;38 Suppl 3:S142–S148.

88. Golding J, Emmett PM, Rogers IS. Gastroenteritis, diarrhoea, and breast feeding. *Early Human Dev* 1997;49:S83–S103.

89. Rowe SY, Rocourt JR, Shiferaw B, Kassenborg HD, Segler SD, Marcus R, Daily PJ, Hardnett FP, Slutsker L, for the Emerging Infections Program FoodNet Working Group. Breast-feeding decreases the risk of sporadic Salmonellosis among infants in FoodNet sites. *Clin Infect Dis* 2004;38 Suppl 3:S262–S270

90. Denneh PH. Rotavirus vaccines: an overview. *Clin Microbiol Rev* 2008;21:198–208.

91. Parashar UD, Holman RC, Cummings KC, Staggs NW, Curns AT, Zimmerman CM et al. Trends in intussusception-associated hospitalizations and deaths among US infants. *Pediatrics* 2000;106:1413–1421.

92. McIntosh EDG, Paradiso PR. Recent progress in the development of vaccines for infants and children. *Vaccine* 2003;21:601–604.

93. Robinson A, Linden MG. *Clinical Genetic Handbook*. Boston: Blackwell Scientific, 1993.

94. Berger KH, Zhu B-P, Copeland G. Mortality throughout early childhood for Michigan children born with congenital anomalies, 1992–1998. *Birth Defects Res A Clin Mol Teratol* 2003;67:656–661.

95. Petrini J, Damus K, Russell R, Poschman K, Davidoff MJ, Mattison D. Contribution of birth defects to infant mortality in the United States. *Teratology* 2002;66 Suppl 1:S3–S6.

96. Christianson A, Howson CP, Modell B. *The March of Dimes Global Report on Birth Defects, The Hidden Toll of Dying and Disabled Children.* White Plains, NY: March of Dimes Birth Defects Foundation, 2006).

97. Watkins ML, Edmonds L, McClearn A, Mullins L, Mulinare J, Khoury M. The surveillance of birth defects: the usefulness of the revised US standard birth certificate. *Am J Public Health* 1996;86:731–734.

98. Hexter AC, Harris JA, Roeper P, Croen LA, Krueger P, Gant D. Evaluation of the hospital discharge diagnoses index and the birth certificate as sources of information on birth defects. *Public Health Rep* 1990;105:296–307.

99. Correa-Villaseñor A, Cragan J, Kucik J, O'Leary L, Siffel C, Williams L. The Metropolitan Atlanta Congenital Defects Program: 35 years of birth defects surveillance at the Centers for Disease Control and Prevention. *Birth Defects Res A Clin Mol Teratol* 2003;67:617–624.

100. Copeland GE, Kirby RS. Using birth defects registry data to evaluate infant and childhood mortality associated with birth defects: an alternative to traditional mortality assessment using underlying cause of death statistics. *Birth Defects Res A Clin Mol Teratol* 2007;79 (11):792–797.

101. Teutsch SM, Churchill RE, Eds. *Principles and Practice of Public Health Surveillance.* 2nd Edition. New York: Oxford University Press, 2000.

102. Lynberg MC, Edmonds LD. Surveillance of birth defects. In Halperin W, Baker E, Editors. *Public Health Surveillance.* New York: Van Nostrand Reinhold, 1992;157–177.

103. Kirby RS. Analytical resources for assessment of clinical genetics services in public health: current status and future prospects. *Teratology* 2000;61:9–16.

104. Jellife-Pawlowski LL, Shaw GM, Nelson V, Harris JA. Risk of mental retardation among children born with birth defects. *Arch Pediatr Adolesc Med* 2003;157:545–550.

105. Kirby RS, Brewster MA, Canino C, Pavin M. Early childhood surveillance of developmental disorders by a birth defects surveillance system: methods, prevalence, and mortality patterns. *J Dev Behav Pediatr* 1995;16:318–326.

106. Kirby RS. Co-occurrence of developmental disabilities with birth defects. *Ment Retard Dev Disabil Res Rev* 2002;8:182–187.

107. National Birth Defects Prevention Network (NBDPN). *Guidelines for Conducting Birth Defects Surveillance.* Sever LE, Ed. Atlanta, GA: National Birth Defects Prevention Network, 2004. Available at http://www.nbdpn.org/current/resources/bdsurveillance.html. Accessed September 6, 2008.

108. International Clearinghouse for Birth Defects Surveillance and Research. *Annual Report 2005 with data for 2003.* Rome, Italy: Centre of the International Clearinghouse for Birth Defects Surveillance and Research, 2006.

109. Besser LM, Williams LJ, Cragan JD. Interpreting changes in the epidemiology of anencephaly and spina bifida following folic acid fortification of the U.S. grain supply in the setting of long-term trends, Atlanta, Georgia, 1968-2003. *Birth Defects Res A Clin Mol Teratol* 2007;79(11):730–736.

110. Salihu HM, Pierre-Louis BJ, Druschel CM, Kirby RS. Omphalocele and gastroschisis in the state of New York, 1992–1999. *Birth Defects Res A Clin Mol Teratol* 2003;67:630–636.

111. Canfield MA, Honein MA, Yuskiv N, Xing J, Mai CT, Collins JS, Devine O, Petrini J, Ramadhani TA, Hobbs CA, Kirby RS. National estimates and race/ethnic-specific variation of selected birth defects in the United States, 1999–2001. *Birth Defects Res A Clin Mol Teratol* 2006;76(11):747–756.

112. Canfield MA, Collins JS, Botto LD, Williams LJ, Mai CT, Kirby RS, Pearson K, Mulinare J, for the National Birth Defects Prevention Network. Changes in the birth prevalence of selected birth defects after flour fortification with folic acid in the United States: findings

from a multi-state population-based study. *Birth Defects Res A Clin Mol Teratol Clin Mol Teratol* 2005;73(10):679–689.

113. Kirby R, Petrini J, Alter C, and the Hispanic Ethnicity Birth Defects Work Group. Collecting and interpreting birth defects surveillance data by hispanic ethnicity: a comparative study. *Teratology* 2000;61:21–27.

114. Resta RG. Changing demographics of advanced maternal age (AMA) and the impact on the predicted incidence of Down syndrome in the United States: implications for prenatal screening and genetic counseling. *Am J Med Genet* 2005;133A:31–36.

115. Reefhuis J, Honein MA. Maternal age and non-chromosomal birth defects – Atlanta 1968–2000: Teenager or thirty-something, who is at risk? *Birth Defects Res A Clin Mol Teratol* 2004;70:572–579.

116. Werler MM, Mitchell AA, Shapiro S. Demographic, reproductive, medical, and environmental factors in relation to gastroschisis. *Teratology* 1992;45:353–360.

117. Fisch H, Hyun G, Golden R, Hensle TW, Olsson CA, Liberson GL. The influence of paternal age on Down syndrome. *J Urol* 2003;169:2275–2278.

118. Li SJ, Ford N, Meister K, Bodurtha J. Increased risk of birth defects among children from multiple births. *Birth Defects Res A Clin Mol Teratol* 2003;67(10):879–885.

119. Derom R, Bryan E, Derom C, Keith L, Vlietinck R. Twins, chorionicity and zygosity. *Twin Res* 2001;4:134–136.

120. Vieira AR. Birth order and neural tube defects: a reappraisal. *J Neurol Sci* 2004;217:65–72.

121. Vieira AR, Orioli IM. Birth order and oral clefts: a meta analysis. *Teratology* 2002;66:209–216.

122. Waller DK, Shaw GM, Rasmussen SA, Hobbs CA, Canfield MA, Siega-Riz AM, Gallaway MS, Correa A. National Birth Defects Prevention Study. Prepregnancy obesity as a risk factor for structural birth defects. *Arch Pediatr Adolesc Med* 2007;161(8):745–750.

123. Shaw GM, Todoroff K, Schaffer DM, Selvin S. Maternal height and prepregnancy body mass index as risk factors for selected congenital anomalies. *Paediatr Perinat Epidemiol* 2000;14:234–239.

124. Watkins ML, Rasmussen SA, Honein MA, Botto LD, Moore CA. Maternal obesity and risk for birth defects. *Pediatrics* 2003;111:1152–1158.

125. Moretti ME, Bar-Oz B, Fried S, Koren G. Maternal hyperthermia and the risk for neural tube defects in offspring: systematic review and meta-analysis. *Epidemiology* 2005;16:216–219.

126. Wyszynski DF, ed. *Cleft Lip and Palate: From Origin to Treatment.* New York: Oxford University Press, 2002.

127. Wyszynski DF, ed. *Neural Tube Defects: From Origin to Treatment.* New York: Oxford University Press, 2005.

128. Schardien JL. *Chemically Induced Birth Defects.* 3rd Edition, Revised and Expanded. New York: Marcel Decker, 2000.

129. Paulozzi LJ, Mercy J, Frazier L Jr, Annest JL. CDC's National Violent Death Reporting System: background and methodology. *Inj Prev* 2004;10:47–52.

130. Danseco ER, Miller TR, Spicer RS. Incidence and costs of 1987–1994 childhood injuries: demographic breakdowns. *Pediatrics* 2000;105:e27.

131. Powell EC, Tanz RR. Adjusting our view of injury risk: the burden of nonfatal injuries in infancy. *Pediatrics* 2002;110:792–796.

132. Tomashek KM, Hsia J, Iyasu S. Trends in postneonatal mortality attributable to injury, United States, 1988–1998. *Pediatrics* 2003;111:1219–1225.

133. WHO *Injury: A Leading Cause of the Global Burden of Disease, 2000.* Geneva: World Health Organization, 2002.

134. Faelker T, Pickett W, Brison RJ. Socioeconomic differences in childhood injury: a population based epidemiologic study in Ontario, Canada. *Inj Prev* 2000;6:203–208.

135. Khambalia A, Joshi P, Brussoni M, Raina P, Morrongiello B, MacArthur C. Risk factors for unintentional injuries due to falls in children aged 0–6 years: a systematic review. *Inj Prev* 2006;12:378–381.

136. Otters H, Schellevis FG, Damen J, van der Wouden JC, Suijlekom-Smit LW, Koes BW. Epidemiology of unintentional injuries in childhood: a population-based survey in general practice. *Br J Gen Pract* 2005;55(517):630–633.
137. Engstrom K, Diderichsen F, Laflamme L. Socioeconomic differences in injury risks in childhood and adolescence: a nation-wide study of intentional and unintentional injuries in Sweden. *Inj Prev* 2002;8:137–142.
138. Agran PF, Anderson C, Winn D, Trent R, Walton-Haynes L, Thayer S. Rates of pediatric injuries by 3-month intervals for children 0 to 3 years of age. *Pediatrics* 2003;111:e683–e692.
139. MMWR Variation in homicide risk during infancy – United States, 1989–1998. *MMWR Morb Mortal Wkly Rep* 2002;51:187–189.
140. Pickett W, Streight S, Simpson K, Brison RJ. Injuries experienced by infant children: a population-based epidemiological analysis. *Pediatrics* 2003;111:e365–e370.
141. Simon HK, Tamura T, Colton K. Reported level of supervision of young children while in the bathtub. *Ambul Pediatr* 2003;3:106–108.
142. de Lourdes DM, Carvalho Leite JC, Marshall T, Anselmo Hess Almaleh CM, Feldens CA, Vitolo MR. Effects of the home environment on unintentional domestic injuries and related health care attendance in infants. *Acta Paediatr* 2007;96:1169–1173.
143. National Center for Injury Prevention and Control. Child Maltreatment: Fact Sheet. 2007.
144. Schnitzer PG, Ewigman BG. Child deaths resulting from inflicted injuries: household risk factors and perpetrator characteristics. *Pediatrics* 2005;116:e687–e693.
145. National Center for Injury Prevention and Control. *CDC Injury Fact Book*. Atlanta, GA: Centers for Disease Control and Prevention, 2006.
146. Gerber P, Coffman K. Nonaccidental head trauma in infants. *Childs Nerv Syst* 2007;23:499–507.
147. Dias MS, Smith K, deGuehery K, Mazur P, Li V, Shaffer ML. Preventing abusive head trauma among infants and young children: a hospital-based, parent education program. *Pediatrics* 2005;115:e470–e477.
148. Newton AW, Vandeven AM. Update on child maltreatment. *Curr Opin Pediatr* 2007;19:223–229.

Chapter 6
The Continuum of Reproductive Loss from Pregnancy Through Infancy

The death of a child is perhaps the most emotionally devastating event a couple can face, invariably permanently altering the course of their lives and their family's life. On a societal level, loss of a child is also damaging because, for both individuals and societies, the loss of a child represents the loss of the future. In this section, we consider pregnancy loss from the conception through the first year of life. We begin by describing epidemiologic measures used to describe rates of loss. We then separately consider the epidemiology of losses during early pregnancy, late pregnancy, and infancy. We end by presenting public health interventions aimed at reducing pregnancy loss and infant mortality.

6.1 Definitions, Measures, Data Sources, and Measurement Issues

Definitions. An *early spontaneous abortion* is the spontaneous loss of an embryo or fetus due to natural causes before the twelfth week of pregnancy. (Weeks of gestation are counted starting from the first day of the last normal menstrual period.) A *late spontaneous abortion* is a spontaneous loss from the twelfth through nineteenth weeks of pregnancy (2).

An *early pregnancy loss* is the spontaneous loss of an embryo or fetus due to natural causes up through 41 days after the first day of the last normal menstrual period. These early losses may occur before implantation, after implantation, or shortly after the next expected menstrual period.

Spontaneous abortions rarely from molar pregnancies. Most of these losses occur as expulsion from the uterus of the products of conception, also termed *miscarriages*. They occur much less frequently as ectopic pregnancies.

Women who experience three or more consecutive spontaneous abortions are considered to have *recurrent or habitual spontaneous abortions* (2). A *threatened abortion* occurs when a woman experiences vaginal bleeding or uterine cramping in

M.M. Adams et al., *Perinatal Epidemiology for Public Health Practice.*
doi: 10.1007/978-0-387-09439-7_6; © Springer Science +Business Media, LLC

WHO definition of a fetal death

"...death before the complete expulsion or extraction from its mother of a product of conception, irrespective of the duration of pregnancy; the death is indicated by the fact that after such separation, the fetus does not breathe or show any other evidence of life, such as beating of the heart, pulsation of the umbilical cord, or definite movement of voluntary muscles." (1)

the first half of pregnancy (2). Less than two-thirds of these women subsequently have a spontaneous abortion. An *incomplete abortion* occurs after the embryo or fetus has died, but the products of conception have not been completely expelled from the uterus.

Fetal deaths are also spontaneous pregnancy losses. In practice, public health workers distinguish between fetal deaths and spontaneous abortions by defining fetal deaths as losses that occur at 20 or more weeks of gestation. *Late fetal deaths* are fetal deaths that occur at 28 or more weeks of gestation. Clinicians further distinguish *antepartum fetal deaths*, which occur before labor, from *intrapartum fetal deaths*, which occur during labor.

The legal requirements for reporting fetal deaths vary among states (Table 6.1) (3, 4) and among countries (5, 6). The U.S. 1992 Model State Vital Statistics Act and Regulation recommends reporting "each fetal death of 350 g or more or if weight is unknown, of 20 completed weeks gestation or more" (7).

WHO's definition of a live birth

"...the complete expulsion or extraction from its mother of a product of conception, regardless of the duration of pregnancy, which, after such separation, breathes or shows any evidence of life, such as beating of the heart, pulsation of the umbilical cord, or definite movement of voluntary muscles, whether or not the umbilical cord has been cut or the placenta is attached; each product of such a birth is considered liveborn" (8)

Babies who die during infancy must have been born alive. Thus, the definition of a live birth influences identification of fetal and infant deaths, especially very early infant deaths. Although many countries use the World Health Organization's (WHO) definition of a live birth, some modify the WHO definition and others use alternate definitions. Beginning in 1988, the United States added the following clarification to WHO's definition: "Heartbeats are to be distinguished from transient cardiac contractions; respirations are to be distinguished from fleeting respiratory efforts or gasps." (3).

International differences in registration practices limit comparability of fetal and perinatal mortality rates (9). Several countries do not register fetuses that are

Table 6.1 Legal standards for vital registration of a fetal death and number of states using them, United States, 1997 (3)

Legal standard for vital registration of a fetal death	Number of states using this standard
All products of conception (i.e., all pregnancy losses reported, regardless of length of gestation when loss occurred)	7
Gestation ≥ 16 weeks	1
Gestation ≥ 20 weeks	25
Birth weight ≥ 350 g	1
Birth weight ≥ 350 g or gestation ≥ 20 weeks	12
Birth weight ≥ 400 g or gestation ≥ 20 weeks	1
Birth weight ≥ 500 g	3
Birth weight ≥ 500 g or gestation ≥ 20 weeks	1

States and the District of Columbia

stillborn before 28 weeks' gestation or babies who are live born, but very small or very preterm and die shortly after birth. These countries require that live born infants with less than a specified length of gestation or birth weight survive at least 24 h (5). Because nearly half of the fetal and infant deaths in the United States occur among babies delivered before 28 weeks' gestation, countries that exclude babies with these very short gestations will have lower fetal and infant mortality rates than those that include them.

The shifting limits of viability

Improvements in resuscitation and neonatal care during the 1990s have led to survival of fetuses delivered after as little as 23 weeks of gestation (see the University of Iowa's registry of "the tiniest babies," http://www.medicine. uiowa.edu/tiniestbabies/index.htm). In additional to substantial risk of death, infants born after gestations of <26 weeks face substantial risks of severe pediatric morbidity, including cerebral palsy and lung disease (10, 11). Their risks for adult morbidity are unknown. Although recent studies show general agreement among European and Australian practitioners regarding lower gestational limits for attempting resuscitation, parental decisions may influence delivery-room actions (12–14). Differences in resuscitation practices may distort temporal and geographic comparisons of fetal and neonatal mortality rates, especially at short gestations.

Infant deaths are deaths that occur from birth through 365 days of life. Researchers often categorize infant deaths by the infant's age when they occur:

Neonatal	0–27 days of life
Early neonatal	0–7 days of life

Table 6.2 Measures of pregnancy loss

Measure	Numerator	Denominator
Fetal death rate	Fetal deaths during a calendar year	Total births (live births plus fetal deaths) during the same year
Conditional fetal death rate	Fetal deaths at a specified gestational age	Live births, fetal deaths and on-going pregnancies at that gestation during the same year
Birth weight-specific fetal death rate	Fetal deaths of a specified birth weight during a calendar year	Live births and fetal deaths at that birth weight during the same year
Perinatal mortality rate	Late fetal and early neonatal (≤ 7 days) deaths during a calendar year	Total births (live births plus fetal deaths) during the same year
Neonatal mortality rate	Neonatal deaths during a calendar year	Live births during the same year
Postneonatal mortality rate	Postneonatal deaths during a calendar year	Live births during the same year
Conditional postneonatal mortality rate	Postneonatal deaths during a calendar year	Neonatal survivors during the same year
Infant mortality rate	Infant deaths during a year	Live births during the same year
Infant death rate	Infant deaths during a calendar year	Estimated mid-year population aged ≤ 1 year for the same year (14)

Late neonatal	8–27 days of life
Postneonatal	28–364 days of life

Perinatal deaths include late fetal deaths and early neonatal deaths.

Measures. Table 6.2 lists the most commonly used measures for spontaneous abortion and fetal and infant mortality.

> The interpretation of a fetal or infant mortality rate depends, in part, on the denominator used to represent the population at risk.

The fetal death rate is the proportion (or percentage) of infants who are born dead among the population at risk of death, i.e., all infants (8). It is the risk of fetal death. The number of infants at risk of death at a specified gestational age is the number of infants who are delivered at that gestation (whether stillborn or liveborn) plus the number of on-going pregnancies at that gestation. Thus, gestation-specific fetal death rates have a denominator that is a subset of all infants. For any week of gestation, the number of infants at risk of fetal death can be estimated by subtracting the number of infants delivered at shorter gestations from the total number of infants. The amount subtracted for very preterm gestations is negligible. However, ignoring the amount at or near term overestimates the denominator, resulting in an underestimate of the true mortality rate. Similar considerations apply to computing birth weight-specific mortality rates. Here, the denominator includes not only infants delivered at specified birth weights, but also fetuses in utero with those birth weights.

The conditional postneonatal mortality rate differs from the commonly used postneonatal mortality rate because the conditional rate includes only infants who are at risk of postneonatal death, i.e., neonatal survivors. The conditional postneonatal mortality rate answers the question, "Among babies who have survived 27 days after birth, how many will die before reaching their first birthday?" Because the denominator for the postneonatal mortality rate includes infants who died as neonates, it overestimates the dominator, falsely decreasing the rate. For term infants or areas with low neonatal mortality rates, the amount of this error is negligible, because neonatal deaths are relatively rare. In areas with high neonatal mortality, or for very preterm (<32 weeks) or very low birth weight (<1,500 g) infants, the error can be substantial. Ignoring it can lead to incorrectly computing trends in postneonatal death and incorrect comparisons between jurisdictions.

Three approaches are commonly used to compute infant mortality. The first and simplest divides the number of infant deaths during a calendar year by the number of live births in that year. This is called *period mortality*, because all deaths occur during a specified period of time. A drawback of period mortality is that its denominator does not include decedents who were born during the preceding year. The second approach, the infant death rate, addresses this shortcoming by using an estimate of the mid-year number of infants during the year when the deaths occurred. A final approach, termed *cohort mortality*, begins with a cohort of infants born alive during a calendar year and then finds the deaths among these infants, whether they occurred during that calendar year or in the following year.

Data sources. In the United States, analysts use certificates for fetal deaths, live births, and infant deaths to compute fetal, perinatal, and infant mortality rates. In consultation with state vital registrars and other stakeholders, the National Center for Health Statistics (NCHS) periodically recommends standard formats for these certificates. Individual states may adopt some or all of these recommendations. Thus, the content of vital certificates varies somewhat among states. Most states implemented certificate revisions in 1989. The newest revision of the birth certificate is being phased in by states beginning in 2003. Appendix 1 presents model certificates. Fetal death certificates combine elements of birth and death certificates.

To supplement information on death certificates, states link certificates for infant deaths with their respective birth certificates. In 1960, the NCHS used state data to compile the first national dataset of linked infant death and birth certificates (16). Analysts next compiled a national linked file in 1980. From 1983 onward, the NCHS annually compiled linked files. Until 1995, these files included deaths that occurred among infants born in a calendar year (cohort files). Beginning in 1995, the files included deaths that occurred during a calendar year and their matching birth certificates (period files).

Analysts have applied linkage methods similar to those used to match birth and death certificates to identify siblings delivered to the same woman, including live or still born sets of twins, triplets, or quadruplets (17, 18). States have linked vital records data to

Medicaid data and hospital discharge data (19–21). The state of Washington has created one of the most extensive perinatal databases by linking each birth certificate to corresponding newborn hospital discharge data, the birth certificates of siblings who were born in Washington and, if death occurred, the death certificate.

Globally, developed countries use systems of registration of fetal and infant deaths that are similar to the United States. Analysts have used these vital record data to create linked databases similar to those in the United States (17). Registration systems also exist in developing countries, but they may be very incomplete, especially for fetal deaths and early neonatal deaths (22). Faced with incomplete vital registration, investigators have used survey techniques – similar to those used for identifying maternal deaths – to obtain a more complete count of fetal and infant deaths (23). Difficulties in adequacy of data severely limit success in linking birth and death certificates in developing countries (23).

> *WHO definition of the underlying cause of death*
>
> "The disease or injury, which initiated the train of morbid events leading directly to death, or the circumstances of the accident or violence which produced fatal injury" (24).

In the United States, the certifier of death provides information about the underlying cause of death, up to three contributing causes, whether an autopsy was performed, and whether the results were available when the death certificate was completed. In 1968, the NCHS began using the Automated Classification of Medical Entities (ACME) method to evaluate the sequence of causes of death and assign an underlying cause of death. Since 1990, nosologists have used the Mortality Medical Indexing, Classification, and Retrieval (MICAR) system to further refine death certificate entries before submitting them to ACME (16, 25). These automated approaches promote consistency in coding among certifiers of death and nosologists.

To promote international consistency in coding, the WHO develops coding guidelines, which the United States uses. From 1979 through 1998, U.S. nosologists applied International Classification of Diseases, Version 9 (ICD-9) codes; in 1999, they switched to ICD-10 codes (the tenth revision). Countries vary in the date when they implemented ICD-10 codes. Changes in the ICD code complicate interpretation of mortality trends and differences among countries (16, 25, 26).

Clinicians and public health analysts have proposed multiple approaches for classifying fetal, perinatal, and infant deaths. The simplest approaches classify deaths by the age of the fetus or infant when they occur or by their frequency, an approach used by the NCHS (27). Many classification schemes aim to promote the use of death data in setting programmatic priorities and evaluating general trends (Table 6.3) (25, 28–33). Thus, the type of intervention needed for prevention rather than their underlying etiology often categorizes deaths. Schemes for categorizing deaths are likely to evolve with experience in their use and the increasing availability of prevention strategies (34).

Table 6.3 Selected schemes for classifying fetal, neonatal, and infant deaths

---

Wigglesworth (28)

Lethal malformation
Death before onset of labor
Asphyxial condition developing in labor
Condition associated with immaturity
Specific condition
Unclassifiable

International Collaborative Effort (ICE) (29)

Congenital anomalies
Asphyxia-related conditions
Immaturity-related conditions
Infections
Sudden death
Deaths due to external causes
Other specific conditions
Other and unclassifiable diagnoses

Neonatal and Intrauterine Death Classification (NICE) (25, 30)

Congenital anomalies
Multiple births
Maternal disease
Specific fetal conditions
Unexplained small-for-dates
Placental abruption
Obstetric complications
Unexplained antepartum stillbirth <37 weeks
Unexplained antepartum stillbirth ≥37 weeks
Specific infant conditions
Unexplained asphyxia
Unexplained immaturity
Unclassifiable cases

Leading causes of infant death, United States (27)

Congenital anomalies
Disorders related to short gestation and low birth weight, not elsewhere classified
Sudden infant death syndrome
Newborn affected by maternal complications of pregnancy
Accidents (unintentional injuries)
Newborn affected by complications of the placenta, cord, and membranes
Respiratory distress of newborn
Bacterial sepsis of newborn
Neonatal hemorrhage
Diseases of the circulatory system

Measurement issues fall into five broad areas:

- Incompletely ascertaining deaths;
- Incorrectly or inconsistently classifying deaths as antepartum, intrapartum, or postpartum;

- Incorrectly assigning the cause or causes of death;
- Changes in schemes used to code the cause of death; and
- Comparing population groups whose mortality data have different percentages of missing information for gestation, birth weight, or other attributes.

Completeness of ascertainment is most problematic for early fetal deaths and neonatal deaths among very small babies (35, 36). A study of registration of fetal deaths weighing <500 g in Canada from 1985 through 1995 showed that the rate of these deaths increased over time and varied geographically, reflecting provincial differences in registration requirements (37). Several investigators using U.S. data from the 1980s have noted underascertainment of fetal deaths (38–40). A more recent study examined the completeness of registration of deaths (i.e., presence or absence of a death certificate when death occurred) among infants with birth weights <750 g who were born in Ohio during the first half of 2006. Seven percent of the deaths among these infants were not registered (41).

A study from a managed care organization in California of neonatal deaths among infants delivered in 1990 and 1991 showed that the computed neonatal mortality rate varied by whether rates included infants born alive but weighing <500 g. Nearly all of these very small infants died. The neonatal mortality rate also varied by whether the neonatal period was computed based on deaths during 27 days after delivery or deaths that occurred within 40 weeks corrected age (i.e., 40 weeks after the last normal menstrual period) plus 27 days (42). Including deaths that occur within 27 days after the corrected age of 40 weeks makes sense biologically, because it puts all infants on a comparable developmental stage. However, it has the disadvantage of being difficult to use when gestational age is uncertain. It also has the disadvantage of allowing different lengths of time after birth for "neonatal" death to occur among infants with short gestations compared with infants born at term.

Underregistration of intentional neonatal deaths

A study of newborns who were killed or left to die from 1985 through 2000 in North Carolina estimated an annual rate of 2.1 deaths per 100,000 live births (43). The lifetime risk of homicide is highest on the first day of life (44) and among newborns killed within 24 h after birth, 95% are not delivered in a hospital (45). Because these babies are deliberately kept outside the medical care system, their births as well as their deaths may not be registered.

To avoid questions about whether an early pregnancy loss meets the criteria for registration as a fetal death, some states require registration of all spontaneous pregnancy losses. This insures that, aside from induced abortions, every pregnancy is counted, either as fetal death or a live birth. In these states, the completeness of ascertainment of first trimester losses has not been described. However, most analysts judge that ascertainment of spontaneous pregnancy losses from the mid-second trimester onward is relatively complete. In states or countries that require registration of only a subset of fetal deaths or live births, registration is often complete only for fetuses that clearly exceed the registration requirements. This is especially true for requirements involving gestational length, which is notoriously difficult to measure accurately (46–48). For example, in states with 20 weeks as the minimum age for registering fetal deaths, many analysts consider registration complete only at gestations of 24 weeks and longer (40).

In many developing countries, incompleteness of civil registration of infant death is a substantial problem. For example, using data from a study of children who died from 1996 through 1998 in part of Kenya, researchers observed that civil registration identified less than half of the neonatal deaths and approximately two-thirds of postneonatal deaths (49).

For infants at the threshold of viability, the decision regarding resuscitation influences whether the fetus is considered a fetal death, a surviving neonate, or a very early neonatal death. Legislation passed by the U.S. Congress in 2002 (Born-Alive Infants' Protection Act) requires that medical care be given to all infants who are born alive (50). As survival of infants born after 21 or 22 weeks of gestation improves, clinicians are likely to register more of these babies as live births rather than fetal deaths. Analyses of international differences in the distribution of fetal deaths and live births among babies with birth weights <750 g suggest that both the completeness of ascertainment of these very small babies and local practices in distinguishing fetal deaths and live births contribute to international differences in infant mortality rates (9). Researchers examining factors associated with death in the first 12 h of life among babies weighing 500–1,000 g observed that decedents were much less likely than survivors to be intubated or receive potentially life-saving surfactant therapy, suggesting a decision by caregivers and parents to let these infants die (51).

Incompleteness of registration of fetal and infant deaths in developing countries is often substantial.

Analyzing perinatal mortality, rather than fetal and neonatal mortality, may be the best approach for comparing data from areas with different practices for registration of fetal deaths and live births. This approach also may be justified in developing countries where skilled attendants do not assist most deliveries. It is less useful in developed countries, however, where skilled attendants who can distinguish antepartum, intrapartum, and early neonatal deaths assist nearly all deliveries and registration practices are comparable (8). Age-specific mortality rates, available only when analysts compute antepartum, intrapartum, and early neonatal rates separately, provide insights to opportunities for prevention. For example, an excess of intrapartum deaths suggest the need for improved delivery services.

A third measurement problem relates to correctly identifying the cause of death. Such identification is especially difficult for antepartum fetal deaths, when maceration of the fetus may limit a pathologist's ability to diagnose abnormalities. Regional differences in autopsy rates and an overall decrease in the autopsy rate affect comparisons of cause-specific mortality rates (52–54). For fetal and neonatal deaths, autopsies are useful in diagnosing congenital malformations of internal organs, particularly malformations that are not apparent from external examination. Clinicians need autopsy results to distinguish between postneonatal deaths from SIDS (Sudden Infant Death Syndrome) and those from intentional or unintentional suffocation. Even when a cause is correctly identified, however, experts may differ on how to correctly categorize the cause of death (34, 55).

A classification quandary: Are congenital anomalies or prematurity and related causes responsible for most infant deaths?

NCHS' classification attributed 21.5% of infant deaths in 1996 to congenital anomalies and 13.7% to short gestation. Using an alternate classification scheme for infant deaths, Sowards attributed 30.9% of deaths in 1996 to prematurity and related causes and 22.4% to congenital anomalies (55).

Such differences can have important consequences in allocation of funds for research and prevention.

A fourth problem is changes over time in the codes used to assign the cause of death. These coding changes can result in apparent changes in cause-specific mortality rates, distorting mortality trends. For example, in the United States in 1999, ICD-10 replaced ICD-9 as the method for coding the cause of death. As a consequence, a smaller portion of deaths were assigned to birth defects than would have occurred if ICD-9 were used (26).

Infants for whom birth weight information is incomplete almost always have higher mortality rates than those for whom information is complete.

A fifth problem relates to the availability of complete information on attributes of the decedent, such as birth weight, gestational age, and race. Information on these attributes is not randomly missing. Infants for whom birth weight information is incomplete almost always have higher mortality rates than those for whom information is complete, consistent with the likelihood that these infants are low birth weight, preterm, or both. If so, the mortality rates for infants <2,500 g or <37 weeks gestation will be biased downward in areas with large proportions of births with missing data on birth weight or gestational age compared with areas with more complete data (56).

6.2 Descriptive Epidemiology: Overall Mortality

The risk of pregnancy loss is highest at the very start of pregnancy.

Occurrence of death. The risk of pregnancy loss is highest at the very start of pregnancy. Differences in the biological criteria for identifying pregnancies, the attributes of the women under study, and the definition of an early pregnancy loss complicate interpretation of reports of early pregnancy loss and spontaneous abortion. The rate of pregnancy loss between fertilization and implantation probably ranges from 30% to 50% (57) (pp. 44–54). After implantation, approximately 22% of pregnancies are lost before the date of next expected menstrual period (58). In the absence of biochemical testing, nearly all losses occurring within the first 6 weeks past the last menstrual period are indistinguishable from menstrual bleeding to women who experience them (58). Of clinically recognized pregnancies (i.e., pregnancies enduring beyond the date of the next expected menstrual period), up to 20–30% may spontaneously abort before 20 weeks' gestation (Table 6.4) (63–65).

In the United States in 1997, fetal deaths accounted for nearly half of the deaths occurring from 20 weeks of gestation through the first year of life.

From 20 weeks of gestation onward, the incidence of fetal death in the United States in 1998 was 6.7 per 1,000 fetal and live births, with nearly equal incidences of death from 20 through 27 completed weeks of gestation and ≥28 completed weeks (4). In the United States in 1997, 12,292 fetal deaths occurred at 20–27 weeks of gestation, 13,039 fetal deaths at 28 weeks or later, and 27,362 infant deaths occurred. Thus, fetal deaths accounted for nearly half of the deaths occurring from 20 weeks of gestation through the first year of life. This substantial contribution highlights the importance of fetal deaths in the spectrum of reproductive loss. Consistent with racial differences in the gestational age distribution of live births, somewhat more fetal deaths occur at term among Whites (in the United States, 1995–1999: 44%) than among Blacks (30%).

Although fetal death may occur during labor and delivery, currently in developed countries, most fetal deaths occur before labor (66). Several investigators have reported that, near term (i.e., 40 weeks of gestation), the conditional risk for fetal death increases as gestation advances (67–69). For example, in Scotland from 1985 to 1996, the conditional risk of antepartum fetal death among singletons increased from 0.4 per 1,000 at 37 and 38 weeks to 1.9 per 1,000 at 42 weeks and 6.3 per 1,000 at 43 weeks. This pattern may not apply to intrapartum death. The conditional risk of intrapartum fetal death observed in Scotland was low overall, ranging from 0.7 per 1,000 at 37 weeks to 0.4 per 1,000 at 42 weeks (70). These risks exclude deaths from congenital anomalies and deaths among multiple gestations. A pattern of increasing risk for fetal death with advancing gestation has been reported for twin gestations (71).

Table 6.4 Selected reports of rates of early pregnancy loss and spontaneous abortion

Study population	Criteria for detecting pregnancy	Number of pregnancies detected	Percent of pregnancies ending in fetal loss
North Carolina, $n = 211$ women (57, 58)	HCG ≥ 0.025 ng/mL × 3 days	189	Loss ≤ 6 weeks after LMP: 25% Total rate of loss: 31%
5 sites within the U.S., 1980–1985, $n = 432$ nondiabetic, pregnant women (59)	HCG increase; measurement of HCG began 2 days after expected menstrual period	432	Loss <20 weeks: 15.4%
Upstate New York, 1989–1992, $n = 217$ women (60)	HCG ≥ 4.0 pmol/L × 3 days, HCG ≥ 5.33 pmol/L × 2 days, or HCG ≥ 6.67 pmol/L × 1 day	115	Loss from 10 days before through 5 days after expected menses: 19.5%
1 site within the U.S., $n = 200$ women attending an OBGYN center (61)	HCG ≥ 0.15 ng/mL × 3 days	116	Loss of occult pregnancies (not clinically recognized): 13% Loss from pregnancy detection through delivery: 31.3%
7 sites within the U.S., $n = 403$ women semiconductor workers aged 18–44 years (62)	HCG ≥ 0.15 ng/mL × 2 or 3 days	52	Loss of clinically unrecognized pregnancies detected only by elevated HCG: 40.4% Loss <20 weeks of clinically recognized pregnancies: 28.6% Loss <20 weeks for all pregnancies: 51.9%
Semiconductor employees, U.S., 1989–1991; $n = 74$ women without fertility problems (63)	HCG ≥ 0.25 ng/mL × 2 days	66	Loss from 7 days before through 5 days after expected menses: 21% Miscarriage[a] among clinically recognized pregnancies: 21.1%
Anhui, China, 1996–1998, $n = 526$ nulliparous nonsmoking women (64)	HCG analysis with no mention of cut-off values	618	Loss <42 days after LMP: 24.6% Loss ≤ 20 weeks: 32.5%

HCG human chorionic gonadotropin; *LMP* last menstrual period
[a]Length of pregnancy when miscarriage occurred not described by authors

Table 6.5 Percentage of deliveries resulting in fetal death, by gestation and plurality, United States, 1995–2002

Weeks of gestation	Plurality	
	Singleton	Multiple
20–27	22.7	11.6
28–36	1.1	0.5
≥37	0.1	0.1

The increasing conditional risk of antepartum fetal death associated with advancing gestational age raises the possibility of averting these deaths by identifying fetuses at risk of death and delivering them. Delivery of fetuses perceived to be at increased risk of death has been practiced widely in the United States. Criteria for diagnosing increased risk are not uniform. None of the systematic reviews in the Cochrane Database of approaches for monitoring fetal well being (e.g., biophysical profiles) have concluded that the potential benefits of early delivery (increased survival) outweigh the potential risks (increased neonatal death and increased maternal and infant morbidity and long-term disability secondary to prematurity).

Fetal death data for the United States from 1995 through 2002 show that the gestation-specific proportion of deliveries resulting in fetal death decreases as gestation advances. Among preterm deliveries, gestation-specific fetal death rates are lower for fetuses in multiple gestations than those in single gestations (Table 6.5).

> The risk of infant death is greatest immediately after transition to extrauterine life.

The risk of infant death is greatest immediately after transition to extrauterine life at delivery and decreases sharply during the first week of life, after which the rate of decrease in the risk slows (Fig. 6.1). For example, among White infants born from 1995 through 1999 in the United States, the risk of death in the first hour after delivery was 81.5 per 100,000 infants. However, the average mortality risk in the following 23 h dropped to 6.0 deaths/h. The rate of decrease in the risk of infant death slows again at about 6 months of age. Thus nodes of elevated risk occur shortly after conception and just before and after delivery.

Cause of death. The proximate causes of early pregnancy loss, spontaneous abortion, and fetal death change as pregnancy advances. Chromosomal anomalies, many of which are incompatible with life, cause the majority of early pregnancy losses and spontaneous abortions during the first trimester. The proportion of losses that are karotypically abnormal peaks at about 60% at 12 weeks' gestation (57, p 110). The striking similarity during the first trimester in the frequency of karyotypically abnormal losses among different populations and during different eras (57) suggests that these events must be related to underlying biological aberrations in human reproduction.

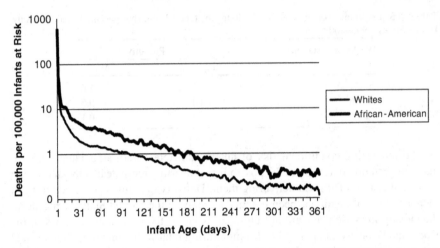

Fig. 6.1 Infant risk of death by age and maternal race, United States, 1995–1999. For deaths at 1–6 days, infant mortality risk equals the number of daily deaths divided by the number of infants surviving the preceding day. To smooth the risks and facilitate visual interpretation, we computed the infant mortality risk at 7–27 days as the 3-day moving average and the risk at 28–362 days as the 5-day moving average

Interpreting data plotted on a logarithmic (log) scale

Log scales are useful for depicting the pace of change in a risk or rate. They show changes in proportion, so that the distance between successive points is equal in proportion (instead of equal in absolute value). For example, on a log scale, the distances between 10, 100, and 1,000 are equal. This is because 100 is 10 times 10 and 1,000 is 10 times 100. When plotted on a log scale, the slope of the line corresponds to the rapidity of change, with nearly horizontal slopes indicating a slow pace of change and nearly vertical slopes indicating a very rapid pace of change.

Although spontaneous abortion of karoytypically abnormal fetuses continues into the second trimester, as gestation advances these abnormal fetuses account for a decreasing proportion of all spontaneous abortions and fetal deaths. After the first trimester, the portion of spontaneous abortions and fetal deaths that are karyotypically abnormal varies substantially among populations (57).

Aside from karotypic abnormalities, spontaneous abortions and fetal deaths are related to fetal factors (e.g., congenital anomalies, plurality, etc), maternal factors, and environmental exposures. The distribution of causes of antepartum death varies by length of gestation. The proportion of deaths attributed to any single cause is population-specific, reflecting the presence or absence of other competing causes of death in the population. A study of fetal deaths occurring in 1998 and 1999 in Stockholm, Sweden, reported that the cause was undetermined for 9% of deaths (72), whereas a study of deaths occurring from 1978 through 1996 in Quebec, Canada, found that the cause could not be determined for 25% of ante-partum fetal deaths (67). A study of late fetal deaths (≥ 28 weeks gestation) from 1982 through 2000 reported that the cause was unknown for about half of all antepartum deaths (73).

The etiologies of infant death also change as the infant ages. In developed countries, the following causes account for most neonatal deaths: immaturity, restricted fetal growth, respiratory distress of the newborn, maternal complications during pregnancy, complications of the placenta, cord, or membranes, and congenital malformations incompatible with life. Thus, the chain of events culminating in neonatal death often originates during pregnancy. In the postneonatal period, congenital malformations, SIDS, infections, and injuries account for the majority of deaths.

A different profile of etiologies for mortality predominates in developing countries, where common causes of intrapartum and neonatal death are intrapartum hypoxia and birth asphyxia and bacterial sepsis of the newborn. These causes are related to the availability of skilled birth attendants, a problem that can be addressed by improving access to health care. Infections cause many deaths throughout infancy. Some of these deaths result from diarrhea and dehydration, which reflect lack of access to clean water and food as well as the absence of adequate rehydration. Other deaths result from respiratory and parasitic infections (e.g., malaria), many of which can be prevented by immunization or effectively treated with medication.

Clearly, early pregnancy losses, spontaneous abortions, fetal deaths, and infant deaths share common etiologies and, to some degree, common patterns of occurrence. These commonalities will be noted in the following three sections, which separately address early pregnancy loss and spontaneous abortion, fetal death, and infant death. Each section begins by presenting the descriptive epidemiology and then considers factors that influence occurrence. The sections on fetal and infant death then address in greater detail the most common causes of death.

6.3   Early Pregnancy Loss and Spontaneous Abortion

Lifetime numbers of pregnancy losses. The number of pregnancy losses an individual woman is likely to experience reflects her fertility: Women who have more pregnancies have more opportunities to experience pregnancy losses. Recent data from the National Survey of Family Growth (NSFG) suggest that, in the United States in 1999, in their lifetimes, women experienced an average of 0.5 fetal losses, most of which were probably early spontaneous abortions (74). Because this number does not include loss of clinically unrecognized pregnancies (i.e., losses before or at the time of expected menses), which occur more frequently than recognized losses, the average number of total pregnancy losses per woman is doubtless higher, perhaps nearly 1.0.

Trends. NSFG data show that, overall, the lifetime likelihood of a fetal loss increased slightly for Hispanics (from 0.5 per woman in 1990 to 0.7 in 1999) and non-Hispanic Whites (from 0.4 in 1990 to 0.5 in 1999), but decreased for non-Hispanic Blacks (from 0.7 in 1990 to 0.6 in 1990) (74). In view of the widespread increasing availability of over-the-counter early pregnancy tests in 1990s, the apparent increases may be an artifact of improved detection of pregnancies at early gestations, when the risk of loss is high.

Demographic variability. Among chromosomally normal pregnancies, male embryos have an approximately 30% higher risk of loss than do females (75). Of all maternal demographic factors, age stands out as having the strongest association with the risk of early pregnancy loss. Furthermore, the association with age is consistent across groups defined by other demographic factors such as race, martial status, and education. Apparent differences in rates of single pregnancy loss among demographic groups defined by these factors are minimal after taking differences in maternal age distributions into account. In contrast, recurrent pregnancy loss has been reported as higher among African-American women as well as those with low socioeconomic status (SES) and education (76).

The association between risk for early pregnancy loss and maternal age is "j-shaped": risks increase somewhat under ages 20 years for women with high gravidity, are lowest at ages 20–24 years, and accelerate rapidly after age 35 years (77, 78). Women who conceive with donor eggs have similar rates of pregnancy loss from age 25 years through their late 40s, after which rates of pregnancy loss increase (79). This observation suggests that much of the increased loss in older women with naturally conceived pregnancies stems from maternal factors. In fact, compared with women in their early 20s, the risk of chromosomally abnormal spontaneous losses increases slightly at maternal ages less than 20 years and increases sharply at ages 35 years and older (57).

Factors influencing occurrence. In general, threats to the conceptus stem from (1) maternal and paternal factors that operate before conception and may manifest as chromosomal or genetic problems or (2) factors that operate during pregnancy through the mother, such as maternal illness or environmental exposures

---

Considerations in studying the causes of spontaneous pregnancy loss

Analysis of demographic and other factors associated with spontaneous pregnancy loss is often limited by:

- Bias in the portion of losses that come to medical attention;
- Lack of information about the presence or absence of chromosomal, genetic, or structural anomalies in the conceptus;
- Variability in gestational ages included in studies.

Many very early losses may not be recognized as such. The mother may instead regard the loss as an irregular menstrual cycle. Losses to women who recognize their pregnancy, but do not seek prenatal care before loss occurs, may never come to medical attention. Such women are more likely to experience barriers to accessing care or unintended pregnancies and thus differ from women who obtain care.

Analysts often do not separate women with karyotypically normal fetuses from those with karyotypically abnormal fetuses. A large portion of early pregnancy losses may be attributable to fetal karyotype abnormalities (80). One study reported that, among spontaneous abortions at <13 weeks, 57% of those in women <35-years old and 82% of those in women >35 years were karyotypically abnormal (81).

Because the contribution of chromosomal abnormalities to spontaneous pregnancy loss diminishes as pregnancy advances, including losses at a wide range of gestations, it increases the probable etiologic heterogeneity of the group. This increased heterogeneity diminishes a researcher's ability to detect risk factors.

(Table 6.6). Chromosomal anomalies in the conceptus are common among spontaneous losses: As many as 69% of first trimester spontaneous losses of clinically recognized pregnancies are chromosomally aberrant (57, 81) (p. 84). Difficulties in obtaining tissue from the conceptus and the cost of karyotyping limit the availability of information on the karyotype of the conceptus. Without knowing the presence or absence of abnormalities in the conceptus, a researcher cannot distinguish pre-and postconception factors. Thus, studies of environmental factors possibly associated with pregnancy loss often have relatively modest relative risks (e.g., 1.5–3.0), because of their inclusion of losses with lethal abnormalities, which would likely have occurred regardless of exposure to the factor under study.

Preconception factors may be maternal or paternal, although distinguishing between the two is usually difficult. An interesting exception is chromosomal trisomies (e.g., trisomy 21, Down's syndrome), where the source of the extra chromosome can be identified as maternal or paternal. Factors operating during pregnancy most frequently are maternal, but paternal exposures may be transmitted through the mother to the conceptus. For example, a conceptus can be exposed to paternal metabolites of cigarette smoke or pesticides through maternal exposure to semen.

6.4 Fetal Death

Temporal trends. In the United States, national vital records data show that the overall rate of fetal death declined modestly from 1990 through 1998 (Fig. 6.2). Nearly all this decline occurred among deaths occurring at ≥28 weeks of gestation (4). Temporal trends for fetal deaths occurring at 20–27 weeks must be interpreted

Table 6.6 Factors influencing early pregnancy loss

Factor	Comments	Selected references
Maternal conditions		
Absence of nausea	Absence of nausea is associated with increased risk	(314)
Antiphospholipid Syndrome	This syndrome is associated with recurrent spontaneous abortion	(315)
Diabetes (Type 1)	Diabetes appears to increase risk for spontaneous loss (316, 317), but the risk may be minimized with adequate control of diabetes (60)	
Fever	Fever in the month preceding the loss was associated with a sixfold increase in risk for spontaneous loss of a euploid fetus (318). However, no association was observed in another study (319)	(318, 319)
Infection	Measles is associated with increased risk for spontaneous abortion	(320)
Infertility and subfertility	Risk depends on cause of infertility	(64)
Interpregnancy Interval	Short and long intervals are associated with increased risk (321)	
Macrophage inhibitory cytokine 1	Low levels at 6–13 weeks' gestation are associated with increased risk. MIC1 may be related to maternal immunomodulatory response to fetus	(322)
Menotropin-induced pregnancies	Use of this assisted reproductive technology increases the risk for early pregnancy loss	(323)
Nutrition	Low level of plasma folate increases risk	(324)
Pregnancy history	Women with history of spontaneous loss have increased risk for another loss	(325, 326)
Pregnancy order	Among women without history of spontaneous abortion, nulliparous women had slightly lower risk at first pregnancy than did parous women (326). Discerning the risk associated with gravidity is complicated by selective fertility (327, 328)	(326)
Thrombophilias		(329)
Uterine abnormalities		(330)
Vascular problems	Spontaneous abortion is associated with 1.5-fold increase in risk for a subsequent maternal cerebrovascular event	(328)
Maternal behaviors		
Alcohol	Prospective study showed that drinking ≥3 drinks per week during the 1st trimester was associated with a 3.9-fold increased risk for spontaneous abortion in the 1st 10 weeks of pregnancy (330)	(332–335)

Caffeine	Some, but not all (336) studies have demonstrated increased risk associated with caffeine consumption. For example, consuming ≥300 mg/day of caffeine was associated with a twofold increase in risk (314). Others found that the risk increased among nonsmokers with fetuses with normal karyotypes and that risk increased for heavy caffeine users who reported nausea and vomiting in early pregnancy (337)	(314, 332, 334–337)
Cigarette smoking	*Active.* Risk increases are proportional to intensity of maternal smoking. One study did not find this association (340)	(334, 341, 342)
	Passive. Increased risk associated with environmental exposure to tobacco smoke (340, 343, 344)	
Diet	Increased risk associated with decreased serum folate (324, 345), decreased preconception serum B6 and folate (345), and iodine deficiency (346)	
Hot tub use	Twofold increase in risk was associated with use in early pregnancy; risk increased with increasing frequency of use	(347)
Maternal environmental exposures		
Contaminated tap water	Contaminants associated with increased risk include arsenic, lead, mercury, potassium, silica	(348–351)
	A study in California showed increased risk associated with consumption of tap water in one region, but not in two other regions (348)	
Organic solvents	Increased risks were observed for percholorethylene, trichloroethylene, and paint thinners	(352, 353)
Maternal occupational exposures		
Cosmetology	Risk increased with number of hours worked per week, number of chemical services performed, and work where nail sculpturing was done	(354)
Dry-cleaning	Exposure to tetrachloroethylene was associated with increased risk. Investigators found increased risk among Finnish dry cleaning workers (355)	(356)
Organic solvents	Organic solvent exposure has been associated with a twofold increased risk for spontaneous abortion	(353)
Standing	Standing for >7 h/day has been associated with relative risks of 1.6–4.3, but only for women with a history of spontaneous abortion	(339, 357)
Toluene, xylene, formaline	Exposure to these chemicals has been associated with a three- to fourfold increased risk for women exposed ≥3 days/week	(358)

(Continued)

Table 6.6 (Continued)

Factor	Comments	Selected references
Embryonic/fetal attributes		
Abnormal karyotypes	The bulk of early pregnancy pregnancy loses are abnormal (81). Embryos and fetuses with abnormal karotypes have a high risk of intrauterine death	
Implantation timing	Implantation 8–10 days after ovulation is associated with lower rates of loss than later implantation	(59)
Multiple gestation	Twinning rate may be as high as 1 out of every 30 spontaneous abortions	(359)
Paternal factors		
Age	Increased risk associated with paternal ages ≥40 years, especially with maternal ages ≥35 years	(77)
Occupational chemical exposures	Pesticides; organic solvents (360), ethylene oxide, rubber chemicals, solvents in refineries, and solvents used in manufacturing rubber products have been associated with increased risk (361)	(360, 361)
Pesticide use		
Other		
Seasonality	Risk peaks in March and August (362) with low rates in summer and autumn. In North Carolina, peaks were found from early September through December (363)	(362–365)

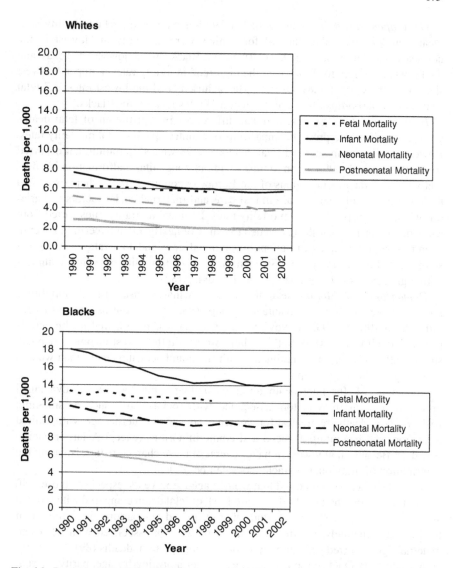

Fig. 6.2 Fetal (deaths ≥20 weeks), infant, neonatal, and postneonatal mortality rates, by maternal race, United States, 1990–2002

cautiously, because improvements in gestational dating and ascertainment have likely influenced ascertainment of these deaths. National vital records data for 1985–1987 and 1995–1998 show that, as the fetal death rate decreased, the preterm delivery rate increased. This pattern is consistent with the possibility that, in recent years, clinicians are inducing labor more frequently in women with fetuses judged to have an elevated risk of antepartum death.

Geographic variability. During the late 1990s, state-specific fetal mortality rates (deaths at ≥ 20 weeks' gestation) for Whites were generally the lowest in the northeast and far west (Fig. 6.3). Rates for Blacks were lowest in Texas and the far west. Of note for Blacks are the high fetal mortality rates in upper Midwest states near the Great Lakes. Overall, Massachusetts had the lowest rates: 3.7 fetal deaths per 1,000 births plus fetal deaths for Whites and 8.6 for Blacks.

International findings. International differences in registration of fetal deaths pose problems in interpreting comparisons of country-specific fetal mortality rates. However, a European study of fetal deaths at ≥ 28 weeks' gestation that occurred from 1993 through 1998 among fetuses without congenital malformation is informative. Using data from regions of ten European countries, researchers examined the contribution of suboptimal clinical care and maternal social factors to variability in country-specific fetal mortality rates. Perinatal mortality rates varied from a low of 4.0 per 1,000 births in Sweden to a high of nearly 9.0 in Greece. In general, countries with low rates of suboptimal clinical care and low rates of maternal smoking had (e.g., Finland and Sweden) lower fetal mortality rates than countries with higher rates of suboptimal care and smoking (82).

Demographic variability. Several reports show that the risk for fetal mortality is highest among socially disadvantaged groups (83, 84). In contrast are results for births from 1988 to 1995 in Nova Scotia, Canada, where essential health care is provided to all women (85). In this cohort, women in the lowest income group had significantly lower risks for perinatal death (fetal and neonatal death) than women in the highest income group.

The high risk for fetal death observed among some socially disadvantaged groups may stem from factors associated with social status, such as smoking. Risks for fetal death are greatest for women at advanced maternal age, with limited education, and belonging to racial and ethnic minorities (except Asian or Pacific Islander). Because many women have several of these characteristics, isolating the contribution of individual characteristics can be difficult.

Several studies have reported that women aged ≥ 35 years, especially those >40 years, have a more than twofold increased risk of fetal death compared with women aged <30 years (67, 86–88). A study that examined antepartum and intrapartum fetal deaths separately reported that the increased risk associated with advanced maternal age occurred for antepartum, but not intrapartum, deaths (89).

A study from Quebec reported that, even after adjusting for age, parity, marital status, and sex, women with <12 years of education had an increased risk for fetal death, compared with those with ≥ 14 years of education (90). An increased risk for fetal death among women with low levels of education has been observed in data from Latin America (88).

Racial disparities in fetal death rates have been consistently observed in the United States and elsewhere, with Black women having two- to threefold higher risks for fetal death than White women (69, 91–96). Using White women as their comparison group, researchers have reported lower rates of fetal death among Chinese women in Canada (97) and Hispanic women who delivered in the United States, but were born in Mexico (91).

A. White

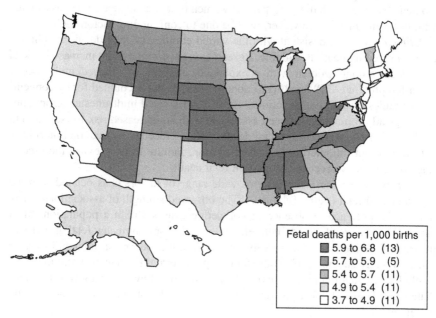

Fetal deaths per 1,000 births
- 5.9 to 6.8 (13)
- 5.7 to 5.9   (5)
- 5.4 to 5.7 (11)
- 4.9 to 5.4 (11)
- 3.7 to 4.9 (11)

B. Blacks

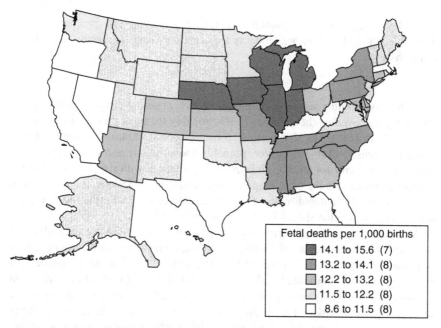

Fetal deaths per 1,000 births
- 14.1 to 15.6 (7)
- 13.2 to 14.1 (8)
- 12.2 to 13.2 (8)
- 11.5 to 12.2 (8)
- 8.6 to 11.5 (8)

Fig. 6.3 State-specific fetal mortality rates (deaths ≥20 weeks), by maternal race, United States, 1999–2000. (**a**) Whites; (**b**) Blacks. Inadequate data to compute stable rates for Alaska, Hawaii, Idaho, Maine, Montana, New Hampshire, New Mexico, North Dakota, South Dakota, Utah, Vermont, and Wyoming

One study reported a higher risk for fetal death among pregnancies of unmarried women compared with those of married women (98). The increased risk associated with not being married, however, may be due to confounding factors (99).

Clinical course. Consistent with the varied etiology of fetal death, the clinical course preceding death is variable. Researchers have reported an increased risk of fetal death among women with unexplained, elevated or reduced midtrimester alpha-fetoprotein (AFP) levels (i.e., abnormal levels not accounted for by congenital anomalies or multiple gestation) (100–102). Elevated midtrimester serum chorionic gonadotropin has also been associated with an increased risk for subsequent fetal death (103). Antepartum fetal death is often preceded by maternal morbidity with or without intrauterine growth restriction. Failure to progress in the second stage of labor may precede intrapartum fetal death.

Factors influencing occurrence. A wide range of factors is associated with the occurrence of fetal death (Table 6.7). The observed strength of associations partly reflects the presence or absence of competing causes within a population. Most causes of fetal death exert their effect through compromising fetal growth or placental function (e.g., maternal hypertension, infection, or thrombophilia). Other causes directly adversely affect the fetus (e.g., maternal Rh sensitization, maternal alcohol use, lethal malformations). Adverse obstetrical events can result in immediate, cataclysmic fetal asphyxia (e.g., placental abruption, compression of the umbilical cord).

> In developed countries, maternal cigarette smoking and preconception overweight and obesity are probably the most prevalent risk factors for fetal death (145).

In developed countries, of all etiologic factors, maternal cigarette smoking and preconception overweight and obesity are probably the most prevalent risk factors for fetal death (145). The risk associated with maternal smoking is proportional to smoking intensity (146). However, probably the strongest and most consistently observed risk factor for fetal death is multiple gestation, with risk increasing as the number of fetuses increases. Compared with singleton gestations, the risk of fetal death is three- to fourfold higher for twin gestations (147). Furthermore, triplets have nearly double the risk of fetal death as twins (148).

Among twins, pairs who are small for gestational age (SGA) or discordant for birth weight have increased risks for fetal death, compared with pairs where each twin has a normal birth weight (149). The risk of fetal death is greater for monozygotic twins compared with dizygotic twins (150). Death of one sibling in a multiple gestation is associated with an increased risk for fetal death in the surviving fetus. Consistent with the shift in gestational age distribution among multiples toward shorter gestations, more fetal deaths among multiples are delivered preterm (90.0% in 1995–1997) than among singletons (77.8%).

Table 6.7 Factors influencing occurrence of fetal death

Factor	Comments and selected references
Maternal attributes	
Chronic illnesses	These disorders include asthma, diabetes, hypertension, thrombophilias, and schizophrenia (88, 104–106). Fetal death may be caused by the disorder itself (e.g., placental abruption associated with hypertension) or treatment for the disorder (e.g., drugs taken for schizophrenia)
Illness acquired during pregnancy	Preeclampsia. In Stockholm County, Sweden 12% of fetal deaths during 1998 and 1999 were attributed to maternal chronic illness and pregnancy-related conditions (72)
Preconception overweight and obesity	Overweight and obesity are associated with an approximately twofold increase in risk for fetal death (109)
Rh sensitization	Maternal Rh sensitization increases the risk for fetal death (88)
Maternal behaviors	
Alcohol	Maternal alcohol use has been associated with fetal death by increasing the risk for placental abruption (108) as well as direct toxic effects on the fetus
Cigarette smoking	Maternal smoking increases the risk for fetal death through fetal growth restriction and placental abruption (68, 109)
Marijuana smoking	Weekly or more frequent maternal marijuana smoking has been associated with a nearly threefold increased risk for fetal death (110)
Fetal attributes	
Growth restriction	Fetal growth restriction is associated with a threefold increase in risk for death (88)
Lethal congenital malformations	In Stockholm County, Sweden, during 1998–1999 10% of the deaths were attributed to congenital malformations (72). The contribution of malformations has likely changed over time, as prenatal diagnosis and termination of affected pregnancies has become more accepted
Multiple gestation	In Stockholm County, Sweden, 5% of all fetal deaths during 1998 and 1999 were due to twin–twin transfusion syndrome (72)
Sex	Males have an increased risk for fetal death of ~20% compared with females (67, 111–118). The increased risk of major malformations among males may partly account for their increased risk of fetal death (119)
Obstetrical factors	
History of fetal death	Women who have experienced one fetal death have a substantially increased risk for a subsequent fetal death (120). The magnitude of this risk is related to the cause of the initial fetal death
Abnormal placentation	

(*Continued*)

Table 6.7 (Continued)

Factor	Comments and selected references
	Placental abnormalities detected during the first 10 weeks of gestation are associated with increased risk for fetal death due to abruption or unexplained death associated with restricted fetal growth (121)
Infections acquired during pregnancy	Infections that increase the risk for fetal death are caused by parvovirus, cytomegalovirus, *Treponema pallidum*, *Toxoplasma gondii*, and *Listeria momocytogenes* (88, 122, 123). In Stockholm County, Sweden, during 1998 and 1999, infections accounted for 24% of all fetal deaths (72)
Interpregnancy interval	Intervals less than 6 months have an increased risk for fetal death (88)
Intrapartum asphyxia	Improved obstetrical care is the most likely explanation for the decrease in intrapartum death that has been observed in industrialized countries during the past two decades. Among fetal deaths in England and Wales during 1992 and 1994, those occurring intrapartum were of higher birth weight and longer gestation than antepartum deaths (124). Intrapartum deaths are associated with cord prolapse and a prolonged second stage of labor in breech presentations (125). In Stockholm County, 5% of all fetal deaths during 1998 and 1999 were due to intrapartum asphyxia (72)
Noncephalic presentation	Noncephalic presentation of the fetus (e.g., breech) increases the risk for fetal death (88). This risk can be nearly eliminated by elective Cesarean delivery
Parity	Primiparas have higher risk than multiparas (68). Some investigators have observed an association between higher parities (e.g., ≥5) and increased risk for fetal death (88, 105, 126, 127). However, others have not observed this association (126)
Placental abruption	Abruption is a frequent cause of fetal death (72, 129, 130). Abruption is commonly associated with maternal hypertension and preeclampsia as well as with high parity and maternal cigarette smoking (131). Abruption may be secondary to blunt abdominal trauma from unintentional injury, such as that occurring in an automobile crash, or intentional injury, such as that occurring from domestic violence (132–135)
Placental insufficiency	Placental insufficiency accounted for 22% of fetal deaths in Stockholm County, Sweden, in 1998 and 1999 (72). Placental problems may be secondary to maternal cigarette smoking, hypertension, thrombophilias, and infections

Prenatal and intrapartum care	Prenatal and intrapartum care decrease the risk for fetal death (88). An increased intensity of obstetrical care is associated with decreased risk of intrapartum death (136)
Trial of labor among women with past Cesarean deliveries	Among women with a previous Cesarean section, a trial of labor is associated with a more than eightfold increase in the risk of perinatal death, regardless of whether the comparison group was other multiparous women or nulliparous women (137)
Umbilical cord complications	Published estimates of the percentage of fetal deaths attributed to umbilical cord abnormalities range from 9% to 15% (72, 138)
Environmental exposures	
Contaminated water, pesticides, water chlorination by-products, and trihalomethanes	Results suggest an increased risk, but not conclusively (139–144)

6.5   Infant Mortality

Temporal trends. In the United States, infant, neonatal, and postneonatal mortality rates declined during 1990s, with the rate of the decline slowing after 1998 (Fig. 6.2). The 1990 infant mortality rate of 9.2 per 1,000 live births, representing 38,351 deaths, dropped to 6.8 in 2001 (27,568 deaths), a decline of 26%. However, preliminary analyses suggest that the national infant mortality rate increased to 7.0 in 2002 (Kochanek DK, Martin JA. Supplemental analyses of recent trends in infant mortality. Health E Stats. 2/13/2004 NCHS). An increase in the early neonatal mortality rate drove this rise. Simultaneously, the late fetal mortality rate decreased, with a net effect of no change between 2001 and 2002 in the perinatal mortality rate.

The drop in the infant mortality rate during the 1990s resulted in large part from decreases in deaths due to congenital anomalies and SIDS. Deaths due to congenital anomalies declined largely because of greater use of prenatal diagnosis and selective pregnancy termination as well as food fortification with folic acid and periconceptional folic acid supplementation. Deaths due to SIDS declined following widespread clinical and public health efforts to encourage the supine sleeping position for infants.

As a result of these changes, the distribution of causes of infant death shifted (Fig. 6.4). In the early 1990s, congenital anomalies and SIDS accounted for more than one-third of all infant deaths and disorders relating to short gestation and low birth weight not elsewhere classified accounted for one-tenth of infant deaths. By 2001, congenital anomalies and SIDS accounted for 28% of all infant deaths while disorders relating to short gestation and low birth weight accounted for 16% of all deaths.

In the United States from 2003 through 2004, compared with White women, a greater percentage of deaths among infants born to Black women occurred neonatally in babies with low birth weight (Table 6.8). Conversely, compared with Black

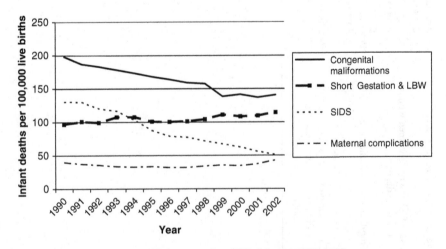

Fig. 6.4 Cause-specific rates of infant mortality, United States, 1990–2002

Table 6.8 Distribution of deaths, by age, birthweight and maternal race, United States, 2003–2004 (Source: 151)

Age at Death (days)	Birthweight (g)	Maternal Race (% of infant deaths)*	
		White	Black
<28	<1,500	45	55
<28	1,500-2,499	10	6
<28	≥2,500	12	7
≥28	<1,500	6	9
≥28	1,500–2,499	6	6
≥28	≥2,500	22	16

*Due to rounding, columns may not sum to 100%

women, a greater portion of deaths among infants born to White women occurred postneonatally in babies with normal birth weight.

Geographic variability. As is evident from these distributions, the state-specific portion of births weighing <1,500 g largely drives a state's infant mortality rate. Although no clinical or public health interventions have been identified to prevent the birth of these very small babies, evidence suggests that the availability of specialty perinatal and neonatal care reduces their risk of death (152–154). Review of state- and race-specific neonatal mortality rates for infants weighing 1,500–2,499 g and ≥2,500 g and postneonatal mortality rates for infants weighing ≥2,500 g shows that rates are generally lowest in California, Florida, Massachusetts, New Jersey, and Texas (Fig. 6.5a–f). A notable exception is the concentration in the Northeast of states with very low rates of postneonatal mortality for White infants with birth weights ≥2,500 g. States with the highest rates vary depending on the measure under consideration. For example, the rates of postneonatal mortality among Black infants with birth weights ≥2,500 g are highest among six contiguous states near the center of the country: Arkansas, Illinois, Indiana, Iowa, Michigan, and Missouri.

International findings. Data from UNICEF estimate a global infant mortality rate of 56 per 1,000 live births for 2002 (UNICEF. State of the world's children, 2004). However, this figure conceals huge international differences in infant mortality rates, which range from a low of 5 per 1,000 live births in industrialized countries to 62 in developing countries and to 99 (equivalent to nearly 10% of live births) in the least-developed countries, which are predominately in sub-Saharan Africa and southeast Asia. Not surprisingly, international disparities in infant mortality are similar to those found for maternal mortality (Chap. 4).

Japan and Scandinavian countries consistently have the lowest infant mortality rates. This occurs despite the markedly lower mean birth weight of Japanese babies.

Data from the WHO and UNICEF shed light on the factors related to the pronounced international differences in infant mortality (Table 6.9). Rates of birth trauma are highest in Cuba, Mexico, and Romania, where access to perinatal

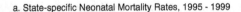

a. State-specific Neonatal Mortality Rates, 1995 - 1999

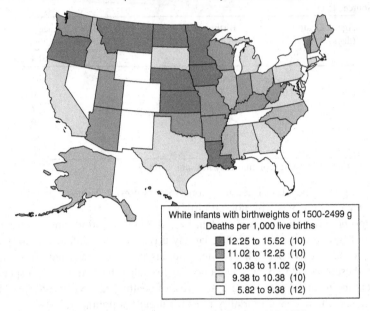

White infants with birthweights of 1500-2499 g
Deaths per 1,000 live births

■ 12.25 to 15.52 (10)
■ 11.02 to 12.25 (10)
▨ 10.38 to 11.02 (9)
☐ 9.38 to 10.38 (10)
☐ 5.82 to 9.38 (12)

b. State-specific Neonatal Mortality Rates, 1995-1999

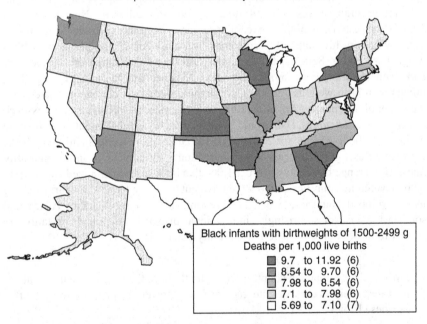

Black infants with birthweights of 1500-2499 g
Deaths per 1,000 live births

■ 9.7 to 11.92 (6)
■ 8.54 to 9.70 (6)
☐ 7.98 to 8.54 (6)
☐ 7.1 to 7.98 (6)
☐ 5.69 to 7.10 (7)

Fig. 6.5 (**a–f**) Inadequate data to compute stable rates for (**a, b**) Alaska, Colorado, Hawaii, Idaho, Iowa, Maine, Montana, Nebraska, New Hampshire, New Mexico, Nevada, North Dakota, Oregon, South Dakota, Utah, Vermont, West Virginia, and Wyoming; (**c, d**) Idaho, Maine, Montana, New Hampshire, North Dakota, Utah, Vermont, and Wyoming; (**e, f**) Alaska, Hawaii, Idaho, Maine, Montana, New Hampshire, New Mexico, Nevada, North Dakota, South Dakota, Utah, Vermont, and West Virginia, and Wyoming

c. State-specific Neonatal Mortality Rates, 1995-1999

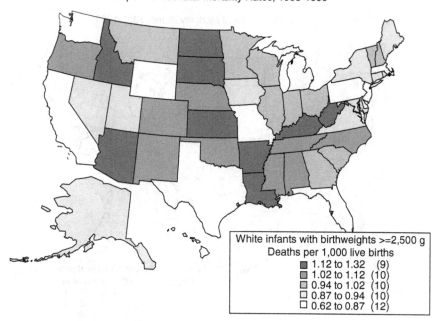

White infants with birthweights >=2,500 g
Deaths per 1,000 live births
■ 1.12 to 1.32 (9)
■ 1.02 to 1.12 (10)
■ 0.94 to 1.02 (10)
□ 0.87 to 0.94 (10)
□ 0.62 to 0.87 (12)

d. State-specific Neonatal Mortality Rates, 1995-1999

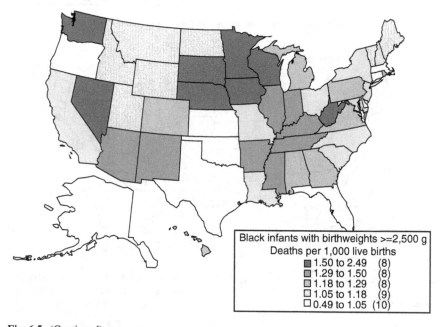

Black infants with birthweights >=2,500 g
Deaths per 1,000 live births
■ 1.50 to 2.49 (8)
■ 1.29 to 1.50 (8)
■ 1.18 to 1.29 (8)
□ 1.05 to 1.18 (9)
□ 0.49 to 1.05 (10)

Fig. 6.5 (Continued)

e. State-specific Postneonatal Mortality Rates, 1995-1999

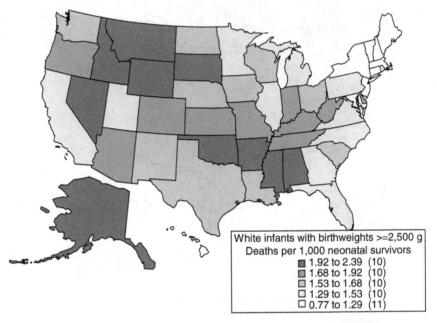

White infants with birthweights >=2,500 g
Deaths per 1,000 neonatal survivors
■ 1.92 to 2.39 (10)
■ 1.68 to 1.92 (10)
□ 1.53 to 1.68 (10)
□ 1.29 to 1.53 (10)
□ 0.77 to 1.29 (11)

f. State-specific Postneonatal Mortality Rates, 1995-1999

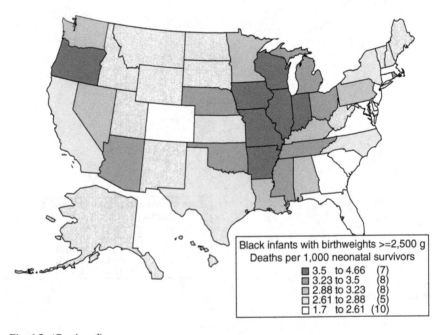

Black infants with birthweights >=2,500 g
Deaths per 1,000 neonatal survivors
■ 3.5 to 4.66 (7)
■ 3.23 to 3.5 (8)
□ 2.88 to 3.23 (8)
□ 2.61 to 2.88 (5)
□ 1.7 to 2.61 (10)

Fig. 6.5 (Continued)

Table 6.9 Age- and cause-specific infant mortality rates for selected countries (Source: 155, 156)

	Cuba, 2000	England & Wales, 1999	Japan, 1999	Mexico, 1999	Romania, 2000	Sweden, 1999	United States, 1999
Infant mortality rate	7.6	5.3	3.2	17.3	26.9	3.5	7.4
Neonatal mortality rate	4.8	1.7	1.5	6.9	8.7	2.3	5.0
Postneonatal mortality rate	2.8	3.6	1.7	10.5	18.2	1.2	2.5
Birth trauma, hypoxia, asphyxia	2.2	0.9	0.5	5.1	3.5	0.6	0.9
Conditions arising in the neonatal period	1.0	1.9	0.5	3.2	2.8	0.8	2.8
Congenital anomalies	2.0	0.9	1.1	3.1	3.6	1.3	1.5
Infectious & parasitic diseases	0.6	0.2	0.1	1.2	0.8	0.0	0.1
Pneumonia and influenza	0.3	0.1	0.1	1.3	5.6	0.1	0.1
SIDS	0.1	0.4	0.3	0.1	0.0	0.3	0.7
Accidents	0.2	0.1	0.2	0.7	0.8	0.0	0.2

specialty care is often limited. Rates of SIDS in some countries, such as Romania and Mexico, are so low that completeness of ascertainment must be questioned.

Demographic variability. Many maternal demographic factors (age, education, social class, marital status, and race) have been associated with the risks for neonatal and postneonatal mortality (Table 6.10). In general, demographic characteristics that represent greater social disadvantage (e.g., fewer years of education) are also associated with greater mortality risks. Low SES is associated with increased risk for infant death, especially perinatal death among infants with birth weights ≥2,500 g and postneonatal death, regardless of birth weight (84, 157, 158).

Exceptions relate to infants with underlying biological factors that strongly increase their risk of death, such as being a twin or a having a very low birth weight (159). Adjusting for intermediate factors, such as use of health care or gestational age distribution, often removes or attenuates the strength of the associations between infant mortality and demographic factors (160–163). For example, a study in Sweden of births from 1973 to 1989 showed that much of the excess risk for neonatal mortality among young teens (aged ≤17 years) stemmed from their increased risk for very preterm deliveries (162).

Table 6.10 Neonatal, postneonatal, and infant mortality by selected maternal, paternal, and infant characteristics and race, United States, 2000–2002

Characteristic	Whites			Blacks		
	Neonatal mortality	Postneonatal mortality	Infant mortality	Neonatal mortality	Postneonatal mortality	Infant mortality
Maternal age (years)						
<17	6.5	3.6	10.1	10.0	5.3	15.3
17–19	4.7	3.3	8.0	8.3	5.3	13.7
20–24	3.6	2.4	6.1	8.2	4.8	12.9
25–29	3.3	1.5	4.9	8.9	3.7	12.6
30–34	3.3	1.2	4.5	9.7	3.5	13.2
35–39	4.0	1.4	5.3	10.5	3.6	14.1
≥40	5.2	2.0	7.2	11.5	4.7	15.3
Maternal education (years)						
0–8	3.8	2.3	6.1	8.5	5.1	13.6
9–11	4.4	3.3	7.6	8.3	6.2	14.5
12	3.9	2.1	6.0	8.6	4.3	12.9
13–15	3.2	1.5	4.7	8.3	3.3	11.6
16	2.8	0.9	3.7	7.9	2.5	10.4
>16	2.6	0.8	3.4	7.2	2.5	9.7
Marital status						
Married	3.3	1.4	4.8	8.4	3.0	11.4
Other	4.6	2.9	7.6	9.1	4.9	14.1
Maternal ethnicity						
Hispanic	3.8	1.8	5.6	7.2	2.6	9.8
Non-Hispanic	3.6	1.9	5.5	8.9	4.4	13.3
Mother's country of birth						
United States	3.7	2.0	5.6	8.8	4.6	13.4
Elsewhere	3.3	1.5	4.8	6.7	2.4	9.1

Paternal race						
White	3.3	1.6	4.9	5.9	2.8	8.7
Black	4.6	3.2	7.8	7.4	3.6	11.0
Unknown	6.5	3.6	10.2	11.7	5.6	17.3
Trimester prenatal care began						
1	3.4	1.7	5.0	8.4	3.8	12.2
2	3.1	2.6	6.0	5.5	4.8	10.3
3	1.8	2.8	4.5	2.2	5.2	7.3
No prenatal care	20.8	5.6	26.4	40.4	11.6	51.9
Gravidity						
1	3.7	1.6	5.3	8.3	3.4	11.8
2	3.2	1.7	5.0	7.9	4.1	12.0
3	3.4	2.0	5.3	8.3	4.5	12.7
>=4	4.7	2.4	7.2	11.0	5.5	16.5
Sex of infant						
Male	4.0	2.1	6.1	9.7	4.7	14.5
Female	3.3	1.6	5.0	8.0	3.9	11.9
Plurality						
Singleton	3.1	1.8	4.8	7.7	4.1	11.8
Twin	20.3	3.9	24.2	41.3	10.9	52.2
Triplet or higher-order	58.7	7.0	65.7	91.7	13.8	105.5

Mortality rates per 1,000 infants. Postneonatal mortality computed as deaths per 1,000 neonatal survivors

How does low socioeconomic status increase infant mortality?

The mechanisms that researchers have proposed to explain the adverse effects of low SES include: psychological effects (e.g., low self-esteem, shame, distrust), material deprivation, income inequity, and inadequate investment in social institutions (164). On a national basis, per capita gross domestic product is positively associated with health (164). Higher per capita GDPs are also associated with greater levels of trust and participation in voluntary organizations.

Although some researchers have observed that increases in the differences of the incomes of the rich and the poor are associated with decreases in overall measures of health, others have not confirmed this relationship (165, 166). In Israel, reductions in income disparities, achieved mainly through transfer payments, correlated with reductions in infant mortality (167). However, evidence from India suggests that, even in the on-going context of low per capita income, sustained investment in the social environment (e.g., gender equality, education) can result in infant mortality rates nearing those of industrialized countries (168).

Clearly, an absolute level of material deprivation has adverse consequences for health. Faced with limited popular support for increasing income transfers (i.e., welfare), American policymakers aiming to improve infant outcomes may find greater support for broadly based programs that invest in human capital and improve the social environment.

Most demographic factors do not act directly as risk factors, but are likely markers for other factors, such as health behaviors, general health status, social support, or access to or use of health care. For example, the absence of paternal information on the birth certificate may reflect lack of paternal support, which in turn may be associated with less advantageous economic or social circumstances for the mother and her infant (169). Of note is that infants whose birth certificates lack information on paternal race have higher mortality than infants of women who are not married, but have named a father on the birth certificate (Table 6.10).

Overall, the risk of infant mortality among singleton infants has a u-shaped relationship with maternal age, increasing moderately for younger women and sharply for older women, compared with those in their twenties. Such is not the case for twins, for whom the risk of mortality is greatest at the youngest maternal ages, decreasing at older ages (170). The finding of an increased risk for postneonatal death among infants of very young mothers (aged ≤15 years) may stem from deficits in the mothers' abilities to care for their infants. However, advanced maternal age (≥35 years) is a biological risk. The increased risk for neonatal mortality among infants of women aged ≥35 likely stems from their greater prevalences of chronic health conditions, such as hypertension and diabetes. These conditions result in inherently greater risks for pregnancy complications and neonatal death. Additionally, women with infertility or previous pregnancy losses likely comprise a larger portion of older gravidas than younger gravidas. A history of infertility or prior pregnancy loss is associated with an increased risk of infant death (171, 172).

The risks for neonatal and postneonatal death vary by birth weight and race (Table 6.11). Extreme deviations from a population's norm for birth weight, either in terms of very low weight or very high weight, are associated with increased risks for death, especially neonatal death (173–176). Similarly, extreme deviations from the weight expected for an individual baby based on his mother's pregnancy history are also associated with increased risks for perinatal mortality (177).

Compared with White infants, overall, Black infants have a higher risk for neonatal death, which is largely – but not totally – driven by the excess of preterm births among Black infants, especially very preterm births (178). Among infants born preterm, however, Black babies have better neonatal survival than do White babies. The associations between maternal race and preterm birth as well as those between race and intrauterine growth restriction are poorly understood, but persistently observed, even when accounting for demographic factors. Preterm birth and growth restriction increase the risk of infant death. Regardless of birth weight, however, Black infants have a higher risk of postneonatal death than do White infants.

The reasons for the Black–White disparities in infant mortality are not understood. Compared with White mothers, as a group, Black mothers have higher prevalences of demographic attributes associated with increased risks for infant mortality. Eliminating these differences, however, is unlikely to eliminate the Black–White disparity in infant mortality. Several studies have shown that disparities in neonatal and postneonatal mortality persist, even among socially advantaged women, such as those with college educations or those residing in nonimpoverished neighborhoods (179).

Infanticide, neglect, and excess mortality among female infants in India and China

Among a cohort of nearly 3,700 pregnancies occurring in a rural county in China in 1999, the early neonatal mortality rate was 69 per 1,000 births among girls and 24 per 1,000 among boys (250).

A recent report from an urban community in India showed infant mortality rates of 72 per 1,000 among girls and 55 per 1,000 among boys (251). Twice as many female infants died from diarrhea (a treatable condition) than did male infants. Among unexplained infant deaths, 75% occurred among females. Because girls usually have a lower infant mortality rate than boys, one can infer that 20 deaths out of every 1,000 births among girls could have been prevented.

Even with smaller female–male differentials in infant mortality than found in these reports, given that China and India accounted for approximately 33% of the world's 133 million births in 2000, the overall impact of the excess mortality among females is staggering.

Table 6.11 Neonatal, postneonatal, and infant mortality rates by birth weight and race, United States, 2000–2002

Birth weight	Neonatal mortality 1			Postneonatal mortality			Infant mortality		
	Blacks	Whites	Black–White ratio	Blacks	Whites	Black–White ratio	Blacks	Whites	Black–White ratio
<1,500	227.9	207.0	1.1	38.8	25.4	1.5	266.7	233.3	1.1
1,500–1,999	14.2	18.5	0.8	11.9	8.7	1.4	26.1	27.2	1.0
2,000–2,499	4.8	6.5	0.7	6.5	4.9	1.3	11.3	11.4	1.0
2,500–3,999	1.1	0.8	1.4	2.7	1.4	1.9	3.9	2.2	1.8
4,000–4,499	0.9	0.5	1.8	1.9	0.8	2.4	2.8	1.3	2.2
≥4,500	3.2	1.1	2.9	2.2	1.0	2.2	5.4	2.1	2.6

Rates per 1,000 line births

Infant characteristics. Short gestation, inadequate intrauterine growth, male sex, and multiple gestation all increase the risk of infant death (Tables 6.10 and 6.12). A substantial portion of the excess risk of death among twins and triplets stems from their greater risks of preterm delivery and intrauterine growth restriction (249). For example, in 1997, 55% of twins were delivered preterm, 14.1% were delivered preterm and SGA, and 20.4% were delivered at term, but were SGA.

Despite their heavier birth weight, male infants consistently have higher mortality than do female infants. The male–female differential is greatest in early pregnancy when the loss rate is 30% higher for male fetuses compared with female fetuses. Males have higher risk of preterm delivery than do females and preterm males are more likely to die than preterm females (75).

Factors influencing occurrence. A comparison of Tables 6.7 and 6.12 shows that many of the same factors influence the risks for both late fetal and neonatal death. Having survived gestation, an infant's fitness for on-going survival is influenced by exposures transmitted during gestation through the mother and by the length of gestation itself (Table 6.12). Gestational length in turn is influenced by maternal health, uterine conditions, and fetal–maternal interactions (see Chap. 7). Maternal antenatal conditions exert their effect by compromising the fetus' growth and/or by prompting clinicians to deliver an infant preterm to rescue him from an adverse intrauterine environment.

After birth, survival is influenced by fitness, environmental exposures (defined in their broadest sense), infant maturation, and care. Although prenatal exposures predominately influence neonatal survival, they also effect postneonatal survival. For example, maternal smoking during pregnancy influences neonatal survival by increasing the risks for preterm delivery and growth restriction, each of which is independently associated with survival. Smoking during pregnancy also appears to influence postneonatal survival through poorly understood mechanisms that increase an infant's risk for SIDS (252).

Environmental exposures range from physical attributes of the environment (for example, temperature and air quality), structural aspects of the environment (such as soft bedding or absence of safety restraints when riding in an auto) and contaminants in the air or water. Environmental exposures also include undefined aspects of season of birth that influence mortality risk. The effects of these exposures tend to be most pronounced after the neonatal period, when many infants with severely compromised fitness have already died.

Physiologic maturation plays an important role in an infant's likelihood of survival. For example, the protection from infection conferred by maternal antibodies passively transferred to the fetus during gestation begins to wane immediately after birth, with rates of infection beginning to increase at about 6 months of age, depending on the amount of antibody transferred. Difficulties in neurological maturation are hypothesized to be responsible in part for the distinctive age at death distribution seen with SIDS.

The nurturing provided to an infant by caregivers and the health care provided to him by clinicians are equally important in determining survival. Before conception, a mother cares for her baby by optimizing her health and nutrition, including folic acid supplementation. For example when women with type 1 diabetes achieve good glycemic control before conception, their risks for perinatal death are reduced (238). During pregnancy, a mother cares for her infant by avoiding adverse exposures (e.g., cigarettes, alcohol, cocaine) and using prenatal care. After delivery, parental care continues through insuring adequate nutrition for the infant, protecting the infant from environmental risks (for example, tobacco smoke), and seeking preventive and therapeutic health care for the infant as indicated.

Health care for the mother during pregnancy and for the infant during and after delivery are generally associated with reduced mortality risks. Some of this reduction is likely due to confounding effects of related maternal behaviors. For example, compared with other women, those who seek early prenatal care are more likely to have intended pregnancies and practice other positive health behaviors. This clustering of behaviors is apparent in the relationship between trimester of initiation of care and postneonatal mortality (Table 6.10).

A number of studies support the notion that, within a country, greater access to both primary care and specialized perinatal or neonatal care is associated with lower infant mortality rates (154, 167, 242). International comparisons, however, do not support this relationship, suggesting that factors other than medical care exert important influences on infant mortality risks (240).

6.5.1   Infant Mortality Due to Sudden Infant Death (SIDS)

In 1991, a panel convened by National Institute of Child Health and Human Development defined SIDS as "the sudden death of an infant under one year of age, which remains unexplained after the performance of a complete postmortem investigation, including an autopsy, examination of the death scene, and review of the case history" (253). Subsequently, investigators have disputed limiting SIDS to deaths during the first year of life, which excludes the small number of apparent SIDS occurring in early childhood. Another concern is that the definition excludes infants for whom a death scene investigation was not conducted.

Because the diagnosis of SIDS is made by excluding other causes of death, it is susceptible to confusion with other causes of postneonatal death, particularly abuse. Researchers examining unexplained infant deaths have observed that their epidemiologic profile included some aspects that were similar to the profile for SIDS, suggesting that some of these unexplained deaths were, in fact, due to SIDS (254). The National Center for Health Statistics recommends that "when sudden infant death syndrome (SIDS) is suspected, a complete investigation should be conducted, typically by a medical examiner. If the infant is under 1 year of age, no cause of death is determined after scene investigation, clinical history is reviewed, and a complete autopsy is performed, then the death can be reported as (SIDS). If the investigation is not complete, the death may be reported as presumed to be (SIDS)." (National Center

Table 6.12 Factors influencing the occurrence of infant death

Factor	Comment and selected references
Maternal attributes	
Diabetes	Women with type 1 or type 2 diabetes before conception have twofold or higher increases in risks for neonatal mortality compared with healthy women (180, 181). Tight periconceptional and prenatal glycemic control among women with type 1 diabetes is not sufficient to avert this increased risk (182, 183)
Nutrition	*Preconception.* Maternal obesity increases the risk for early neonatal death, with the amount of increase proportional to the severity of obesity (184)
	Prenatal. Although some investigators have concluded that participation in the federal Special Supplementation Program for Women, Infants and Children (WIC) lowers the risk for infant mortality (185), others have found that WIC's impact is uncertain (186, 187)
Maternal behaviors	
Alcohol	Binge or heavy drinking during pregnancy can increase the risk of infant death secondary to alcohol-induced fetal malformations. Parental drinking during infancy can impair care-giving abilities, as suggested by the finding that siblings of infants with fetal alcohol syndrome (FAS) have an increased risk of death, compared with siblings of non-FAS infants (188)
Breastfeeding	In a sample of infants born in the United States in 1988, infants who were ever breastfed had 20% lower risk of postneonatal death than those never breastfed. Longer duration of breastfeeding conferred greater reductions in risk for postneonatal death (189)
Changing partner	Infants born to women who conceived with a different man than their previous pregnancy have an 80% higher adjusted risk of infant mortality (190)
Child abuse	Among infants identified as abused in Alaska from 1994 to 2000, the mortality rate was 12.3 per 1,000 (191)
Domestic violence	A study of police-reported partner violence in Washington State (1995–1999) found that infants born to women who had experienced violence had a three-and-a-half-fold increase in their risk for neonatal death (192). Increased rates of very low birth weight babies and very preterm deliveries accounted for part of this increase. Studies in developing countries support the association between prenatal physical or sexual abuse and increased risk for infant mortality (193, 194)
Drug use	Maternal prenatal heroin use appears to increase the risk for neonatal mortality (195). In one study, newborns weighing <2,500 g and screening positive for cocaine and opiates had a sixfold higher risk of death during the first 2 years of life than screen-negative newborns (196). Maternal prenatal polydrug use is associated with an increased risk for the Sudden Infant Death Syndrome (SIDS) (197)

(*Continued*)

Table 6.12 (Continued)

Factor	Comment and selected references
Smoking	A study of infants born in the United States in 1997 found that, overall, maternal smoking is associated with a 40% increase in risk for infant death (198). The effect of smoking was greatest among American Indians. The hazard for smoking increases with gestation and is greatest for term deliveries (199). In general, effect of smoking is strongest for postneonatal, rather than neonatal deaths. In the United States in 1997, 14% of the postneonatal deaths among Whites, 9% among Blacks, and 13% among American Indians were attributed to maternal prenatal smoking (198)
Sleep practices for infant	*Prone position.* A study in Tasmania from 1988 to 1995 found that infants placed in the prone position for sleeping had a more than tenfold higher risk of postneonatal death than those placed supine (200). Other researchers have found that infants who routinely sleep on their stomach (prone) have a two-or-greater-fold increased risk for SIDS than those placed to sleep on their back (201, 202) Co-sleeping. Some, but not all, studies suggest that infants who sleep with an adult have an increased risk for SIDS or accidental postneonatal death (203–206). The risk appears to be mediated by location of sleep (bed vs. sofa), adult fatigue, parental smoking, and other factors.
Use of prenatal care	*Delayed entry to prenatal care.* In unadjusted analyses, neonatal mortality is higher among infants of women who start prenatal care in the first trimester compared with infants whose mothers begin later. In contrast, postneonatal mortality is lower among infants of women with first-trimester entry to prenatal care (Table 6.10). *No prenatal care.* Lack of prenatal care is associated with twofold higher risk for neonatal mortality and a slightly smaller increase in risk for postneonatal mortality. The protective effect of prenatal care in averting neonatal death is evident for both White and Black infants and is most pronounced for infants delivered at or after 36 weeks of gestation. The protective effect of prenatal care in averting postneonatal deaths is most pronounced for infants delivered with selected risk factors, such as postterm pregnancy or small for dates (207, 208)
Fetal/infant attributes Birth defects	Overall in the United States, birth defects are leading cause of infant mortality, accounting for nearly 20% of infant deaths in 1999. Among Black infants, however, prematurity is the leading cause of infant death (209)
Gestation, birth weight, and fetal growth	*Short gestation,* measured either directly by weeks in utero or low birth weight is consistently associated with increased neonatal and postneonatal mortality, with the magnitude of the increase inversely proportional to the length of gestation *Prolonged gestation* increases the risk for neonatal and postneonatal death, largely due to increased frequency of small for gestational age (210, 211) *Inadequate or excessive fetal growth* is associated with increased risk for infant death (161, 173)

Infection	Group B streptococcal infection increases the risk for neonatal death and is a key pathogen associated with infection-related neonatal mortality in the United States (212, 213). In developing countries, bacterial infections are the most common reason for neonatal hospital admission (214)
Length at birth	A study in Norway showed that, within birth weight strata, perinatal mortality is lowest slightly below the median length, sharply rising as the z-score for length deviated from the mean length (215)
Plurality, birth order, and weight discrepancy	Overall, singletons have lower infant mortality than infants from multiple gestations, largely due to excess preterm delivery among multiple deliveries (Table 6.10). Among twins, infants born second have higher mortality compared with those born first (216). Differences in birth weight of >15% in same-sex twins or >30% in different-sex twins are associated with increased risk of neonatal death, with the magnitude of the difference proportional to the increase in risk (217, 218)
Sex	Neonatal and postneonatal mortality rates are higher for boys than for girls (Table 6.10), and this relationship persists across all birth weight strata (219)
Obstetrical factors	
First and second trimester vaginal bleeding	Threatened miscarriage during the first or second trimester increases the risk for neonatal mortality (220, 221)
Placental problems	Placenta previa is associated with a three- to fourfold increased risk for neonatal death, resulting mainly from preterm delivery (222, 223). Even at term, placenta previa doubles the risk of neonatal death
Exposure to labor	Among small-for-gestational age infants delivered at <32 weeks, exposure labor increases the risk of neonatal mortality by 80%. At all gestational ages, exposure to labor decreases the risk of late neonatal and postneonatal death (224)
Obstetrical intervention	Increasing rates of induced delivery, particularly at gestations near term (17, 20, 21), is associated with decreasing rates of stillbirth and infant death. Despite the contribution to rising rates of preterm delivery, induction near term may have the overall benefit of reducing perinatal mortality (148, 225)
Method of delivery	Among very low birth weight (VLBW) infants with breech presentation, Cesarean delivery may be associated with halving the risk of neonatal mortality. Among VLBW infants with vertex presentation and no obstetrical risk factors, a protective effect of Cesarean delivery is not observed (226–228). Among term deliveries of breech infants without malformations, elective Cesarean delivery reduces infant mortality by more than half, compared with vaginal delivery (229)
Short or long interpregnancy interval	In Sweden, 1983–1997, intervals >72 months increased the risk for neonatal death by 30% (OR 1.3; 95% CI 0.9–2.1). Short intervals were not associated with the risk for neonatal death (230). In contrast, in Scotland, from 1992 to 1998, among women whose first pregnancy ended in a term live birth, an interpregnancy interval <6 months was associated with a 3.5-fold increase in the risk for neonatal death unrelated to birth defects, after adjusting for confounders (231)

(Continued)

Table 6.12 (Continued)

Factor	Comment and selected references
Preeclampsia and eclampsia	Most, but not all, studies show that severe preeclampsia and prenatal eclampsia increase the risk for neonatal death, largely due to induced very preterm delivery (233–235)
Health care	
Immunizations	Maternal tetanus immunization, before or during pregnancy, can nearly eliminate neonatal mortality due to tetanus (236, 237)
Neonatal vitamin supplementation	In India, newborn supplementation with oral Vitamin A reduced mortality up to 6 months of age by 22% (238)
Preconception care	Preconception care aimed at optimizing maternal health can reduce adverse pregnancy outcomes. For example, preconception and early pregnancy care reduced perinatal deaths among women with type 1 diabetes (239)
Perinatal specialty hospital care	For VLBW infants, maternal residence in either a county with a hospital providing subspeciality perinatal care or in a county adjacent to one with such a hospital is associated with reduced risk of neonatal death (240)
Specialized neonatal care	Among infants ≤32 weeks gestation delivered in France in 1997, in-hospital mortality for those delivered in hospitals with primary or secondary neonatal care was 8 times higher than for those delivered in hospitals with tertiary neonatal care (154)
	However, international comparisons suggest that "greater neonatal intensive care facilities are not consistently associated with lower birth-weight specific infant mortality" (240). Thompson et al. speculate that "Provision of preconception and prenatal care may be important in explaining international differences in neonatal mortality."
	Data from the United States for 1995 showed that areas with 4.3 neonatologists per 10,000 live births had 7% lower rates of infant mortality than areas with 2.7 neonatologists per 10,000 births. The number of neonatal intensive care beds per 10,000 live births was not associated with neonatal mortality (152). Although the risk of neonatal mortality did not decline as the regional supply of neonatologists rose above 4.3 per 10,000 live births, 60% of infants were born in areas with such an excess
	In another study, which examined babies weighing <2,000 g who were born in California in 1992 and 1993, it was found that those born in a hospital without a regional neonatal intensive care unit (NICU) had a more than twofold increased risk of neonatal death (153)

Primary care access	Analysis of U.S. births from 1985 through 1995 showed that, after adjusting for confounders, states with higher numbers of primary care providers had lower infant mortality rates (163)
Weekday of delivery	Although fewer babies are born on weekends (Saturday and Sunday) than on weekdays, several studies have shown that infants born on weekends have a 10% or higher risk of early neonatal death (241, 242). Some investigators attribute the higher risk to an excess of preterm deliveries on the weekends (241); however, other investigators have not confirmed this relationship (243)

Environmental exposures

Air pollution	Data from Great Britain show that residential proximity to industrial cokeworks is not associated with neonatal or postneonatal mortality (247). Data from the United States show an association between ambient SO_4^{2-} and infant mortality (245)
Seasonality	A greater portion of infant deaths occur in the winter (December–February) than in the summer (June–August). Except for deaths due to trauma, the ratio of winter–summer deaths is greater for postneonatal deaths than for neonatal deaths (246)
Passive smoking	Passive exposure to tobacco smoke increases the risk for SIDS, a leading cause of postneonatal mortality (247)
Weekday	Some, but not all, studies show an increased risk for SIDS on weekend days, especially Sunday (248)

for Health Statistics: Possible solutions to common problems in death certification. http://www.cdc.gov/nchs/about/major/dvs/brief.htm, accessed October 28, 2004.)

A defining feature of SIDS is the association between age and risk. Risk peaks from 60 through 90 days of life among term infants, but at later ages among infants delivered preterm (255).

Ascertainment. In the United States, SIDS is usually ascertained from death certificates, which may be supplemented by reports from medical examiners. A difficulty in using death certificates is that, although they may indicate that an autopsy was performed, one cannot assume that complete results of the autopsy were available when the cause of death was recorded on the certificate.

Incidence. In the United States in 2004, 2,246 deaths were attributed to SIDS. These deaths comprised 8% of all infant deaths and occurred at an annual rate of 54.6 per 100,000 infants (27). SIDS incidence varies widely by geographic location, demographic attributes, season, and prenatal and postnatal exposures and practices (256). For example, during the 1980s in the United States, among Native Americans

The interpretation of a fetal or infant mortality rate depends, in part, on the denominator used to represent the population at risk.The "Back to Sleep" campaign in the United States during the early 1990s reduced the incidence of SIDS by nearly half. Other countries who also promoted the prone sleeping position for infants experienced decreases in SIDS incidence of similar magnitude.

and Alaskan Natives, the incidence was 4.6 per 1,000 live births, but much lower among Native Americans in the Southwest (257). Most areas that have aggressively promoted supine sleeping position for infants have observed substantial declines in SIDS incidence (Fig. 6.4) (258, 259).

Demographic factors. SIDS incidence is lowest for infants of Asian women and highest in those of African-American and Native American mothers. In 2000 in the United States, rates per 1,000 live births ranged from 1.2 for Blacks and American Indians to 0.5 for Whites and 0.3 for Hispanics, Asians, and Pacific Islanders. In 2000, 26% of the excess mortality of American Indians compared with Whites can be attributed to SIDS. Incidence in Hispanics is slightly higher than that of Whites, which is about half the rate of African-Americans. Markedly higher incidences have been observed in indigenous populations outside of the United States (e.g., Native Americans in Canada and Aborigines in Australia) (260–262).

Increased risk for SIDS is experienced in infants of mothers who are of lower socio-economic status, teenaged, and unmarried, whose partners are unemployed and who have fewer years of education (263–267).

Factors associated with occurrence. Maternal behaviors play an important role in the incidence of SIDS (Table 6.13). Risks are reduced with breastfeeding, but increased with smoking and/or drinking alcohol during pregnancy. A recent study among Northern Plains Indians reported a high adjusted odds ratio for prenatal binge drinking (OR 8.2; 1.9–35.3). The association with binge drinking has not been recognized by other investigators, perhaps because of methodologic problems in correctly ascertaining binge drinking (295).

Table 6.13 Selected risk factors influencing the occurrence of SIDS

Factor	Comments and selected references
Maternal attributes	
Weight	Infants of women with high preconception weights have increased risks for SIDS, but only when they sleep with their mother (268)
Maternal behaviors	
Breastfeeding	Compared with exclusive breastfeeding for ≥16 weeks, exclusive breastfeeding for <4 weeks was associated with a fivefold increased risk for SIDS, with smaller increases in risk associated with longer durations of exclusive breastfeeding (269)
Drinking	Binge drinking during pregnancy is associated with increased risk for SIDS. Maternal binge drinking (≥5 drinks) on the day before or the day of SIDS is associated with sixfold increase in the risk of SIDS, compared with women who did not drink or drank moderately (270)
Sleeping practices for infant	Increased incidence is associated with prone or side sleeping position, bed sharing, soft bedding, sleeping on a previously used bed, especially if the bed came from another household, and overheating secondary to excessive bedcovers or clothing (201, 266, 271–279)
Smoking	Prenatal smoking is associated with a three- to fourfold increase in the risk for SIDS (248). Neither paternal smoking during or after pregnancy nor maternal smoking after pregnancy are associated with increased risk for SIDS (252)
Fetal/infant attributes	
Family history of SIDS	"SIDS deaths showed strong sibship aggregation consistent with genetic susceptibility in subsets of SIDS that may interact with environmental factors." (280)
Gestation, birth weight, and fetal growth	Low birth weight, whether due to preterm delivery, fetal growth restriction, or both, is associated with increased risks for SIDS (281, 282)
Infection	SIDS is often preceded by a non–life-threatening respiratory infection. The presence of the infection per se may be less important than the inflammatory response to it (283–285)
Plurality	Twins have a higher risk for SIDS than singletons (282), but this increase appears because of the increased proportion of twins who are preterm or low birth weight (286, 287)
Sex	Males have a higher risk for SIDS than do females (282, 288)
Obstetrical factors	
Parity	Infants delivered to women with higher parities have an increased risk of SIDS (288)
Preeclampsia/eclampsia	Preeclampsia and eclampsia have been associated with a 50% increase in risk for SIDS (289)

(Continued)

Table 6.13 (Continued)

Factor	Comments and selected references
Health care	
Inadequate prenatal care	Fewer visits for prenatal care are associated with increased risk for SIDS (281, 290)
Environment	
Altitude	The risk of SIDS increases with increasing altitude (291)
Season of birth	Even after accounting for season of death, risk of death from SIDS is 37% higher among infants born in August than those born in April (292)
Season of death	Death rates are twofold higher in winter than in summer, possibly due to higher exposure to infectious diseases in the winter (Mage, Malloy). The seasonal relationship persists in Hawaii, where the temperature is nearly constant throughout the year (Mage). Since the "Back to Sleep" campaign in the United States, the magnitude of the winter–summer differential has diminished (Malloy). Similar changes have been observed elsewhere as SIDS rates dropped (293). Seasonality is more pronounced among infants who die from SIDS at younger ages (294)

Postnatally, factors under the control of the infant's caregivers influence his risk of death from SIDS. Increased incidence is associated with prone or side sleeping position, bed sharing, soft bedding, sleeping on a previously used bed, especially if the bed came from another household, and overheating secondary to excessive bedcovers or clothing (201, 266, 271–279). Infants born at higher parities and those who are first-born, males, low birth weight (by virtue of growth restriction or preterm delivery), or from a multiple gestation have an elevated risk for SIDS (265, 266). Incidence is highest in the winter and during the night. One study suggests that deaths occurring during the night are etiologically distinct from those occurring during the day (296).

The magnitude of relative risks associated with many of the risk factors for SIDS is in the range of 2–3, varying among populations, over time, and by the adequacy of accounting for confounding factors and effect modifiers. No single factor seems to account for a substantial portion of the occurrences of SIDS. In seeking to explain the etiology of SIDS, researchers (297, 298) have supported the hypothesis that SIDS results from three factors: (1) intrinsic vulnerability (e.g., prenatal brain stem damage); (2) age-specific (developmental) factors; and (3) immediate precipitating factors (e.g., minor infections). Others judge that the wide range of factors associated with SIDS is more consistent with a multifactorial etiology that does not require the presence of intrinsic vulnerability (299). Evidence of interactions between risk factors, such as season of death, and attributes of SIDS victims, such as age at death, suggest that multiple etiologies may have a common final manifestation as SIDS (294).

6.6 Public Health Interventions, Their Availability, and Use

In this section, we consider public health interventions aimed at preventing fetal and infant death. These interventions include actions to improve access to clinical services and remove barriers to and demand for them. They also include actions to promote specific behaviors in either women or their health-care providers.

We judge an intervention to be public health in nature when it applies broadly to a health-care system (e.g., immunization registries that automatically generate reminder and recall notices) or population (e.g., laws mandating use of infant car seats).

Although a wide range of interventions (Table 6.14) have been proposed for reducing fetal and infant mortality, strong evidence for the effectiveness of many of these interventions is lacking. The fact that many of these interventions have become routine practice – despite the absence of evidence – complicates conduct of intervention trials to evaluate them. Such trials require a control group that does not receive the intervention, a condition that potential participants may refuse to accept for practices they view as routine. Because of this, observational studies, rather than experimental studies, may be the only feasible way to assess interventions.

Table 6.14 Selected objectives and actions for reducing fetal and infant mortality and their related public health intervention, by quality of evidence.

Objectives and actions	PH intervention to achieve objective	Quality of evidence[a]
Before pregnancy, reduce fetal and infant deaths due to birth defects and low birthweight by: • Encouraging pregnancy intendedness; • Promoting interpregnancy intervals 6 months; • Optimizing maternal health; • Ceasing tobacco and alcohol use; and • Insuring adequate maternal intake of folic acid.	1. Contraceptive equity legislation 2. Government subsidies of family planning services (300) 3. Legislation requiring insurance coverage of preconception care 4. Media campaigns to promote cessation of smoking with interventions (301) 5. Increasing the unit price for tobacco products (301) 6. Provider reminder systems regarding patient's smoking status and provider education (301) 7. For smoking cessation, quitter telephone support with related interventions (301) 8. Media campaigns to promote cessation of alcohol use before conception and during pregnancy 9. Food fortification with folic acid (302, 303) 10. Media campaigns to encourage use of folic acid supplements among reproductive age women	1. none 2. + 3. none 4. +++ 5. +++ 6. +++ 7. +++ 8. none 9. +++ 10. ++
During pregnancy, prevent stillbirth by: • Encouraging maternal smoking cessation; • Treating maternal pregnancy-related illnesses; and • Monitoring fetal health through prenatal care.	1. Government subsidies for prenatal care (304, 305) 2. Presumptive eligibility for subsidized prenatal care 3. Community outreach programs to encourage women to obtain prenatal care	1. ++ 2. ++ 3. ++
At delivery, improve neonatal survival of high risk infants (e.g., very preterm infants) by • Insuring receipt of specialty neonatal services.	1. Regionalization of neonatal care (306)	1. ++
In the neonatal period, reduce deaths due to neonatal tetanus by • Insuring adequate immunity among pregnant women.	1. Immunization programs for pregnant women.(307)	
In the postneonatal period, prevent infant death from SIDS by • Delaying pregnancy for teens;	1. Media campaigns to encourage supine infant sleeping position (308) 2. Extending postpartum maternity leave to facilitate breastfeeding 3. Worksite childcare facilities where mothers can breastfeed	1. ++ 2. none 3. none

- Decreasing maternal smoking during pregnancy;
- encouraging breastfeeding; and
- encouraging supine infant sleeping position and beneficial infant sleep practices

4. Worksite rooms where women can pump breast milk — 4. none
5. Media campaigns to promote the benefits of breastfeeding — 5. none

During infancy, prevent death from motor vehicle injuries by
- Insuring that infants ride in safety seats

1. Child safety seat laws (309) — 1. +++
2. Distribution plus education programs (309) — 2. +++
3. Community-wide education plus enhanced enforcement campaigns (309) — 3. ++
4. Incentive plus education programs — 4. ++

During infancy, prevent death from diphtheria, pertussis, and tetanus by
- Insuring adequate infant immunization

1. Client recall/reminder (310) — 1. +++
2. Multicomponent interventions with education (310) — 2. +++
3. Regulations requiring immunizations for childcare attendance (310) — 3. ++
4. Subsidies or insurance to reduce out-of-pocket costs (310) — 4. +++
5. Multicomponent interventions to expand access (310) — 5. +++
6. Provider reminder/recall systems (310) — 6. +++
7. Assessment and feedback for providers (310) — 7. +++

During infancy, prevent death from diarrheal diseases by
- Providing clean drinking water
- providing oral rehydration solution

1. Water and sewer systems (307) — 1. +++
2. Improve access to primary care — 2. ++

ᵃQuality of evidence supporting PH action:
None = no evidence
+ = Suggestive evidence
++ = Moderately strong evidence
+++ = Strong evidence

Possibly one of the most important objectives related to the overall goal of decreasing fetal and infant mortality is increasing pregnancy intendedness. Although intendedness per se is not directly related to mortality, it directly effects whether women receive preconception care, which ultimately influences infant health. The impact on infant of improving contraceptive access is most pronounced in developing countries, where contraceptive use is often very low. Experience in the United States suggests that removing financial barriers to nonpermanent contraception increases its use. Because publicly funded contraceptive services are managed at the state level, financial criteria for receiving subsidized contraceptive services vary among states, leaving gaps in availability (311).

One investigator has judged that the two most important goals of public health interventions aimed at reducing fetal and neonatal mortality in industrialized countries are normalization of maternal preconception weight and elimination of maternal prenatal smoking (312). The prevalence of overweight has increased in the United States, despite a plethora of diet foods and commercial diet programs. Although the health risks of overweight for chronic illnesses have been well publicized, little has been done to heighten public awareness of the adverse effect of preconception overweight on pregnancy outcome. Evidence regarding effective public health interventions to normalize maternal weight before conception is virtually absent.

In contrast, substantial evidence exists about cost-effective public health interventions to promote smoking cessation. In light of this evidence, many states have aggressively applied these interventions, with observable decreases in the overall prevalence of smoking in their populations and in the prevalence of smoking during pregnancy (313).

Remarkable success has been achieved during the past century in reducing infant mortality. The observation of an increase in infant mortality in the United States in 2002, continuing disparities in fetal and infant mortality rates within the United States, and the poor ranking of the U.S. infant mortality rate relative to other industrialized countries suggest that substantial opportunities remain for further reductions in infant mortality. Developing, evaluating, and applying public health interventions can play an important role in achieving this reduction.

Discussion Topics

1. An investigator divides the number of fetal deaths at a specified gestation by the total number of fetal deaths and live births at that gestation. How should this measure be interpreted? What additional information would expand the interpretation?

2. Given the differences in fertility, access to medical care, and attitudes toward induced abortion between many developed and developing countries, how could one obtain valid, comparable measures of the rates of first-trimester spontaneous pregnancy loss?

3. What could explain why women who start prenatal care after the first trimester have lower neonatal mortality rates than women starting care during the first trimester? Why do women who obtain no prenatal care have high rates of neonatal mortality?

4. Your boss, the director of the Health Department in your state, asks you to identify the factor or factors that account for the most infant deaths in your state. How would you approach this assignment? In answering this question, focus on primary causes and potentially preventable intermediate and proximal causes. For example, Chlamydia infection (a primary cause) may lead to infertility, which prompts the use of assisted reproductive technologies (an intermediate cause), which in turn lead to multiple gestations and preterm delivery (proximal causes) and, ultimately, neonatal death.

5. For one of the factors you identified in Question 4, describe potential interventions, the percentage of infant deaths they could avert, and, if possible, the groups most affected by the intervention (e.g., younger women, uninsured women). What factors could increase or reduce the effectiveness of these interventions? Why?

6. You are the director of the Family Planning Program in your state. What evidence can you present to your state legislature that demonstrates the impact of family planning services on reducing fetal and infant mortality?

Promising Areas for Future Research

1. Developing methods for unbiased and more complete surveillance of spontaneous pregnancy losses and fetal deaths.

2. Assessing the impact of improved access to and content of prenatal care on the rate of fetal death.

3. Assessing public health interventions that reduce variation in cause-specific infant mortality rates.

4. Assessing the relationship between fetal death rates, the preterm delivery rates of live born infants, and neonatal mortality.

5. Assess the cost-effectiveness of public health interventions to reduce feto-infant mortality.

Abbreviations

ACME	Automated Classification of Medical Entities
AFP	Alpha-Fetoprotein
GDP	Gross Domestic Product
HCG	Human Chorionic Gonadatropin
ICD	International Classification of Disease
LMP	Last Menstrual Period

MICAR　　Mortality Medical Indexing, Classification, and Retrieval
NCHS　　National Center for Health Statistics
NSFG　　National Survey of Family Growth
SES　　　Socioeconomic Status
SGA　　　Small for Gestational Age
SIDS　　　Sudden Infant Death Syndrome
UNICEF　United Nations International Children's Emergency Fund
WHO　　 World Health Organization

References

1. Fetal Death (2007). Retrieved July 15, 2008, from http://www.cdc.gov/nchs/datawh/nchsdefs/fetaldeath.htm
2. Beers MH, Berkow R, editors. Gynecology and Obstetrics. STAT!Ref Online Electronic Medical Library. Section 18. West Point, PA: Merck & Co, 1999.
3. Kowaleski J. State defintions and reporting requirements for live births, fetal deaths, and induced terminations of pregnancy (1997 revision). Hyattsville, Maryland: National Center for Health Statistics, 1997.
4. Martin JA, Hoyert DL. The national fetal death file. Semin Perinatol 2002; 26(1):3–11.
5. Gourbin G, Masuy-Stroobant G. Registration of vital data: are live births and stillbirths comparable all over Europe? Bull World Health Organ 1995; 73(4):449–460.
6. Graafmans WC, Richardus JH, Macfarlane A, Rebagliato M, Blondel B, Verloove-Vanhorick SP, et al. Comparability of published perinatal mortality rates in Western Europe: the quantitative impact of differences in gestational age and birthweight criteria. BJOG 2001; 108(12):1237–1245.
7. Model State Vital Statistics Act and Regulations, 1992 Revision. DHHS Pub No. (PHS) 94–1115, 1994.
8. Kramer MS, Liu S, Luo Z, Yuan H, Platt RW, Joseph KS. Analysis of perinatal mortality and its components: time for a change? Am J Epidemiol 2002; 156(6):493–497.
9. Kramer MS, Platt RW, Yang H, Haglund B, Cnattingius S, Bergsjo P. Registration artifacts in international comparisons of infant mortality. Paediatr Perinat Epidemiol 2002; 16(1):16–22.
10. ACOG Practice Bulletin: Clinical Management Guidelines for Obstetrician-Gynecologists: Number 38, September 2002. Perinatal care at the threshold of viability. Obstet Gynecol 2002; 100(3):617–624.
11. Regev RH, Lusky A, Dolfin T, Litmanovitz I, Arnon S, Reichman B. Excess mortality and morbidity among small-for-gestational-age premature infants: a population-based study. J Pediatr 2003; 143(2):186–191.
12. Mulvey S, Partridge JC, Martinez AM, Yu VY, Wallace EM. The management of extremely premature infants and the perceptions of viability and parental counselling practices of Australian obstetricians. Aust NZ J Obstet Gynaecol 2001; 41(3):269–273.
13. Anderson RN, Smith BL. Deaths: leading causes for 2001. Natl Vital Stat Rep 2003; 52(9):1–85.
14. De Leeuw R, Cuttini M, Nadai M, Berbik I, Hansen G, Kucinskas A, et al. Treatment choices for extremely preterm infants: an international perspective. J Pediatr 2000; 137(5):608–616.
15. Arias E, Anderson RN, Kung HC, Murphy SL, Kochanek KD. Deaths: final data for 2001. Natl Vital Stat Rep 2003; 52(3):1–115.
16. Hetzel AM. History and organization of the vital statistics system. National Center for Health Statistics, 1997.

17. Croft ML, Read AW, de Klerk N, Hansen J, Kurinczuk JJ. Population based ascertainment of twins and their siblings, born in Western Australia 1980 to 1992, through the construction and validation of a maternally linked database of siblings. Twin Res 2002; 5(5):317–323.

18. Herman AA, McCarthy BJ, Bakewell JM, Ward RH, Mueller BA, Maconochie NE, et al. Data linkage methods used in maternally-linked birth and infant death surveillance data sets from the United States (Georgia, Missouri, Utah and Washington State), Israel, Norway, Scotland and Western Australia. Paediatr Perinat Epidemiol 1997; 11(Suppl 1):5–22.

19. Buescher PA. Method of linking Medicaid records to birth certificates may affect infant outcome statistics. Am J Public Health 1999; 89(4):564–566.

20. Herrchen B, Gould JB, Nesbitt TS. Vital statistics linked birth/infant death and hospital discharge record linkage for epidemiological studies. Comput Biomed Res 1997; 30 (4):290–305.

21. Gyllstrom ME, Jensen JL, Vaughan JN, Castellano SE, Oswald JW. Linking birth certificates with Medicaid data to enhance population health assessment: methodological issues addressed. J Public Health Manag Pract 2002; 8(4):38–44.

22. Mahapatra P, Shibuya K, Lopez AD, Coullare F, Notzon FC, Rao C, et al. Civil registration systems and vital statistics: successes and missed opportunities. Lancet 2007; 370 (9599):1653–1663.

23. Shamsuddin K, Lieberman E. Linking death reports from the Malaysian Family Life Survey-2 with birth and death certificates. Med J Malaysia 1998; 53(4):343–353.

24. World Health Organization. International Statistical Classification of Diseases and Related Health Problems, 10th Revision. Geneva: World Health Organization, 1992.

25. Hoyert DL, Arias E, Smith BL, Murphy SL, Kochanek KD. Deaths: final data for 1999. Natl Vital Stat Rep 2001; 49(8):1–113.

26. Hoyert DL. Mortality associated with birth defects: influence of successive disease classification revisions. Birth Defects Res, Part A: Clin Mol Teratol 2003; 67(9):651–655.

27. Heron M. Deaths: leading causes for 2004. Natl Vital Stat Rep 2007; 56(5):1–95.

28. Wigglesworth JS. Monitoring perinatal mortality. A pathophysiological approach. Lancet 1980; 2(8196):684–686.

29. Cole S, Hartford RB, Bergsjo P, McCarthy B. International collaborative effort (ICE) on birth weight, plurality, perinatal, and infant mortality. III: A method of grouping underlying causes of infant death to aid international comparisons. Acta Obstet Gynecol Scand 1989; 68(2):113–117.

30. Winbo IG, Serenius FH, Dahlquist GG, Kallen BA. NICE, a new cause of death classification for stillbirths and neonatal deaths. Neonatal and Intrauterine Death Classification according to Etiology. Int J Epidemiol 1998; 27(3):499–504.

31. Baird D, Walker J, Thomson AM. The causes and prevention of stillbirths and first week deaths. III. A classification of deaths by clinical cause; the effect of age, parity and length of gestation on death rates by cause. J Obstet Gynaecol Br Emp 1954; 61(4):433–448.

32. Alberman E, Botting B, Blatchley N, Twidell A. A new hierarchical classification of causes of infant deaths in England and Wales. Arch Dis Child 1994; 70(5):403–409.

33. Dollfus C, Patetta M, Siegel E, Cross AW. Infant mortality: a practical approach to the analysis of the leading causes of death and risk factors. Pediatrics 1990; 86(2):176–183.

34. Keeling JW, MacGillivray I, Golding J, Wigglesworth J, Berry J, Dunn PM. Classification of perinatal death. Arch Dis Child 1989; 64(10, Spec No):1345–1351.

35. Anthony S, van der Pal-de Bruin KM, Graafmans WC, Dorrepaal CA, Borkent-Polet M, van Hemel OJ, et al. The reliability of perinatal and neonatal mortality rates: differential under-reporting in linked professional registers vs. Dutch civil registers. Paediatr Perinat Epidemiol 2001; 15(3):306–314.

36. Heck KE, Schoendorf KC, Parker J. Are very low birthweight births among American Indians and Alaska Natives underregistered? Int J Epidemiol 1999; 28(6):1096–1101.

37. Joseph KS, Allen A, Kramer MS, Cyr M, Fair M. Changes in the registration of stillbirths <500 g in Canada, 1985–95. Fetal-Infant Mortality Study Group of the Canadian Perinatal Surveillance System. Paediatr Perinat Epidemiol 1999; 13(3):278–287.
38. Greb AE, Pauli RM, Kirby RS. Accuracy of fetal death reports: comparison with data from an independent stillbirth assessment program. Am J Public Health 1987; 77(9):1202–1206.
39. Goldhaber MK. Fetal death ratios in a prospective study compared to state fetal death certificate reporting. Am J Public Health 1989; 79(9):1268–1270.
40. Harter L, Starzyk P, Frost F. A comparative study of hospital fetal death records and Washington State fetal death certificates. Am J Public Health 1986; 76(11):1333–1334.
41. Unregistered deaths among extremely low birthweight infants – Ohio, 2006. MMWR 2007; 56(42):1101–1103.
42. Escobar GJ, Gardner MN, Chellino M, Fireman B, Verdi J, Yanover M. Identification of neonatal deaths in a large managed care organisation. Paediatr Perinat Epidemiol 1997; 11(1):93–104.
43. Herman-Giddens ME, Smith JB, Mittal M, Carlson M, Butts JD. Newborns killed or left to die by a parent: a population-based study. JAMA 2003; 289(11):1425–1429.
44. Variation in homicide risk during infancy – United States, 1989–1998. MMWR 2002; 51(9):187–189.
45. Overpeck MD, Brenner RA, Trumble AC, Trifiletti LB, Berendes HW. Risk factors for infant homicide in the United States. N Engl J Med 1998; 339(17):1211–1216.
46. Kramer MS, McLean FH, Boyd ME, Usher RH. The validity of gestational age estimation by menstrual dating in term, preterm, and postterm gestations. JAMA 1988; 260(22):3306–3308.
47. Yang H, Kramer MS, Platt RW, Blondel B, Breart G, Morin I, et al. How does early ultrasound scan estimation of gestational age lead to higher rates of preterm birth? Am J Obstet Gynecol 2002; 186(3):433–437.
48. Dietz PM, England LJ, Callaghan WM, Pearl M, Wier ML, Kharrazi M. A comparison of LMP-based and ultrasound-based estimates of gestational age using linked California live-birth and prenatal screening records. Paediatr Perinat Epidemiol 2007; 21(Suppl 2):62–71.
49. Arudo J, Gimnig JE, ter Kuile FO, Kachur SP, Slutsker L, Kolczak MS, et al. Comparison of government statistics and demographic surveillance to monitor mortality in children less than five years old in rural western Kenya. Am J Trop Med Hyg 2003; 68(4, Suppl):30–37.
50. Sayeed SA. Baby doe redux? The Department of Health and Human Services and the Born-Alive Infants Protection Act of 2002: a cautionary note on normative neonatal practice. Pediatrics 2005; 116(4):e576–e585.
51. Shankaran S, Fanaroff AA, Wright LL, Stevenson DK, Donovan EF, Ehrenkranz RA, et al. Risk factors for early death among extremely low-birth-weight infants. Am J Obstet Gynecol 2002; 186:796–802.
52. Khong TY. Falling neonatal autopsy rates. BMJ 2002; 324(7340):749–750.
53. Brodlie M, Laing IA, Keeling JW, McKenzie KJ. Ten years of neonatal autopsies in tertiary referral centre: retrospective study. BMJ 2002; 324(7340):761–763.
54. Okah FA. The autopsy: experience of a regional neonatal intensive care unit. Paediatr Perinat Epidemiol 2002; 16(4):350–354.
55. Sowards KA. What is the leading cause of infant mortality? A note on the interpretation of official statistics. Am J Public Health 1999; 89(11):1752–1754.
56. Wen SW, Chen LM, Li CY, Kramer MS, Allen AC. The impact of missing birth weight in deceased versus surviving fetuses and infants in the comparison of birth weight-specific feto-infant mortality. Chronic Dis Can 2002; 23(4):146–151.
57. Kline J, Stein Z, Susser M. Conception to birth. Epidemiology of prenatal development. New York: Oxford University Press, 1989.
58. Wilcox AJ, Weinberg CR, O'Connor JF, Baird DD, Schlatterer JP, Canfield RE, et al. Incidence of early loss of pregnancy. N Engl J Med 1988; 319(4):189–194.
59. Wilcox AJ, Baird DD, Weinberg CR. Time of implantation of the conceptus and loss of pregnancy. N Engl J Med 1999; 340(23):1796–1799.

60. Mills JL, Simpson JL, Driscoll SG, Jovanovic-Peterson L, Van Allen M, Aarons JH, et al. Incidence of spontaneous abortion among normal women and insulin-dependent diabetic women whose pregnancies were identified within 21 days of conception. N Engl J Med 1988; 319(25):1617–1623.

61. Ellish NJ, Saboda K, O'Connor J, Nasca PC, Stanek EJ, Boyle C. A prospective study of early pregnancy loss. Hum Reprod 1996; 11(2):406–412.

62. Zinaman MJ, Clegg ED, Brown CC, O'Connor J, Selevan SG. Estimates of human fertility and pregnancy loss. Fertil Steril 1996; 65(3):503–509.

63. Eskenazi B, Gold EB, Lasley BL, Samuels SJ, Hammond SK, Wight S, et al. Prospective monitoring of early fetal loss and clinical spontaneous abortion among female semiconductor workers. Am J Ind Med 1995; 28(6):833–846.

64. Hakim RB, Gray RH, Zacur H. Infertility and early pregnancy loss. Am J Obstet Gynecol 1995; 172(5):1510–1517.

65. Wang X, Chen C, Wang L, Chen D, Guang W, French J. Conception, early pregnancy loss, and time to clinical pregnancy: a population-based prospective study. Fertil Steril 2003; 79 (3):577–584.

66. Kramer MS, Liu S, Luo Z, Yuan H, Platt RW, Joseph KS. Analysis of perinatal mortality and its components: time for a change? Am J Epidemiol 2002; 156(6):493–497.

67. Huang DY, Usher RH, Kramer MS, Yang H, Morin L, Fretts RC. Determinants of unexplained antepartum fetal deaths. Obstet Gynecol 2000; 95(2):215–221.

68. Raymond EG, Cnattingius S, Kiely JL. Effects of maternal age, parity, and smoking on the risk of stillbirth. Br J Obstet Gynaecol 1994; 101(4):301–306.

69. Ferguson R, Myers SA. Population study of the risk of fetal death and its relationship to birthweight, gestational age, and race. Am J Perinatol 1994; 11(4):267–272.

70. Smith GC. Life-table analysis of the risk of perinatal death at term and post term in singleton pregnancies. Am J Obstet Gynecol 2001; 184(3):489–496.

71. Sairam S, Costeloe K, Thilaganathan B. Prospective risk of stillbirth in multiple-gestation pregnancies: a population-based analysis. Obstet Gynecol 2002; 100(4):638–641.

72. Karin P, Katarina B, Roger B, Alexandra H, Ingela HV, Marius K, et al. Diagnostic evaluation of intrauterine fetal deaths in Stockholm 1998–99. Acta Obstet Gynecol Scand 2002; 81 (4):284–292.

73. Bell R, Parker L, MacPhail S, Wright C. Trends in the cause of late fetal death, 1982–2000. BJOG 2004; 111(12):1400–1407.

74. Ventura SJ, Abma JC, Mosher WD, Henshaw S. Revised pregnancy rates, 1990–97, and new rates for 1998–99: United States. Natl Vital Stat Rep 2003; 52(7):1–14.

75. Ingemarsson I. Gender aspects of preterm birth. BJOG 2003; 110(Suppl 20):34–38.

76. Price SK. Prevalence and correlates of pregnancy loss history in a national sample of children and families. Matern Child Health J 2006; 10(6):489–500.

77. de La RE, Thonneau P. Paternal age and maternal age are risk factors for miscarriage; results of a multicentre European study. Hum Reprod 2002; 17(6):1649–1656.

78. Osborn JF, Cattaruzza MS, Spinelli A. Risk of spontaneous abortion in Italy, 1978–1995, and the effect of maternal age, gravidity, marital status, and education. Am J Epidemiol 2000; 151:98–105.

79. Toner JP, Grainger DA, Frazier LM. Clinical outcomes among recipients of donated eggs: an analysis of the U.S. national experience, 1996–1998. Fertil Steril 2002; 78(5):1038–1045.

80. Cramer DW, Wise LA. The epidemiology of recurrent pregnancy loss. Semin Reprod Med 2000; 18(4):331–339.

81. Hogge WA, Byrnes AL, Lanasa MC, Surti U. The clinical use of karyotyping spontaneous abortions. Am J Obstet Gynecol 2003; 189(2):397–400.

82. Richardus JH, Graafmans WC, Verloove-Vanhorick SP, Mackenbach JP. Differences in perinatal mortality and suboptimal care between 10 European regions: results of an international audit. BJOG 2003; 110(2):97–105.

83. Haglund B, Cnattingius S, Nordstrom ML. Social differences in late fetal death and infant mortality in Sweden 1985–86. Paediatr Perinat Epidemiol 1993; 7(1):33–44.
84. Guildea ZE, Fone DL, Dunstan FD, Sibert JR, Cartlidge PH. Social deprivation and the causes of stillbirth and infant mortality. Arch Dis Child 2001; 84(4):307–310.
85. Joseph KS, Liston RM, Dodds L, Dahlgren L, Allen AC. Socioeconomic status and perinatal outcomes in a setting with universal access to essential health care services. CMAJ 2007; 177 (6):583–590.
86. Cnattingius S, Berendes HW, Forman MR. Do delayed childbearers face increased risks of adverse pregnancy outcomes after the first birth? Obstet Gynecol 1993; 81(4):512–516.
87. Fretts RC, Schmittdiel J, McLean FH, Usher RH, Goldman MB. Increased maternal age and the risk of fetal death. N Engl J Med 1995; 333(15):953–957.
88. Conde-Agudelo A, Belizan JM, Diaz-Rossello JL. Epidemiology of fetal death in Latin America. Acta Obstet Gynecol Scand 2000; 79(5):371–378.
89. Kiely JL, Paneth N, Susser M. An assessment of the effects of maternal age and parity in different components of perinatal mortality. Am J Epidemiol 1986; 123(3):444–454.
90. Chen J, Fair M, Wilkins R, Cyr M. Maternal education and fetal and infant mortality in Quebec. Fetal and Infant Mortality Study Group of the Canadian Perinatal Surveillance System. Health Rep 1998; 10(2):53–64.
91. Guendelman S, Chavez G, Christianson R. Fetal deaths in Mexican-American, Black, and White non-Hispanic women seeking government-funded prenatal care. J Community Health 1994; 19(5):319–330.
92. Kallan JE. Rates of fetal death by maternal race, ethnicity, and nativity: New Jersey, 1991–1998. JAMA 2001; 285(23):2978–2979.
93. Kliewer EV, Stanley FJ. Stillbirths, neonatal and post-neonatal mortality by race, birth-weight and gestational age. J Paediatr Child Health 1993; 29(1):43–50.
94. Naeye R. Causes of fetal and neonatal mortality by race in a selected U.S. population. Am J Public Health 1979; 69(9):857–861.
95. van Coeverden de Groot HA. Trends in perinatal mortality in Cape Town, 1967–1977. S Afr Med J 1979; 56(25):1087–1092.
96. Vintzileos AM, Ananth CV, Smulian JC, Scorza WE, Knuppel RA. Prenatal care and Black–White fetal death disparity in the United States: heterogeneity by high-risk conditions. Obstet Gynecol 2002; 99(3):483–489.
97. Wen SW, Kramer MS. A comparison of perinatal mortality between ethnic Chinese and ethnic Whites: why the Chinese rate was lower. Ethn Health 1997; 2(3):177–182.
98. Lammer EJ, Brown LE, Anderka MT, Guyer B. Classification and analysis of fetal deaths in Massachusetts. JAMA 1989; 261(12):1757–1762.
99. Arntzen A, Moum T, Magnus P, Bakketeig LS. Marital status as a risk factor for fetal and infant mortality. Scand J Soc Med 1996; 24(1):36–42.
100. Brazerol WF, Grover S, Donnenfeld AE. Unexplained elevated maternal serum alpha-fetoprotein levels and perinatal outcome in an urban clinic population. Am J Obstet Gynecol 1994; 171(4):1030–1035.
101. Krause TG, Christens P, Wohlfahrt J, Lei U, Westergaard T, Norgaard-Pedersen B, et al. Second-trimester maternal serum alpha-fetoprotein and risk of adverse pregnancy outcome. Obstet Gynecol 2001; 97(2):277–282.
102. Wenstrom KD, Owen J, Davis RO, Brumfield CG. Prognostic significance of unexplained elevated amniotic fluid alpha-fetoprotein. Obstet Gynecol 1996; 87(2):213–216.
103. Walton DL, Norem CT, Schoen EJ, Ray GT, Colby CJ. Second-trimester serum chorionic gonadotropin concentrations and complications and outcome of pregnancy. N Engl J Med 1999; 341(27):2033–2038.
104. Modrzewska K. The offspring of schizophrenic parents in a North Swedish isolate. Clin Genet 1980; 17(3):191–201.
105. Chek K, Kerr GR. Factors associated with fetal mortality in the triethnic population in Texas, 1993 through 1995. Tex Med 1999; 95(12):78–83.
106. Wen SW, Demissie K, Liu S. Adverse outcomes in pregnancies of asthmatic women: results from a Canadian population. Ann Epidemiol 2001; 11(1):7–12.

107. Cnattingius S, Bergstrom R, Lipworth L, Kramer MS. Prepregnancy weight and the risk of adverse pregnancy outcomes. N Engl J Med. 1998;338(3):147–152.
108. Kaminski M, Rumeau C, Schwartz D. Alcohol consumption in pregnant women and the outcome of pregnancy. Alcohol Clin Exp Res 1978; 2(2):155–163.
109. Walles B, Tyden T, Herbst A, Ljungblad U, Rydhstrom H. Maternal health care program and markers for late fetal death. Acta Obstet Gynecol Scand 1994; 73(10):773–778.
110. Williams MA, Lieberman E, Mittendorf R, Monson RR, Schoenbaum SC. Risk factors for abruptio placentae. Am J Epidemiol 1991; 134(9):965–972.
111. Feitosa MF, Krieger H. Demography of the human sex ratio in some Latin American countries, 1967–1986. Hum Biol 1992; 64(4):523–530.
112. Imaizumi Y. Perinatal mortality in single and multiple births in Japan, 1980–1991. Paediatr Perinat Epidemiol 1994; 8(2):205–215.
113. Jakobovits A, Jakobovits AA, Viski A. Sex ratio of the stillborn fetuses and neonates dying in the first week. Early Hum Dev 1987; 15(3):131–135.
114. Luna F, Polo V, Fernandez-Santander A, Moral P. Stillbirth pattern in an isolated mediterranean population: La Alpujarra, Spain. Hum Biol 2001; 73(4):561–573.
115. McMillen MM. Differential mortality by sex in fetal and neonatal deaths. Science 1979; 204 (4388):89–91.
116. Smith GC. Sex, birth weight, and the risk of stillbirth in Scotland, 1980–1996. Am J Epidemiol 2000; 151(6):614–619.
117. Waldron I. Sex differences in human mortality: the role of genetic factors. Soc Sci Med 1983; 17(6):321–333.
118. Zhang J, Cai WW. Risk factors associated with antepartum fetal death. Early Hum Dev 1992; 28(3):193–200.
119. Lary JM, Paulozzi LJ. Sex differences in the prevalence of human birth defects: a population-based study. Teratology 2001; 64(5):237–251.
120. Samueloff A, Xenakis EM, Berkus MD, Huff RW, Langer O. Recurrent stillbirth. Significance and characteristics. J Reprod Med 1993; 38(11):883–886.
121. Smith GCS, Crossley JA, Aitken DA, Pell JP, Cameron AD, Connor JM, et al. First-trimester placentation and the risk of antepartum stillbirth. JAMA 2004; 292(18):2249–2254.
122. Gust DA, Levine WC, St Louis ME, Braxton J, Berman SM. Mortality associated with congenital syphilis in the United States, 1992–1998. Pediatrics 2002; 109(5):E79.
123. Gibbs RS. The origins of stillbirth: infectious diseases. Semin Perinatol 2002; 26(1):75–78.
124. Alberman E, Blatchley N, Botting B, Schuman J, Dunn A. Medical causes on stillbirth certificates in England and Wales: distribution and results of hierarchical classifications tested by the Office for National Statistics. Br J Obstet Gynaecol 1997; 104(9):1043–1049.
125. Chandra S, Ramji S, Thirupuram S. Perinatal asphyxia: multivariate analysis of risk factors in hospital births. Indian Pediatr 1997; 34(3):206–212.
126. Oron T, Sheiner E, Shoham-Vardi I, Mazor M, Katz M, Hallak M. Risk factors for antepartum fetal death. J Reprod Med 2001; 46(9):825–830.
127. Abu-Heija AT, Chalabi HE. Great grand multiparity: is it a risk? Int J Gynaecol Obstet 1997; 59(3):213–216.
128. Babinszki A, Kerenyi T, Torok O, Grazi V, Lapinski RH, Berkowitz RL. Perinatal outcome in grand and great-grand multiparity: effects of parity on obstetric risk factors. Am J Obstet Gynecol 1999; 181(3):669–674.
129. Ananth CV, Berkowitz GS, Savitz DA, Lapinski RH. Placental abruption and adverse perinatal outcomes. JAMA 1999; 282(17):1646–1651.
130. Copper RL, Goldenberg RL, DuBard MB, Davis RO. Risk factors for fetal death in White, Black, and Hispanic women. Collaborative Group on Preterm Birth Prevention. Obstet Gynecol 1994; 84(4):490–495.
131. Abu-Heija A, al Chalabi H, el Iloubani N. Abruptio placentae: risk factors and perinatal outcome. J Obstet Gynaecol Res 1998; 24(2):141–144.
132. Connolly AM, Katz VL, Bash KL, McMahon MJ, Hansen WF. Trauma and pregnancy. Am J Perinatol 1997; 14(6):331–336.

133. Rogers FB, Rozycki GS, Osler TM, Shackford SR, Jalbert J, Kirton O, et al. A multi-institutional study of factors associated with fetal death in injured pregnant patients. Arch Surg 1999; 134(11):1274–1277.
134. Schiff MA, Holt VL, Daling JR. Maternal and infant outcomes after injury during pregnancy in Washington State from 1989 to 1997. J Trauma 2002; 53(5):939–945.
135. Schiff MA, Holt VL. The injury severity score in pregnant trauma patients: predicting placental abruption and fetal death. J Trauma 2002; 53(5):946–949.
136. Kiely JL, Paneth N, Susser M. Fetal death during labor: an epidemiologic indicator of level of obstetric care. Am J Obstet Gynecol 1985; 153(7):721–727.
137. Smith GC, Pell JP, Cameron AD, Dobbie R. Risk of perinatal death associated with labor after previous cesarean delivery in uncomplicated term pregnancies. JAMA 2002; 287 (20):2684–2690.
138. Collins JH. Umbilical cord accidents: human studies. Semin Perinatol 2002; 26(1):79–82.
139. Arbuckle TE, Sever LE. Pesticide exposures and fetal death: a review of the epidemiologic literature. Crit Rev Toxicol 1998; 28(3):229–270.
140. Bell EM, Hertz-Picciotto I, Beaumont JJ. Case-cohort analysis of agricultural pesticide applications near maternal residence and selected causes of fetal death. Am J Epidemiol 2001; 154(8):702–710.
141. Bove FJ, Fulcomer MC, Klotz JB, Esmart J, Dufficy EM, Savrin JE. Public drinking water contamination and birth outcomes. Am J Epidemiol 1995; 141(9):850–862.
142. Dodds L, King W, Woolcott C, Pole J. Trihalomethanes in public water supplies and adverse birth outcomes. Epidemiology 1999; 10(3):233–237.
143. King WD, Dodds L, Allen AC. Relation between stillbirth and specific chlorination by-products in public water supplies. Environ Health Perspect 2000; 108(9):883–886.
144. White FM, Cohen FG, Sherman G, McCurdy R. Chemicals, birth defects and stillbirths in New Brunswick: associations with agricultural activity. CMAJ 1988; 138(2):117–124.
145. Cnattingius S, Stephansson O. The epidemiology of stillbirth. Semin Perinatol 2002; 26 (1):25–30.
146. Little RE, Weinberg CR. Risk factors for antepartum and intrapartum stillbirth. Am J Epidemiol 1993; 137(11):1177–1189.
147. Warner BB, Kiely JL, Donovan EF. Multiple births and outcome. Clin Perinatol 2000; 27 (2):347–361.
148. Joseph KS, Marcoux S, Ohlsson A, Liu S, Allen AC, Kramer MS, et al. Changes in stillbirth and infant mortality associated with increases in preterm birth among twins. Pediatrics 2001; 108(5):1055–1061.
149. Demissie K, Ananth CV, Martin J, Hanley ML, MacDorman MF, Rhoads GG. Fetal and neonatal mortality among twin gestations in the United States: the role of intrapair birth weight discordance. Obstet Gynecol 2002; 100(3):474–480.
150. Imaizumi Y. Perinatal mortality in twins and factors influencing mortality in Japan, 1980–98. Paediatr Perinat Epidemiol 2001; 15(3):298–305.
151. United States Department of Health and Human Services (US DHHS), Centers of Disease Control and Prevention (CDC), National Center for Health Statistics (NCHS), Office of Analysis and Epidemiology (OAE), Division of Vital Statistics (DVS), Linked Birth / Infant Death Records 2003-2004 on CDC WONDER On-line Database. Retrieved September 20, 2008 from http://wonder.cdc.gov/lbd-icd10.html.
152. Goodman DC, Fisher ES, Little GA, Stukel TA, Chang CH, Schoendorf KS. The relation between the availability of neonatal intensive care and neonatal mortality. N Engl J Med 2002; 346(20):1538–1544.
153. Cifuentes J, Bronstein J, Phibbs CS, Phibbs RH, Schmitt SK, Carlo WA. Mortality in low birth weight infants according to level of neonatal care at hospital of birth. Pediatrics 2002; 109(5):745–751.

154. Empana JP, Subtil D, Truffert P. In-hospital mortality of newborn infants born before 33 weeks of gestation depends on the initial level of neonatal care: the EPIPAGE study. Acta Paediatr 2003; 92(3):346–351.

155. World Health Organization. WHO Mortality Database. Geneva: World Health Organization. Available at: http://www.who.int/whosis/menu.cfm?path=whosis,mort&language=english

156. United Nations Children's Fund. Official Summary: The State of the World's Children 2002. New York: Oxford University Press, 2002.

157. Geronimus AT, Korenman S. Maternal youth or family background? On the health disadvantages of infants with teenage mothers. Am J Epidemiol 1993; 137(2):213–225.

158. Bambang S, Spencer NJ, Logan S, Gill L. Cause-specific perinatal death rates, birth weight and deprivation in the West Midlands, 1991–93. Child Care Health Dev 2000; 26(1):73–82.

159. Rolett A, Kiely JL. Maternal sociodemographic characteristics as risk factors for preterm birth in twins versus singletons. Paediatr Perinat Epidemiol 2000; 14(3):211–218.

160. Sharma RK. Causal pathways to infant mortality: linking social variables to infant mortality through intermediate variables. J Health Soc Policy 1998; 9:15–28.

161. Alexander GR, Kogan MD, Himes JH, Mor JM, Goldenberg R. Racial differences in birthweight for gestational age and infant mortality in extremely-low-risk US populations. Paediatr Perinat Epidemiol 1999; 13:205–217.

162. Olausson PO, Cnattingius S, Haglund B. Teenage pregnancies and risk of late fetal death and infant mortality. Br J Obstet Gynaecol 1999; 106(2):116–121.

163. Shi L, Macinko J, Starfield B, Xu J, Regan J, Politzer R, et al. Primary care, infant mortality, and low birth weight in the states of the USA. J Epidemiol Community Health 2004; 58 (5):374–380.

164. Lynch JW, Smith GD, Kaplan GA, House JS. Income inequality and mortality: importance to health of individual income, psychosocial environment, or material conditions. BMJ 2000; 320(7243):1200–1204.

165. Hales S, Howden-Chapman P, Salmond C, Woodward A, Mackenbach J. National infant mortality rates in relation to gross national product and distribution of income. Lancet 1999; 354:2047.

166. Bremberg S. Does an increase of low income families affect child health inequalities? A Swedish case study. J Epidemiol Community Health 2003; 57:584–588.

167. Shmueli A. Population health and income inequality: new evidence from Israeli time–series analysis. Int J Epidemiol 2004; 33(2):311–317.

168. Kabir N, Krishnan TN. Social intermediation and health change: Lessons from Kerala. In: Das Gupta M, Chen LC, Krishnan TN, editors. Health, poverty, and development in India. Delhi: Oxford University Press, 1996.

169. Gaudino JA, Jr., Jenkins B, Rochat RW. No fathers' names: a risk factor for infant mortality in the State of Georgia, USA. Soc Sci Med 1999; 48:253–265.

170. Misra DP, Ananth CV. Infant mortality among singletons and twins in the United States during 2 decades: effects of maternal age. Pediatrics 2002; 110(6):1163–1168.

171. Draper ES, Kurinczuk JJ, Abrams KR, Clarke M. Assessment of separate contributions to perinatal mortality of infertility history and treatment: a case-control analysis. Lancet 1999; 353:1746–1749.

172. Jivraj S, Anstie B, Cheong YC, Fairlie FM, Laird SM, Li TC. Obstetric and neonatal outcome in women with a history of recurrent miscarriage: a cohort study. Hum Reprod 2001; 16 (1):102–106.

173. Boulet SL, Alexander GR, Salihu HM, Pass M. Macrosomic births in the United States: determinants, outcomes, and proposed grades of risk. Am J Obstet Gynecol 2003; 188 (5):1372–1378.

174. Wilcox AJ, Russell IT. Birthweight and perinatal mortality: III. Towards a new method of analysis. Int J Epidemiol 1986; 15:188–196.

175. Wilcox AJ, Russell IT. Birthweight and perinatal mortality: II. On weight-specific mortality. Int J Epidemiol 1983; 12:319–325.

176. Wilcox AJ, Russell IT. Birthweight and perinatal mortality: I. On the frequency distribution of birthweight. Int J Epidemiol 1983; 12:314–318.
177. Skjaerven R, Wilcox AJ, Russell D. Birthweight and perinatal mortality of second births conditional on weight of the first. Int J Epidemiol 1988; 17:830–838.
178. Kerr GR, Ying J, Spears W. Ethnic differences in causes of infant mortality: Texas births, 1989 through 1991. Tex Med 1995; 91(9):50–56.
179. Papacek EM, Collins JW, Jr., Schulte NF, Goergen C, Drolet A. Differing postneonatal mortality rates of African-American and White infants in Chicago: an ecologic study. Matern Child Health J 2002; 6(2):99–105.
180. Cundy T, Gamble G, Townend K, Henley PG, MacPherson P, Roberts AB. Perinatal mortality in Type 2 diabetes mellitus. Diabet Med 2000; 17(1):33–39.
181. Dunne F, Brydon P, Smith K, Gee H. Pregnancy in women with Type 2 diabetes: 12 years outcome data 1990–2002. Diabet Med 2003; 20(9):734–738.
182. Evers IM, de Valk HW, Visser GH. Risk of complications of pregnancy in women with type 1 diabetes: nationwide prospective study in the Netherlands. BMJ 2004; 328(7445):915.
183. Penney GC, Mair G, Pearson DW. Outcomes of pregnancies in women with type 1 diabetes in Scotland: a national population-based study. BJOG 2003; 110(3):315–318.
184. Cedergren MI. Maternal morbid obesity and the risk of adverse pregnancy outcome. Obstet Gynecol 2004; 103(2):219–224.
185. Moss N, Carver K. The effect of WIC and Medicaid on infant mortality in the United States. Am J Public Health 1998; 88:1354–1361.
186. Besharov DJ, Germanis P. Evaluating WIC. Eval Rev 2000; 24(2):123–190.
187. Rush D, Leighton J, Sloan NL, Alvir JM, Garbowski GC. The National WIC Evaluation: evaluation of the Special Supplemental Food Program for Women, Infants, and Children. II. Review of past studies of WIC. Am J Clin Nutr 1988; 48:394–411.
188. Burd L, Wilson H. Fetal, infant, and child mortality in a context of alcohol use. Am J Med Genet 2004; 127C(1):51–58.
189. Chen A, Rogan WJ. Breastfeeding and the risk of postneonatal death in the United States. Pediatrics 2004; 113(5):e435–439.
190. Vatten LJ, Skjaerven R. Effects on pregnancy outcome of changing partner between first two births: prospective population study. BMJ 2003; 327(7424):1138.
191. Gessner BD, Moore M, Hamilton B, Muth PT. The incidence of infant physical abuse in Alaska. Child Abuse Negl 2004; 28(1):9–23.
192. Lipsky S, Holt VL, Easterling TR, Critchlow CW. Impact of police-reported intimate partner violence during pregnancy on birth outcomes. Obstet Gynecol 2003; 102(3):557–564.
193. Asling-Monemi K, Pena R, Ellsberg MC, Persson LA. Violence against women increases the risk of infant and child mortality: a case-referent study in Nicaragua. Bull World Health Organ 2003; 81(1):10–16.
194. Jejeebhoy SJ. Associations between wife-beating and fetal and infant death: impressions from a survey in rural India. Stud Fam Plann 1998; 29:300–308.
195. Hulse GK, Milne E, English DR, Holman CD. Assessing the relationship between maternal opiate use and neonatal mortality. Addiction 1998; 93:1033–1042.
196. Ostrea EM, Jr., Ostrea AR, Simpson PM. Mortality within the first 2 years in infants exposed to cocaine, opiate, or cannabinoid during gestation. Pediatrics 1997; 100:79–83.
197. Fares I, McCulloch KM, Raju TN. Intrauterine cocaine exposure and the risk for sudden infant death syndrome: a meta-analysis. J Perinatol 1997; 17:179–182.
198. Salihu HM, Aliyu MH, Pierre-Louis BJ, Alexander GR. Levels of excess infant deaths attributable to maternal smoking during pregnancy in the United States. Matern Child Health J 2003; 7(4):219–227.
199. Platt RW, Joseph KS, Ananth CV, Grondines J, Abrahamowicz M, Kramer MS. A proportional hazards model with time-dependent covariates and time-varying effects for analysis of fetal and infant death. Am J Epidemiol 2004; 160(3):199–206.

200. Dwyer T, Ponsonby AL, Couper D, Cochrane J. Short-term morbidity and infant mortality among infants who slept supine at 1 month of age – a follow-up report. Paediatr Perinat Epidemiol 1999; 13(3):302–315.
201. Beal SM, Finch CF. An overview of retrospective case-control studies investigating the relationship between prone sleeping position and SIDS. J Paediatr Child Health 1991; 27(6):334–339.
202. Hauck FR, Moore CM, Herman SM, Donovan M, Kalelkar M, Christoffel KK, et al. The contribution of prone sleeping position to the racial disparity in sudden infant death syndrome: the Chicago Infant Mortality Study. Pediatrics 2002; 110(4):772–780.
203. Blair PS, Fleming PJ, Smith IJ, Platt MW, Young J, Nadin P, et al. Babies sleeping with parents: case-control study of factors influencing the risk of the sudden infant death syndrome. CESDI SUDI Research Group. BMJ 1999; 319(7223):1457–1461.
204. Klonoff-Cohen H, Edelstein SL. Bed sharing and the sudden infant death syndrome. BMJ 1995; 311(7015):1269–1272.
205. Scragg R, Mitchell EA, Taylor BJ, Stewart AW, Ford RP, Thompson JM, et al. Bed sharing, smoking, and alcohol in the sudden infant death syndrome. New Zealand Cot Death Study Group. BMJ 1993; 307(6915):1312–1318.
206. Beal SM, Byard RW. Sudden infant death syndrome in South Australia 1968–97. Part 3: is bed sharing safe for infants? J Paediatr Child Health 2000; 36(6):552–554.
207. Vintzileos A, Ananth CV, Smulian JC, Scorza WE, Knuppel RA. The impact of prenatal care on postneonatal deaths in the presence and absence of antenatal high-risk conditions. Am J Obstet Gynecol 2002; 187(5):1258–1262.
208. Vintzileos AM, Ananth CV, Smulian JC, Scorza WE, Knuppel RA. The impact of prenatal care on neonatal deaths in the presence and absence of antenatal high-risk conditions. Am J Obstet Gynecol 2002; 186(5):1011–1016.
209. Petrini J, Damus K, Russell R, Poschman K, Davidoff MJ, Mattison D. Contribution of birth defects to infant mortality in the United States. Teratology 2002; 66(Suppl 1):S3–S6.
210. Clausson B, Cnattingius S, Axelsson O. Outcomes of post-term births: the role of fetal growth restriction and malformations. Obstet Gynecol 1999; 94:758–762.
211. Hilder L, Costeloe K, Thilaganathan B. Prolonged pregnancy: evaluating gestation-specific risks of fetal and infant mortality. Br J Obstet Gynaecol 1998; 105:169–173.
212. Mullaney DM. Group B streptococcal infections in newborns. J Obstet Gynecol Neonatal Nurs 2001; 30(6):649–658.
213. Embleton N, Wariyar U, Hey E. Mortality from early onset group B streptococcal infection in the United Kingdom. Arch Dis Child Fetal Neonatal Ed 1999; 80:F139–F141.
214. Osrin D, Vergnano S, Costello A. Serious bacterial infections in newborn infants in developing countries. Curr Opin Infect Dis 2004; 17:217–224.
215. Melve KK, Gjessing HK, Skjaerven R, Oyen N. Infants' length at birth: an independent effect on perinatal mortality. Acta Obstet Gynecol Scand 2000; 79(6):459–464.
216. Shinwell ES, Blickstein I, Lusky A, Reichman B. Effect of birth order on neonatal morbidity and mortality among very low birthweight twins: a population based study. Arch Dis Child Fetal Neonatal Ed 2004; 89(2):F145–F148.
217. Ananth CV, Demissie K, Hanley ML. Birth weight discordancy and adverse perinatal outcomes among twin gestations in the United States: the effect of placental abruption. Am J Obstet Gynecol 2003; 188(4):954–960.
218. Branum AM, Schoendorf KC. The effect of birth weight discordance on twin neonatal mortality. Obstet Gynecol 2003; 101:570–574.
219. Stevenson DK, Verter J, Fanaroff AA, Oh W, Ehrenkranz RA, Shankaran S, et al. Sex differences in outcomes of very low birthweight infants: the newborn male disadvantage. Arch Dis Child Fetal Neonatal Ed 2000; 83(3):F182–F185.
220. Mulik V, Bethel J, Bhal K. A retrospective population-based study of primigravid women on the potential effect of threatened miscarriage on obstetric outcome. J Obstet Gynaecol 2004; 24(3):249–253.

221. Williams MA, Mittendorf R, Lieberman E, Monson RR. Adverse infant outcomes associated with first-trimester vaginal bleeding. Obstet Gynecol 1991; 78:14–18.
222. Salihu HM, Li Q, Rouse DJ, Alexander GR. Placenta previa: neonatal death after live births in the United States. Am J Obstet Gynecol 2003; 188(5):1305–1309.
223. Ananth CV, Smulian JC, Vintzileos AM. The effect of placenta previa on neonatal mortality: a population-based study in the United States, 1989 through 1997. Am J Obstet Gynecol 2003; 188(5):1299–1304.
224. Kinzler WL, Ananth CV, Smulian JC, Vintzileos AM. The effects of labor on infant mortality among small-for-gestational-age infants in the USA. J Matern Fetal Neonatal Med 2002; 12(3):201–206.
225. Joseph KS, Demissie K, Kramer MS. Obstetric intervention, stillbirth, and preterm birth. Semin Perinatol 2002; 26(4):250–259.
226. Paul DA, Sciscione A, Leef KH, Stefano JL. Caesarean delivery and outcome in very low birthweight infants. Aust NZ J Obstet Gynaecol 2002; 42(1):41–45.
227. Jain L, Ferre C, Vidyasagar D. Cesarean delivery of the breech very-low-birth-weight infant: does it make a difference? J Matern Fetal Med 1998; 7:28–31.
228. Jonas HA, Lumley JM. The effect of mode of delivery on neonatal mortality in very low birthweight infants born in Victoria, Australia: Caesarean section is associated with increased survival in breech-presenting, but not vertex-presenting, infants. Paediatr Perinat Epidemiol 1997; 11:181–199.
229. Roman J, Bakos O, Cnattingius S. Pregnancy outcomes by mode of delivery among term breech births: Swedish experience 1987–1993. Obstet Gynecol 1998; 92(6):945–950.
230. Stephansson O, Dickman PW, Cnattingius S. The influence of interpregnancy interval on the subsequent risk of stillbirth and early neonatal death. Obstet Gynecol 2003; 102(1):101–108.
231. Smith GC, Pell JP, Dobbie R. Interpregnancy interval and risk of preterm birth and neonatal death: retrospective cohort study. BMJ 2003; 327(7410):313.
232. Hauth JC, Ewell MG, Levine RJ, Esterlitz JR, Sibai B, Curet LB, et al. Pregnancy outcomes in healthy nulliparas who developed hypertension. Calcium for Preeclampsia Prevention Study Group. Obstet Gynecol 2000; 95(1):24–28.
233. Chen CL, Cheng Y, Wang PH, Juang CM, Chiu LM, Yang MJ, et al. Review of pre-eclampsia in Taiwan: a multi-institutional study. Zhonghua Yi Xue Za Zhi (Taipei) 2000; 63(12):869–875.
234. Hall DR, Odendaal HJ, Kirsten GF, Smith J, Grove D. Expectant management of early onset, severe pre-eclampsia: perinatal outcome. BJOG 2000; 107:1258–1264.
235. Greenwood B. Maternal immunisation in developing countries. Vaccine 2003; 21(24):3436–3441.
236. Neonatal tetanus: the final countdown. CVI Forum 1994; 6–9.
237. Rahmathullah L, Tielsch JM, Thulasiraj RD, Katz J, Coles C, Devi S, et al. Impact of supplementing newborn infants with vitamin A on early infant mortality: community based randomised trial in southern India. BMJ 2003; 327(7409):254.
238. McElvy SS, Miodovnik M, Rosenn B, Khoury JC, Siddiqi T, Dignan PS, et al. A focused preconceptional and early pregnancy program in women with type 1 diabetes reduces perinatal mortality and malformation rates to general population levels. J Matern Fetal Med 2000; 9:14–20.
239. Samuelson JL, Buehler JW, Norris D, Sadek R. Maternal characteristics associated with place of delivery and neonatal mortality rates among very-low-birthweight infants, Georgia. Paediatr Perinat Epidemiol 2002; 16(4):305–313.
240. Thompson LA, Goodman DC, Little GA. Is more neonatal intensive care always better? Insights from a cross-national comparison of reproductive care. Pediatrics 2002; 109 (6):1036–1043.
241. Luo ZC, Liu S, Wilkins R, Kramer MS. Risks of stillbirth and early neonatal death by day of week. CMAJ 2004; 170(3):337–341.
242. Gould JB, Qin C, Marks AR, Chavez G. Neonatal mortality in weekend vs weekday births. JAMA 2003; 289(22):2958–2962.

243. Hamilton P, Restrepo E. Weekend birth and higher neonatal mortality: a problem of patient acuity or quality of care? J Obstet Gynecol Neonatal Nurs 2003; 32(6):724–733.
244. Dolk H, Pattenden S, Vrijheid M, Thakrar B, Armstrong B. Perinatal and infant mortality and low birth weight among residents near cokeworks in Great Britain. Arch Environ Health 2000; 55(1):26–30.
245. Lipfert FW, Zhang J, Wyzga RE. Infant mortality and air pollution: a comprehensive analysis of U.S. data for 1990. J Air Waste Manag Assoc 2000; 50(8):1350–1366.
246. Spiers PS, Guntheroth WG. The seasonal distribution of infant deaths by age: a comparison of sudden infant death syndrome and other causes of death. J Paediatr Child Health 1997; 33:408–412.
247. Milerad J, Vege A, Opdal SH, Rognum TO. Objective measurements of nicotine exposure in victims of sudden infant death syndrome and in other unexpected child deaths. J Pediatr 1998; 133:232–236.
248. Mooney JA, Helms PJ, Jolliffe IT. Higher incidence of SIDS at weekends, especially in younger infants. Arch Dis Child 2004; 89(7):670–672.
249. Kogan MD, Alexander GR, Kotelchuck M, MacDorman MF, Buekens P, Martin JA, et al. Trends in twin birth outcomes and prenatal care utilization in the United States, 1981–1997. JAMA 2000; 284(3):335–341.
250. Wu Z, Viisainen K, Wang Y, Hemminki E. Perinatal mortality in rural China: retrospective cohort study. BMJ 2003; 327(7427):1319.
251. Khanna R, Kumar A, Vaghela JF, Sreenivas V, Puliyel JM. Community based retrospective study of sex in infant mortality in India. BMJ 2003; 327(7407):126.
252. Alm B, Milerad J, Wennergren G, Skjaerven R, Oyen N, Norvenius G, et al. A case-control study of smoking and sudden infant death syndrome in the Scandinavian countries, 1992 to 1995. The Nordic Epidemiological SIDS Study. Arch Dis Child 1998; 78(4):329–334.
253. Willinger M, James LC, Catz C. Defining the sudden infant death syndrome (SIDS): deliberations of an expert panel convened by the National Institute of Child Health and Human Development. Pediatr Pathol 1991; 11:677–684.
254. Overpeck MD, Brenner RA, Cosgrove C, Trumble AC, Kochanek K, MacDorman M. National underascertainment of sudden unexpected infant deaths associated with deaths of unknown cause. Pediatrics 2002; 109(2):274–283.
255. Adams MM, Rhodes PH, McCarthy BJ. Are race and length of gestation related to age at death in the sudden infant death syndrome? Paediatr Perinat Epidemiol 1990; 4(3):325–339.
256. Dwyer T, Ponsonby AL. SIDS epidemiology and incidence. Pediatr Ann 1995; 24(7):350–356.
257. Bulterys M. High incidence of sudden infant death syndrome among northern Indians and Alaska natives compared with southwestern Indians: possible role of smoking. J Community Health 1990; 15(3):185–194.
258. Ponsonby AL, Dwyer T, Cochrane J. Population trends in sudden infant death syndrome. Semin Perinatol 2002; 26(4):296–305.
259. Dwyer T, Ponsonby AL, Blizzard L, Newman NM, Cochrane JA. The contribution of changes in the prevalence of prone sleeping position to the decline in sudden infant death syndrome in Tasmania. JAMA 1995; 273(10):783–789.
260. Panaretto KS, Whitehall JF, McBride G, Patole S, Whitehall JS. Sudden infant death syndrome in Indigenous and non-Indigenous infants in north Queensland, 1990–1998. J Paediatr Child Health 2002; 38(2):135–139.
261. Luo ZC, Wilkins R, Platt RW, Kramer MS. Risks of adverse pregnancy outcomes among Inuit and North American Indian women in Quebec, 1985–97. Paediatr Perinat Epidemiol 2004; 18(1):40–50.
262. Alessandri LM, Read AW, Burton PR, Stanley FJ. Sudden infant death syndrome in Australian aboriginal and non-aboriginal infants: an analytical comparison. Paediatr Perinat Epidemiol 1996; 10(3):309–318.

263. Sullivan FM, Barlow SM. Review of risk factors for sudden infant death syndrome. Paediatr Perinat Epidemiol 2001; 15(2):144–200.
264. Daltveit AK, Irgens LM, Oyen N, Skjaerven R, Markestad T, Alm B, et al. Sociodemographic risk factors for sudden infant death syndrome: associations with other risk factors. The Nordic Epidemiological SIDS Study. Acta Paediatr 1998; 87:284–290.
265. Leach CE, Blair PS, Fleming PJ, Smith IJ, Platt MW, Berry PJ, et al. Epidemiology of SIDS and explained sudden infant deaths. CESDI SUDI Research Group. Pediatrics 1999; 104(4): e43.
266. Iyasu S, Randall LL, Welty TK, Hsia J, Kinney HC, Mandell F, et al. Risk factors for sudden infant death syndrome among northern plains Indians. JAMA 2002; 288(21):2717–2723.
267. Mehanni M, Cullen A, Kiberd B, McDonnell M, O'Regan M, Matthews T. The current epidemiology of SIDS in Ireland. Ir Med J 2000; 93(9):264–268.
268. Carroll-Pankhurst C, Mortimer EA, Jr. Sudden infant death syndrome, bedsharing, parental weight, and age at death. Pediatrics 2001; 107(3):530–536.
269. Alm B, Wennergren G, Norvenius SG, Skjaerven R, Lagercrantz H, Helweg-Larsen K, et al. Breast feeding and the sudden infant death syndrome in Scandinavia, 1992–95. Arch Dis Child 2002; 86(6):400–402.
270. Alm B, Wennergren G, Norvenius G, Skjarven R, Oyen N, Helweg-Larsen K, et al. Caffeine and alcohol as risk factors for sudden infant death syndrome. Arch Dis Child 1999; 81 (2):107–111.
271. Dwyer T, Ponsonby AL, Gibbons LE, Newman NM. Prone sleeping position and SIDS: evidence from recent case-control and cohort studies in Tasmania. J Paediatr Child Health 1991; 27(6):340–343.
272. Gessner BD, Ives GC, Perham-Hester KA. Association between sudden infant death syndrome and prone sleep position, bed sharing, and sleeping outside an infant crib in Alaska. Pediatrics 2001; 108(4):923–927.
273. Irgens LM, Markestad T, Baste V, Schreuder P, Skjaerven R, Oyen N. Sleeping position and sudden infant death syndrome in Norway 1967–91. Arch Dis Child 1995; 72(6):478–482.
274. James C, Klenka H, Manning D. Sudden infant death syndrome: bed sharing with mothers who smoke. Arch Dis Child 2003; 88(2):112–113.
275. Jonville-Bera AP, Autret-Leca E, Barbeillon F, Paris-Llado J. Sudden unexpected death in infants under 3 months of age and vaccination status – a case-control study. Br J Clin Pharmacol 2001; 51(3):271–276.
276. Oyen N, Markestad T, Skaerven R, Irgens LM, Helweg-Larsen K, Alm B, et al. Combined effects of sleeping position and prenatal risk factors in sudden infant death syndrome: the Nordic Epidemiological SIDS Study. Pediatrics 1997; 100(4):613–621.
277. Taylor JA, Krieger JW, Reay DT, Davis RL, Harruff R, Cheney LK. Prone sleep position and the sudden infant death syndrome in King County, Washington: a case-control study. J Pediatr 1996; 128(5, Pt 1):626–630.
278. Unger B, Kemp JS, Wilkins D, Psara R, Ledbetter T, Graham M, et al. Racial disparity and modifiable risk factors among infants dying suddenly and unexpectedly. Pediatrics 2003; 111 (2):E127–E131.
279. Wilson CA, Taylor BJ, Laing RM, Williams SM, Mitchell EA. Clothing and bedding and its relevance to sudden infant death syndrome: further results from the New Zealand Cot Death Study. J Paediatr Child Health 1994; 30(6):506–512.
280. Oyen N, Skjaerven R, Irgens LM. Population-based recurrence risk of sudden infant death syndrome compared with other infant and fetal deaths. Am J Epidemiol 1996; 144(3):300–305.
281. Stewart AJ, Williams SM, Mitchell EA, Taylor BJ, Ford RP, Allen EM. Antenatal and intrapartum factors associated with sudden infant death syndrome in the New Zealand Cot Death Study. J Paediatr Child Health 1995; 31(5):473–478.
282. Fujita T. Sudden infant death syndrome in Japan 1995–1998. Forensic Sci Int 2002; 130 (Suppl):S71–S77.

283. Blackwell CC, Moscovis SM, Gordon AE, Al Madani OM, Hall ST, Gleeson M, et al. Ethnicity, infection and sudden infant death syndrome. FEMS Immunol Med Microbiol 2004; 42(1):53–65.

284. Blackwell CC, Weir DM, Busuttil A. Infection, inflammation and sleep: more pieces to the puzzle of sudden infant death syndrome (SIDS). APMIS 1999; 107(5):455–473.

285. Goldwater PN. SIDS pathogenesis: pathological findings indicate infection and inflammatory responses are involved. FEMS Immunol Med Microbiol 2004; 42(1):11–20.

286. Malloy MH, Freeman DH, Jr. Sudden infant death syndrome among twins. Arch Pediatr Adolesc Med 1999; 153(7):736–740.

287. Platt MJ, Pharoah PO. The epidemiology of sudden infant death syndrome. Arch Dis Child 2003; 88(1):27–29.

288. Millar WJ, Hill GB. Prevalence of and risk factors for sudden infant death syndrome in Canada. CMAJ 1993; 149(5):629–635.

289. Li DK, Wi S. Maternal pre-eclampsia/eclampsia and the risk of sudden infant death syndrome in offspring. Paediatr Perinat Epidemiol 2000; 14(2):141–144.

290. Buck GM, Cookfair DL, Michalek AM, Nasca PC, Standfast SJ, Sever LE. Timing of prenatal care and risk of sudden infant death syndrome. Int J Epidemiol 1990; 19(4):991–996.

291. Kohlendorfer U, Kiechl S, Sperl W. Living at high altitude and risk of sudden infant death syndrome. Arch Dis Child 1998; 79(6):506–509.

292. Douglas AS, Gupta R, Helms PJ, Jolliffe IT. Month of birth as an independent variable in the sudden infant death syndrome. Paediatr Perinat Epidemiol 1997; 11(1):57–66.

293. Alm B, Norvenius SG, Wennergren G, Skjaerven R, Oyen N, Milerad J, et al. Changes in the epidemiology of sudden infant death syndrome in Sweden 1973–1996. Arch Dis Child 2001; 84(1):24–30.

294. Douglas AS, Helms PJ, Jolliffe IT. Seasonality of sudden infant death syndrome (SIDS) by age at death. Acta Paediatr 1998; 87(10):1033–1038.

295. Kesmodel U. Binge drinking in pregnancy – frequency and methodology. Am J Epidemiol 2001; 154(8):777–782.

296. Williams SM, Mitchell EA, Taylor BJ. Are risk factors for sudden infant death syndrome different at night? Arch Dis Child 2002; 87(4):274–278.

297. Rognum TO, Saugstad OD. Biochemical and immunological studies in SIDS victims. Clues to understanding the death mechanism. Acta Paediatr Suppl 1993; 82(Suppl 389):82–85.

298. Filiano JJ, Kinney HC. A perspective on neuropathologic findings in victims of the sudden infant death syndrome: the triple-risk model. Biol Neonate 1994; 65:194–197.

299. Guntheroth WG, Spiers PS. The triple risk hypotheses in sudden infant death syndrome. Pediatrics 2002 Nov;110(5):e64.

300. Gold RB. Doing more for less: study says state Medicaid family planning expansions are cost-effective. The Guttmacher Report 2004; 7(1).

301. Centers for Disease Control and Prevention. Strategies for reducing exposure to environmental tobacco smoke, increasing tobacco-use cessasation, and decreasing initiation in communities and health care systems. MMWR 2000; 49(RR-12):1–20.

302. Ray JG, Meier C, Vermeulen MJ, Boss S, Wyatt PR, Cole DE. Association of neural tube defects and folic acid food fortification in Canada. Lancet 2002; 360(9350):2047–2048.

303. Williams LJ, Mai CT, Edmonds LD, Shaw GM, Kirby RS, Hobbs CA, et al. Prevalence of spina bifida and anencephaly during the transition to mandatory folic acid fortification in the United States. Teratology 2002; 66(1):33–39.

304. van der Pal-de Bruin KM, de Walle HE, Jeeninga W, de Rover C, Cornel MC, de Jong-van den Berg LT, et al. The Dutch 'Folic Acid Campaign' – have the goals been achieved? Paediatr Perinat Epidemiol 2000; 14(2):111–117.

305. Folic acid campaign and evaluation – southwestern Virginia, 1997–1999. MMWR 1999; 48:914–917.

306. Bode MM, O'shea TM, Metzguer KR, Stiles AD. Perinatal regionalization and neonatal mortality in North Carolina, 1968–1994. Am J Obstet Gynecol 2001; 184(6):1302–1307.
307. Jones G, Steketee RW, Black RE, Bhutta ZA, Morris SS. How many child deaths can we prevent this year? Lancet 2003; 362(9377):65–71.
308. Hill SA, Hjelmeland B, Johannessen NM, Irgens LM, Skjaerven R. Changes in parental risk behaviour after an information campaign against sudden infant death syndrome (SIDS) in Norway. Acta Paediatr 2004; 93(2):250–254.
309. Zaza S, Sleet DA, Thompson RS, Sosin DM, Bolen JC. Reviews of evidence regarding interventions to increase use of child safety seats. Am J Prev Med 2001; 21(4, Suppl):31–47.
310. Briss PA, Rodewald LE, Hinman AR, Shefer AM, Strikas RA, Bernier RR, et al. Reviews of evidence regarding interventions to improve vaccination coverage in children, adolescents, and adults. The Task Force on Community Preventive Services. Am J Prev Med 2000; 18(1, Suppl):97–140.
311. Preventing unintended pregnancy in the U.S. Issues Brief (Alan Guttmacher Institute). 2004; 3:1–4.
312. Cnattingius S, Lambe M. Trends in smoking and overweight during pregnancy: prevalence, risks of pregnancy complications, and adverse pregnancy outcomes. Semin Perinatol 2002; 26(4):286–295.
313. Smoking during pregnancy – United States, 1990–2002. MMWR 2004; 53(39):911–915.
314. Giannelli M, Doyle P, Roman E, Pelerin M, Hermon C. The effect of caffeine consumption and nausea on the risk of miscarriage. Paediatr Perinat Epidemiol 2003; 17(4):316–323.
315. Gezer S. Antiphospholipid syndrome. Dis Mon 2003; 49(12):696–741.
316. Dorman JS, Burke JP, McCarthy BJ, Norris JM, Steenkiste AR, Aarons JH, et al. Temporal trends in spontaneous abortion associated with Type 1 diabetes. Diabetes Res Clin Pract 1999; 43(1):41–47.
317. Lorenzen T, Pociot F, Johannesen J, Kristiansen OP, Nerup J. A population-based survey of frequencies of self-reported spontaneous and induced abortions in Danish women with Type 1 diabetes mellitus. Danish IDDM Epidemiology and Genetics Group. Diabet Med 1999; 16 (6):472–476.
318. Kline J, Stein Z, Susser M, Warburton D. Fever during pregnancy and spontaneous abortion. Am J Epidemiol 1985; 121(6):832–842.
319. Andersen AM, Vastrup P, Wohlfahrt J, Andersen PK, Olsen J, Melbye M. Fever in pregnancy and risk of fetal death: a cohort study. Lancet 2002; 360(9345):1552–1556.
320. Chiba ME, Saito M, Suzuki N, Honda Y, Yaegashi N. Measles infection in pregnancy. J Infect 2003; 47(1):40–44.
321. Casterline JB. Maternal age, gravidity, and pregnancy spacing effects on spontaneous fetal mortality. Soc Biol 1989; 36(3–4):186–212.
322. Tong S, Marjono B, Brown DA, Mulvey S, Breit SN, Manuelpillai U, et al. Serum concentrations of macrophage inhibitory cytokine 1 (MIC 1) as a predictor of miscarriage. Lancet 2004; 363(9403):129–130.
323. Ransom MX, Bohrer M, Blotner MB, Kemmann E. The difference in miscarriage rates between menotropin-induced and natural cycle pregnancies is not surveillance related. Fertil Steril 1993; 59(3):567–570.
324. George L, Mills JL, Johansson AL, Nordmark A, Olander B, Granath F, et al. Plasma folate levels and risk of spontaneous abortion. JAMA 2002; 288(15):1867–1873.
325. Alberman E, Elliott M, Creasy M, Dhadial R. Previous reproductive history in mothers presenting with spontaneous abortions. Br J Obstet Gynaecol 1975; 82(5):366–373.
326. Andersen AMN, Wohlfahrt J, Christens P, Olsen J, Melbye M. Maternal age and fetal loss: population based register linkage study. BMJ 2000; 320(7251):1708–1712.
327. Roman E. Fetal loss rates and their relation to pregnancy order. J Epidemiol Community Health 1984; 38(1):29–35.
328. Golding J, Vivian S, Newcombe RG. Fetal loss, gravidity and pregnancy order: is the truncated cascade analysis valid? Early Hum Dev 1982; 6(1):71–76.

329. Brenner B. Inherited thrombophilia and pregnancy loss. Best Pract Res Clin Haematol 2003; 16(2):311–320.

330. Procter JA, Haney AF. Recurrent first trimester pregnancy loss is associated with uterine septum but not with bicornuate uterus. Fertil Steril 2003; 80(5):1212–1215.

331. Pell JP, Smith GC, Walsh D. Pregnancy complications and subsequent maternal cerebrovascular events: a retrospective cohort study of 119,668 births. Am J Epidemiol 2004; 159 (4):336–342.

332. Windham GC, Von Behren J, Fenster L, Schaefer C, Swan SH. Moderate maternal alcohol consumption and risk of spontaneous abortion. Epidemiology 1997; 8(5):509–514.

333. Abel EL. Maternal alcohol consumption and spontaneous abortion. Alcohol Alcohol 1997; 32(3):211–219.

334. Armstrong BG, McDonald AD, Sloan M. Cigarette, alcohol, and coffee consumption and spontaneous abortion. Am J Public Health 1992; 82(1):85–87.

335. Kline J, Shrout P, Stein Z, Susser M, Warburton D. Drinking during pregnancy and spontaneous abortion. Lancet 1980; 2(8187):176–180.

336. Fenster L, Hubbard AE, Swan SH, Windham GC, Waller K, Hiatt RA, et al. Caffeinated beverages, decaffeinated coffee, and spontaneous abortion. Epidemiology 1997; 8(5):515–523.

337. Fenster L, Eskenazi B, Windham GC, Swan SH. Caffeine consumption during pregnancy and spontaneous abortion. Epidemiology 1991; 2(3):168–174.

338. Cnattingius S, Signorello LB, Anneren G, Clausson B, Ekbom A, Ljunger E, et al. Caffeine intake and the risk of first-trimester spontaneous abortion. N Engl J Med 2000; 343 (25):1839–1845.

339. Fenster L, Hubbard AE, Windham GC, Waller KO, Swan SH. A prospective study of work-related physical exertion and spontaneous abortion. Epidemiology 1997; 8(1):66–74.

340. Windham GC, Swan SH, Fenster L. Parental cigarette smoking and the risk of spontaneous abortion. Am J Epidemiol 1992; 135(12):1394–1403.

341. Kline J, Levin B, Kinney A, Stein Z, Susser M, Warburton D. Cigarette smoking and spontaneous abortion of known karyotype. Precise data but uncertain inferences. Am J Epidemiol 1995; 141(5):417–427.

342. Kline J, Stein ZA, Susser M, Warburton D. Smoking: a risk factor for spontaneous abortion. N Engl J Med 1977; 297(15):793–796.

343. Lindbohm ML, Sallmen M, Taskinen H. Effects of exposure to environmental tobacco smoke on reproductive health. Scand J Work Environ Health 2002; 28(Suppl 2):84–96.

344. Venners SA, Wang X, Chen C, Wang L, Chen D, Guang W, et al. Paternal smoking and pregnancy loss: a prospective study using a biomarker of pregnancy. Am J Epidemiol 2004; 159(10):993–1001.

345. Ronnenberg AG, Goldman MB, Chen D, Aitken IW, Willett WC, Selhub J, et al. Preconception folate and vitamin B(6) status and clinical spontaneous abortion in Chinese women. Obstet Gynecol 2002; 100(1):107–113.

346. Dillon JC, Milliez J. Reproductive failure in women living in iodine deficient areas of West Africa. BJOG 2000; 107(5):631–636.

347. Li DK, Janevic T, Odouli R, Liu L. Hot tub use during pregnancy and the risk of miscarriage. Am J Epidemiol 2003; 158(10):931–937.

348. Swan SH, Waller K, Hopkins B, Windham G, Fenster L, Schaefer C, et al. A prospective study of spontaneous abortion: relation to amount and source of drinking water consumed in early pregnancy. Epidemiology 1998; 9(2):126–133.

349. Hertz-Picciotto I. The evidence that lead increases the risk for spontaneous abortion. Am J Ind Med 2000; 38(3):300–309.

350. Aschengrau A, Zierler S, Cohen A. Quality of community drinking water and the occurrence of spontaneous abortion. Arch Environ Health 1989; 44(5):283–290.

351. Deane M, Swan SH, Harris JA, Epstein DM, Neutra RR. Adverse pregnancy outcomes in relation to water consumption: a re-analysis of data from the original Santa Clara County Study, California, 1980–1981. Epidemiology 1992; 3(2):94–97.

352. Windham GC, Shusterman D, Swan SH, Fenster L, Eskenazi B. Exposure to organic solvents and adverse pregnancy outcome. Am J Ind Med 1991; 20(2):241–259.

353. Lindbohm ML, Taskinen H, Sallmen M, Hemminki K. Spontaneous abortions among women exposed to organic solvents. Am J Ind Med 1990; 17(4):449–463.

354. John EM, Savitz DA, Shy CM. Spontaneous abortions among cosmetologists. Epidemiology 1994; 5(2):147–155.

355. Olsen J, Hemminki K, Ahlborg G, Bjerkedal T, Kyyronen P, Taskinen H, et al. Low birthweight, congenital malformations, and spontaneous abortions among dry-cleaning workers in Scandinavia. Scand J Work Environ Health 1990; 16(3):163–168.

356. Kyyronen P, Taskinen H, Lindbohm ML, Hemminki K, Heinonen OP. Spontaneous abortions and congenital malformations among women exposed to tetrachloroethylene in dry cleaning. J Epidemiol Community Health 1989; 43(4):346–351.

357. Eskenazi B, Fenster L, Wight S, English P, Windham GC, Swan SH. Physical exertion as a risk factor for spontaneous abortion. Epidemiology 1994; 5(1):6–13.

358. Taskinen H, Kyyronen P, Hemminki K, Hoikkala M, Lajunen K, Lindbohm ML. Laboratory work and pregnancy outcome. J Occup Med 1994; 36(3):311–319.

359. Uchida IA, Freeman VC, Gedeon M, Goldmaker J. Twinning rate in spontaneous abortions. Am J Hum Genet 1983; 35(5):987–993.

360. Taskinen H, Anttila A, Lindbohm ML, Sallmen M, Hemminki K. Spontaneous abortions and congenital malformations among the wives of men occupationally exposed to organic solvents. Scand J Work Environ Health 1989; 15(5):345–352.

361. Lindbohm ML, Hemminki K, Bonhomme MG, Anttila A, Rantala K, Heikkila P, et al. Effects of paternal occupational exposure on spontaneous abortions. Am J Public Health 1991; 81(8):1029–1033.

362. Kallan JE, Enneking EA. Seasonal patterns of spontaneous abortion. J Biosoc Sci 1992; 24(1):71–75.

363. Weinberg CR, Moledor E, Baird DD, Wilcox AJ. Is there a seasonal pattern in risk of early pregnancy loss? Epidemiology 1994; 5(5):484–489.

364. Eriksson AW, Fellman J. Seasonal variation of livebirths, stillbirths, extramarital births and twin maternities in Switzerland. Twin Res 2000; 3(4):189–201.

365. Weerasinghe DP, MacIntyre RC. Seasonality of births and abortions in New South Wales, Australia. Med Sci Monit 2003; 9(12):CR534–CR540.

Chapter 7
Birth Weight, Gestational Duration, and Fetal Growth[1]

Joseph was so unlike my best friend's first child, Mary. Mary was born right on time and weighed 8 pounds. She was an alert and happy baby with a plump round face and chubby thighs. She was so easy to care for and grew quickly. My pregnancy with Joseph was very different. I was barely half way through my pregnancy when I started having trouble. I wasn't eating well and was still struggling to stop smoking. There were serious concerns about how well the baby was growing and then the pains started. At 30 weeks, my Obstetrician said he should intervene. Delivered by c-section, Joseph was so small and thin. He weighed only 2 pounds at birth and stayed in the Neonatal Intensive Care Unit at the hospital for over two months. Who knows what it will all cost and the bills are still coming. When we finally got him home, Joseph was very fragile and fussy. I had to give up my job to stay home and care for him. At six and nine months of age, he wasn't able to do the same things that Mary did. He couldn't sit up or crawl when Mary did. My pediatrician says he is going to refer him for special help. I worry about whether he will ever be all right. I don't know what I did wrong.

7.1 Introduction

Many factors influence birth weight, the most proximate being length of gestation and rate of fetal growth. Thus, when evaluating changes in the distribution of birth weight, without additional information, one cannot be sure if changes reflect changes in gestational length, fetal growth rates, or both.

Being born too soon and/or too small is a significant risk factor for early mortality, newborn and later morbidity, as well as developmental delay. The birth weight of

---

[1] Excerpts of this chapter are reprinted with permission from the National Academies Press, Copyright 2007, National Academy of Sciences.

M.M. Adams et al., *Perinatal Epidemiology for Public Health Practice.*
doi: 10.1007/978-0-387-09439-7_7; © Springer Science + Business Media, LLC 2009

an infant is a function of both the length of pregnancy duration (the gestational age) and the extent of fetal growth. Combined, these factors are powerful predictors of newborn viability, early survival, and the need for extended medical care and ongoing support services. This chapter explores these three interrelated indicators of the degree of fetal development and maturation at birth. We begin with birth weight, the most readily determined measure at birth, and then turn to its two immediate precursors, gestational duration and fetal growth. As will become apparent, these measures are not interchangeable even though they are highly correlated. They have different risk factors, etiologies, and consequences. Equally importantly, there are complex measurement issues that complicate their use and interpretation. Although there is a common appreciation by the public that being born too soon or too small can result in some fairly severe adverse outcomes, much confusion remains about the causes of extreme variation in birth weight, gestational age, and fetal growth and potential prevention by mothers, clinicians, public health professionals, and policy makers.

7.2 Birth Weight

7.2.1 Definitions, Measures, Data Sources, and Measurement Issues

Definition: Birth weight is the weight of the fetus or infant at delivery, exclusive of other byproducts of the delivery, e.g., amniotic fluid or the placenta, and is traditionally recorded in either metric (grams) or avoirdupois (pounds and ounces) weight units. Because of the widespread use of external standardized scales of measurement, birth weight is generally considered a very reliably measured indicator in developed nations.

Although birth weight is actually no more than a measure of fetal or infant mass at delivery, it is conceptually employed as an important indicator of the approximate degree of maturity and extent of physical development of a fetus or newborn infant. Moreover, it is highly predictive of the ability of a newborn infant to survive and to be relatively free of serious early morbidity.

The birth weight of an infant or fetus is immediately dependent on: (1) the duration of the pregnancy, i.e., the amount of time the fetus has to grow in utero, and (2) the rate and extent of fetal growth (1, 2). In addition, birth weight may be influenced by genetic predisposition and environmental exposures (3). Infants who are delivered earlier than normal are expected to be of smaller birth weight than average, as they have had less time to develop and increase their overall size and mass, assuming a normal rate of fetal development. Delay in delivery beyond the normal length of pregnancy is also a problem with potential consequences for birth weight. Additionally, infants who had slower or faster fetal growth can also have a birth weight that is lower or higher than would be average for their length of gestational duration.

Birth Weight Conversion and Round-off:

Both gram and avoirdupois scales continue to be used to measure birth weight in the United States. As parents often want to know their infant's birth weight in pounds and ounces, measures of birth weight in grams may be converted to pounds and ounces and later reconverted to grams. Accompanying this conversion process, rounding off to the nearest quarter pound or 100-g interval often occurs. The combination of using and converting between the two measurement scales and the practice of round-off creates notable anomalies in the birth weight distribution (see Fig. 7.1).

Scale conversion:

$$1 \text{ oz} = 28.349523 \text{ g}$$
$$4 \text{ oz} = 113.3981 \text{ g}$$
$$1 \text{ lb} = 453.5924 \text{ g}$$
$$5.5 \text{ lb} = 2494.7579 \text{ g}$$
$$7.5 \text{ lb} = 3401.9427 \text{ g}$$
$$1 \text{ g} = 0.03527 \text{ oz}$$
$$125 \text{ g} = 4.4093 \text{ oz}$$
$$250 \text{ g} = 8.8185 \text{ oz}$$
$$500 \text{ g} = 17.637 \text{ oz}$$
$$1,500 \text{ g} = 3.3066 \text{ lb}$$
$$2,500 \text{ g} = 5.5116 \text{ lb}$$
$$3,350 \text{ g} = 7.3855 \text{ lb}$$
$$4,000 \text{ g} = 8.8175 \text{ lb}$$

Measures: Individual birth weight values from each member of a population are used to generate an overall population distribution of birth weights for a variety of statistical comparisons. Because of measurement problems (described in a following section), the birth weight distribution is typically based on categories of birth weight, typically 500-g intervals, but also 250 and 125-g intervals depending on the number of cases available throughout the range of birth weights. When avoirdupois weights are used, ½ or 1-lb intervals of birth weight are generally employed for creating birth weight distributions. The 125-g birth weight interval closely compares with the quarter pound interval (4.4 oz) but will still result in a slightly different distribution (Fig. 7.1).

Using year 2001–2002 live births and fetal deaths to US resident mothers, the distribution of birth weight values measured in 250-g intervals is provided in Fig. 7.2. The distribution of birth weights for live births approximates a bell-shaped distribution with most (~80%) births concentrated between 2,750 and 4,250 g. Although not a truly normal distribution, as noted by the left-hand tail, the median birth weight for US singleton, full-term (40-weeks gestation) live births is 3,487 g and the mean birth weight is 3,303 g. The birth weight distribution is slightly skewed (skewness: −0.90). The birth weight distribution of fetal deaths is quite

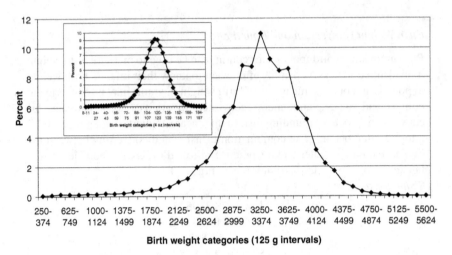

Fig. 7.1 Birth weight distribution of live births, United States, 2001–2002

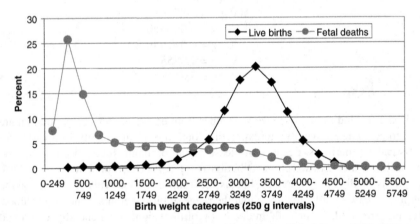

Fig. 7.2 Birth weight distribution of live births and fetal deaths, United States, 2001–2002

distinct, reflecting myriad etiologies that result in a high proportion of early and small deliveries and a trailing tail of heavier stillbirths delivered closer to term.

Birth weight categories: Birth weight is typically categorized for use by researchers and policy makers as a means to identify the proportion of the population that falls within high to low-risk birth weight groupings. The most common categorization of birth weight is low birth weight (LBW), which is a term used to describe infants born at the lower extreme of the birth weight distribution. In 1948, the World Health Assembly recommended that a single definition of LBW be established for consistent reporting of vital statistics and other public policy purposes (4). The current definition, weighing less than 2,500 g (approximately 5 lbs 8 oz), was derived from earlier recommendations by Ethel Dunham and Arvo Ylppo (5–7). The decision to use *less than* 2,500 g in part reflected a problem of recording rounded-off birth weight values. A review of the history of the development of the LBW measure reveals that the criterion of 2,500 g per 5.5 lb was originally selected not only as a means to identify higher risk infants but also to facilitate the comparison of data between countries using metric and avoirdupois scales. The original proposition that 2,500 g denoted higher risk was based on an early 1900 analysis of German infants by Ylppo (6, 7). Nevertheless, the criterion has been widely used in divergent populations as a *one-size-fits-all* measures of risk even though there is little evidence to support the appropriateness of such applications.

Marked advances in medical technology and practice have occurred since the 2,500-g criterion for LBW was established. These developments have resulted in vastly improved survival rates for LBW infants, which lead to the need for further classifications of LBW to better identify high-risk infants (8). Very small infants are now further categorized as very low birth weight (VLBW: <1,500 g; ~3 lbs 5 oz) and extremely low birth weight (ELBW: <1,000 g; ~2 lbs 3 oz). Moderately low birth weight (MLBW: 1,500–2,499 g) is presently used to denote those infants who are still at moderate risk due to their lower than average birth weight but not at the extreme risk of the VLBW group. This birth weight category has taken on greater significance in recent years as interest has grown in investigating potential changes in clinical practice with regard to earlier intervention for high-risk pregnancy. Clinicians are able to identify high-risk conditions earlier in pregnancy and, with the aid of advances in neonatal technology, can provide effective extra-utero support. This ability to intervene may be reflected by increases in the proportion of moderately low birth weight infants and may be a means of assessing trends in the use of earlier intervention therapies, i.e., c-section, to reduce the risk of fetal and infant death.

Birth Weight Categories:
Low birth weight: <2,500 g
  Moderately low birth weight: 1,500–2,499 g
  Very low birth weight: <1,500 g
  Extremely low birth weight: <1,000 g
Macrosomia (high birth weight): >4,000 g
  Grade I: 4,000–4,499 g
  Grade II: 4,500–4,999 g
  Grade III: 5,000+ g

At the other extreme of the birth weight distribution are births characterized by being heavier than average. High birth weight (HBW) or macrosomia (large body) in an infant is related to increased mortality and morbidity risk to both infant and mother. A widely agreed upon definition of macrosomia has yet to be established, but often used definitions include birth weights equal to or exceeding 4,000; 4,500; or 5,000 g, as well as births weighing at or above the 90th percentile of birth weights for the infant's gestational age (also known as: large-for-gestational age). Most recently there has been a proposal to categorize macrosomic births into three grades: grade I (4,000–4,499 g), grade II (4,500–4,999 g), and grade III (5,000+ g) (9). Grade I macrosomia has been proposed for use in studies seeking to identify increased risks of labor and newborn complications, while grade II and III are touted for use in investigating predictors of neonatal morbidity and infant mortality risk, respectively (10).

Table 7.1 depicts the proportion of 2001–2002 live births and fetal deaths to US resident mothers that fall within each of the commonly used birth weight risk categories. The risks of mortality for these typically used categories of birth weight are also provided (Table 7.2). For this time period, 7.7% of live births were LBW and 1.4% of live births were VLBW. However, LBW and VLBW infants made up 67 and 53%, respectively, of the infant deaths. The infant mortality rate for LBW infants was 57.8 deaths per 1,000 live-born LBW infants and was 245.4 deaths per 1,000 for VLBW infants. Macrosomic infants (4,000+ g) comprised over 9% of live births, while contributing only 2.1% of the infant deaths. The risk of an infant death rose sharply for birth greater than 5,000 g. In addition, it is important to consider the extreme racial and ethnic variations in these outcomes. For this time period, 13.2% of all black infants were LBW and 3.1% were VLBW. LBW and VLBW infants made up 75 and 63.6%, respectively, of the deaths among black infants. The infant mortality rate among LBW black infants was 74.4 per 1,000 live births compared with 51.4 among whites.

The close relationship between an infant's birth weight and the risk of dying within the first year of life has long been recognized, and birth weight is often used by researchers as a measure of mortality risk (11). At light and heavy birth weights, an infant's risk of mortality soars (Fig. 7.3), although in recent decades, heavier infant births have become less associated with high mortality risks, probably due to medical intervention. Nevertheless, VLBW infants continue to be at grave risk of mortality, morbidity, and long-term developmental problems (12–15). Birth-weight-specific neonatal, postneonatal, and infant mortality rates for live births are provided in Fig. 7.3. This figure employs a log scale for mortality rates, which is a typical convention to display these data. Clearly evident are the higher rates of mortality at the extremes of birth weight with a wide nadir of mortality found for infant in the 3,500–4,000-g interval. For LBW and Grade III macrosomic infants, there is a higher rate of neonatal mortality (death in the first month of life) compared with postneonatal mortality (death in months 2–11). This pattern is reversed for normal birth weight infants.

Additionally, the patterns of birth weight-specific mortality rates vary substantially among non-Hispanic White, non-Hispanic Black, Hispanic, and infants of

Table 7.1 Percentages of live births, fetal deaths, and infant deaths by birth weight categories and by race, United States, 2001–2002

	Live Birth (%)					Fetal Death (%)					Infant Death (%)				
	All	W	B	His	O	All	W	B	His	O	All	W	B	His	O
Low birth weight (LBW: <2500 g)	7.7	6.7	13.2	6.5	7.6	80.4	78.2	86.6	77.8	79.5	67.3	63.3	75.0	66.1	65.8
Very low birth weight (VLBW: <1500 g)	1.4	1.1	3.1	1.2	1.2	64.1	61.6	71.4	60.7	62.9	53.3	48.5	63.6	50.0	50.1
Moderately LBW (MLBW: 1500–2499 g)	6.3	5.6	10.1	5.3	6.4	16.3	16.6	15.2	17.1	16.6	14.1	14.8	10.1	16.1	15.1
Normal birth weight (NBW: 2500–3999 g)	83.0	82.3	81.8	84.9	85.6	17.5	19.8	12.0	19.4	18.1	30.5	34.1	23.8	31.7	31.7
Macrosomia (High Birth Weight: 4000+ g)	9.3	10.9	5.0	8.6	6.8	2.1	2.1	1.5	2.8	2.4	2.1	2.6	1.2	2.2	2.5
Macrosomia Grade I: 4000–4499 g	7.9	9.3	4.3	7.4	5.8	1.3	1.4	0.9	1.8	1.5	1.6	2.1	0.9	1.5	1.8
Macrosomia Grade II: 4500–4999 g	1.2	1.5	0.6	1.1	0.9	0.5	0.5	0.4	0.6	0.5	0.4	0.4	0.2	0.5	0.6
Macrosomia Grade III: 5000+ g	0.1	0.2	0.1	0.1	0.1	0.3	0.3	0.2	0.4	0.4	0.1	0.1	0.1	0.2	0.1

All = All races; W = White; B = Black; His = Hispanic; O = Other

Table 7.2 Fetal, neonatal, and postneonatal mortality rates by birth weight categories, United States, 2001–2002

	FMR					NMR					Post NMR					IMR				
	All	W	B	His	O	All	W	B	His	O	All	W	B	His	O	All	W	B	His	O
Low birth weight (LBW: <2500 g)	56.9	50.4	64.3	58.1	74.7	47.0	42.4	59.2	44.8	42.0	10.8	9.0	15.2	10.3	8.9	57.8	51.4	74.4	55.2	50.9
Very low birth weight (VLBW: <1500 g)	202.7	194.7	192.2	212.2	290.7	215.1	208.4	228.7	204.6	225.9	30.4	24.7	39.1	29.7	28.5	245.4	233.1	267.8	234.3	254.4
Moderately LBW (MLBW: 1500–2499 g)	14.9	13.5	15.6	16.2	19.6	8.6	8.7	7.0	10.2	8.5	6.3	5.8	7.8	6.1	5.3	14.9	14.5	14.7	16.4	13.8
Normal birth weight (NBW: 2500–3999 g)	1.2	1.1	1.5	1.2	1.6	0.8	0.8	1.1	0.8	0.8	1.6	1.4	2.7	1.3	1.4	2.4	2.3	3.8	2.0	2.2
Macrosomia (High birth weight: 4000+ g)	1.3	0.9	3.1	1.7	2.7	0.6	0.5	1.2	0.6	0.7	0.9	0.8	2.0	0.8	1.5	1.5	1.3	3.3	1.4	2.2
Macrosomia Grade I: 4000–4499g	0.9	0.6	2.1	1.2	2.0	0.5	0.5	0.8	0.4	0.5	0.9	0.7	2.0	0.7	1.3	1.4	1.2	2.8	1.1	1.8
Macrosomia Grade II: 4500–4999g	2.3	1.6	6.4	2.7	4.2	1.0	0.6	2.5	1.3	2.0	1.1	0.9	2.5	1.0	2.0	2.1	1.5	4.9	2.3	3.9
Macrosomia Grade III: 5000+g	12.7	8.7	25.7	15.9	22.8	3.8	2.6	10.4	5.0	1.6	2.2	1.8	2.1	2.5	4.8	5.9	4.3	12.5	7.5	6.4

FMR = Fetal Mortality Rate (fetal deaths per 1,000 live births plus fetal deaths)

NMR = Neonatal Mortality Rate (deaths less than 28 days per 1,000 live births)

PNMR = Postneonatal Mortality Rate (deaths 28–365 days per 1,000 live births)

IMR = Infant Mortality Rate (death less than one year per 1,000 live births)

All = All races; W = White; B = Black; His = Hispanic; O = Other

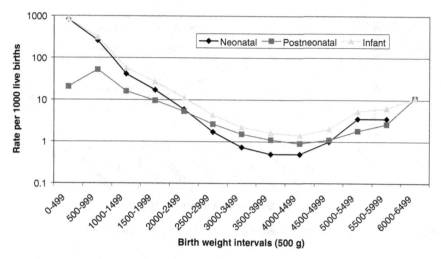

Fig. 7.3 Birth weight-specific mortality rates, 2001–2002

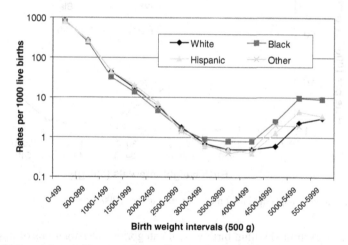

Fig. 7.4 Birth-weight-specific neonatal mortality rates by race, 2001–2002

other races. Figures 7.4 –7.6 present birth weight-specific mortality rates by race. Postneonatal mortality rates are consistently higher among Blacks; for neonatal and infant mortality rates, the rate of mortality is higher for Blacks beginning at roughly 2,500 g.

Populations with more infants born at very high or very low birth weights predictably have higher infant mortality rates. Therefore, it is an established procedure to take birth weight into account when making comparisons of mortality among newborn populations. Whether the comparison involves temporal, geographic, socioeconomic, hospital or other contrasts, infant mortality differences

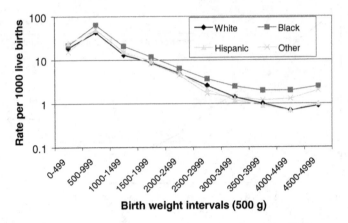

Fig. 7.5 Birth weight-specific postneonatal mortality rates by race, 2001–2002

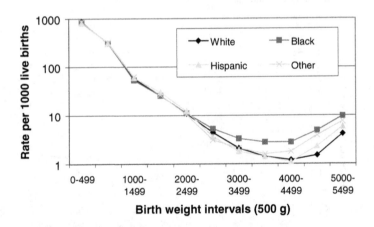

Fig. 7.6 Birth weight-specific infant mortality rates by race, 2001–2002

are typically examined within birth weight categories. Investigations of improving trends in infant mortality rates often start with an examination of the extent to which any changes are related to improvements in the distribution of birth weights within categories (i.e., fewer births at extreme birth weights), as opposed to reductions in birth weight-specific mortality rates (i.e., infants in specific birth weight categories having better survival).

Data Sources: Birth certificate data compiled by state vital record offices are the basic source of population-based birth weight information in the United States. State vital record data are further compiled by the National Center for Health Statistics (NCHS) and are made publicly available on CD-ROMS (16). Data from these public-access data files have been extensively used throughout this book for examples. Hospital-based perinatal data systems are increasingly being implemented and represent another source of birth weight information on regional, local, and hospital catchment populations.

Measurement Issues: Various studies have confirmed the validity and reliability of birth weight collected on the birth certificate by comparing hospital data to birth certificate data (17–22). However, a host of measurement problems have been noted with the collection of birth weight data. The initial source of error involves the accurate recording of the scale reading on the birth certificate data collection form and then entering that on the actual birth certificate or automated birth registry system. Commonly cited recording errors include transposed numbers, dropped digits, and other problems stemming for inaccurate reading and transcribing birth weight values onto data collection forms, certificates, or data files (23).

Although still commonly reported on U.S. birth certificates in pounds and ounces, the original birth weight is increasingly measured using gram-based scales in U.S. hospitals, which then may be converted to an avoirdupois weight for reporting to parents and then reconverted back to grams for centralized statistical use by state public health agencies. In addition to recording and calculation errors that may occur during this conversion process, slightly different conversion procedures may be employed, e.g., using 28.3495 vs. 28.3 to convert ounces to grams, which may result in modest changes from the original birth weight value. Moreover, original birth weight values may be initially rounded off and then rounded-off again during this process of converting birth weight values. Grams may be rounded off to the nearest 10, 50, or 100 g, and avoirdupois weights may be rounded to the nearest quarter pound with rounding procedures varying among hospitals and even among staff within hospitals. Added to the universal problem of imprecisely calibrated scales, these recording and conversion processes conceivably may result in systematic measurement biases as well as creating other problems for researchers who aggregate birth weight values into categories for analysis.

The accurate reporting of live births less than 500 g is yet another source of measurement error that continues to plague perinatal researchers. It has been suggested that trends toward the increased reporting of deliveries of less than 500 g as live births, rather than as fetal deaths or not reporting them at all, may partially underlie the apparent lack of improvement in preterm and LBW rates in many parts of the United States (24). Ignoring considerations about accurately measuring an infant's weight, a more liberal definition of what is considered a live birth will cause the live birth distribution to include more very tiny babies and lower the mean for the entire population's birth weight distribution of all live births. The issue regarding variations in live births vs. fetal death definitions is discussed further in Chapter 6.

7.2.2 Descriptive Epidemiology

Temporal Trends: Figure 7.7 depicts US trends in LBW, VLBW, and high birth weight from 1980 to 2002. Although the proportion of live births with birth weights 4,000+ g has declined since 1990, the percent of LBW and VLBW infants has risen

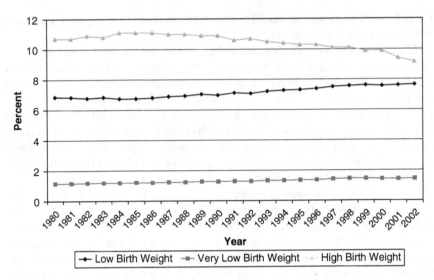

Fig. 7.7 US trends in low birth weight, very low birth weight, and high birth weight, 1980–2002

fairly steadily. Since 1980, the proportion of VLBW has risen from 1.15% to 1.44%, a 25% increase. At the same time LBW rates have increased nearly 12%. The most recent data from the 2000s provide little evidence to suggest that this trend has reversed or even stopped. Nearly all of the decline in infant mortality rates in the USA in the last quarter of the twentieth century was due to improvements in survival rather than any betterment in the birth weight distribution (25–27). Better survival within birth weight groups has been attributed to advances in obstetric and newborn medical care (25–27). However, the increasing medical care costs that have accompanied these advances raise concerns about overly relying on medical technology to reduce infant death rates. Accordingly, research attention has been directed at finding the determinants of LBW in order to develop more cost-effective, population-wide programs to further diminish infant mortality.

Geographic variability: VLBW and LBW rates historically have been higher in the southeastern USA. As evident in Figs. 7.8 and 7.9, with the exception of Colorado, likely due to its high altitude, the highest rates of VLBW and LBW are clustered in the states from Louisiana and Maryland. The northeastern industrialized states tend to have the next highest rates, a pattern that has persisted over the past 50 years. Conversely, northwestern states exhibited the lowest rates of LBW and VLBW, along with the northern New England states.

In addition, there are international differences in LBW percentages. The overall LBW percentage around the world is 15.5%. In more developed countries, the average is 7.7% and in less developed countries, 16.5%, and those least developed countries have a LBW percentage of 18.6%. Figure 7.10 presents the percentages of LBW from 2000 in the six United Nations world regions. The highest proportion of LBW infants was noted in Asia (18.3%) with the proportion for South-Central Asia at 27.1% (28).

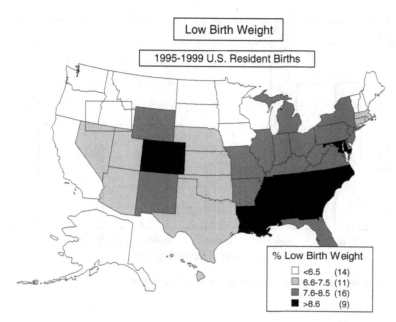

Fig. 7.8 State-specific low birth weight rates (<2500 g), United States, 1995–1999

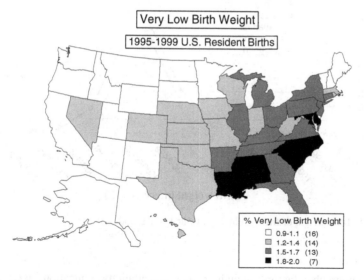

Fig. 7.9 State-specific rates of very low birth rates (<1500 g), United States, 1995–1999

Demographic Variability: Birth weight distribution variations, involving differences in mean birth weight and percentages of high risk births at both tails of the distribution, have been associated with infant gender, multiple birth, maternal

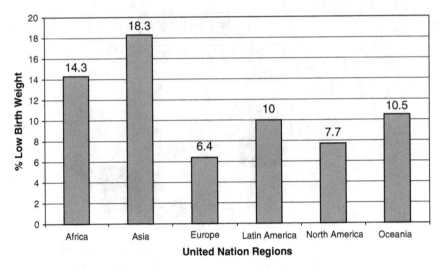

Fig. 7.10 Low birth weight percentages by United Nation regions, 2000

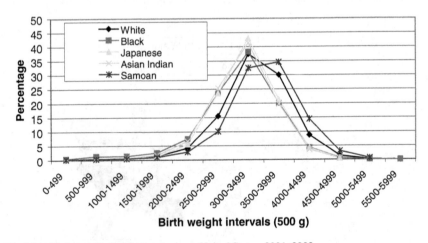

Fig. 7.11 Birth weight distribution by race, United States, 2001–2002

sociodemographic factors, including race and ethnicity, education, age, marital status, maternal anthropometry, behavior factors, including substance use and nutrition, and current and previous pregnancy medical risk characteristics, e.g., parity (29–33). In Fig. 7.11, a comparison of the birth weight distributions in race and ethnic groups reflects more subtle differences with both a shift in mean birth weight and a difference in the skewness of the very low birth weight tail.

One of the unresolved questions among researchers is whether there is a single common average human birth weight or whether there are normal variations in average birth weight among population subgroups. This question entails important medical care, public health policy, and political aspects as it engenders deliberation about what is a *normal* birth weight and in contrast a *high-risk* birth weight. There is ongoing debate regarding whether a single *one-size-fits-all* criterion for high-risk birth weights, e.g., a single 2,500-g criterion for LBW, is equally valid for all infants (8). These discussions are fueled by the continuing inability of researchers to adequately explain population subgroup disparities in birth weight using available sociodemographic risk factors (31).

7.2.3 Factors Influencing Birth Weight Distribution

This section reviews selected factors influencing birth weight. The role of unwed marital status on increasing LBW is still poorly defined but is likely to work in

Risk Factors and Attributable Risks: Risk Factors for LBW

Demographic risks:
- Maternal race
- Maternal age
- SES
- Maternal education
- Marital status

Medical risks:
- Parity
- Previous pregnancy outcome
- Multiple birth
- Hypertension
- Infections

Behavioral and environmental risks:
- Substance use
- Nutrition
- High altitude
- Physical labor

Health care risks:
- Prenatal care

Evolving risks:
- Stress
- Contextual factors

association with poverty (30). Poverty is associated with reduced access to health care, poor nutrition, lower education, and inadequate housing. It is also generally linked with poorer average health status and is concentrated in a number of minority racial and ethnic populations. These poverty-related factors may work in combination to increase the risk of delivering a LBW infant (30–35). Furthermore, socioeconomic status is linked to individual behaviors, such as cigarette smoking and alcohol consumption and also varies markedly by race and ethnicity (36). While socioeconomic status and race/ethnicity cannot be termed *causes* of LBW, they serve as indicators of complex links between environmental, psychological, and physiological factors that may result in higher risks of LBW (30). Figure 7.12 depicts the marked shift in the birth weight distributions among singleton and multiple births. The deviation among multiple births in median birth weight is clearly evident.

Much attention has been given to delineating the precursors of LBW. Nevertheless, the number of identified risk factors that are actually modifiable during pregnancy is still few. At the other extreme of the birth weight distribution, one-third of macrosomic births are still unexplained. Several factors are known to contribute to excessive fetal size, including large size of parents (especially the mother), multiparity, diabetes in the mother, and prolonged gestation (37–47). Older maternal age, male infants, and previous delivery of a high birth weight infant also seem to be indicative of macrosomic births (37–47). Babies of diabetic women are usually large at birth but they behave clinically as if they are immature (48–52). These infants are not longer in average length but have increased fetal weight (52). Because glucose, a substance necessary for fetal growth, is elevated in both diabetic and obese women, these mothers are more likely to have macrosomic births (51–53).

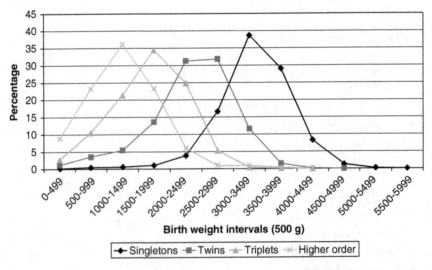

Fig. 7.12 Birth weight distribution by plurality, United States, 2001–2002

Risks for birth injuries rise rapidly for heavier babies, with vaginal deliveries being related to higher morbidity and mortality for both the infant and the mother (37, 39, 41, 42). Lacerations of the birth canal and hemorrhaging may occur to the mother; fetal death may occur due to asphyxia, and infants may suffer broken clavicles and neurologic damage (42, 43). While cesarean section has been pre-scribed as the best delivery method to prevent fetal death or injury, others suggest that vaginal birth is still possible for some macrosomic infants (37, 42).

Tables 7.3 and 7.4 detail the risk factors for VLBW and LBW births that are commonly available on vital records. These risk factors are provided for 5-years intervals from 1980 to 1999. Risk characteristics include age of mother (often grouped as teenaged mothers, <18 years, and older mothers, 30+ years), maternal education (groups may delineate less than high school, high school, and more than high school education), marital status, parity (first birth and a high number of previous births for age), and race of mother.

As seen in Table 7.3, the total percentage of live births to teen mothers in the United States has stayed fairly constant (between 4.8 and 5.3%) over this period. For VLBW infants, the proportion born to teenaged mothers has however fallen from 9.5% in 1980–1984 to 7.1% in 1995–1999. The proportion of VLBW infants born to teen mothers was 2.1% throughout the 20-year period, during which VLBW percentages increased from 1.2% in 1980–1984 to 1.4% in 1995–1999. The VLBW odds ratio for teens, indicating the risk of having a VLBW infant if the mother is a teen compared with a mother 18–29 years of age, declined from 1.16 to 1.04. Similarly the attributable risk fraction for teens also declined from 4.3 to 2.8%, suggesting that the impact of teenage pregnancy on the VLBW problems is modest and dwindling.

For both LBW and VLBW infants, three risk characteristics stand out: multiple birth, marital status, and black race of mother. The number and proportion of multiple births has risen dramatically in the United States in recent years (53). This trend has important implications given the higher risk of VLBW and LBW for twins, triplets, and higher order multiple births.

7.3 Gestational Duration and Fetal Growth

7.3.1 Definitions, Measures, Data Sources, and Measurement Issues

Definition: The definition of prematurity has evolved in the literature of the last century. Initially used to designate an infant born too early or too small, it was often defined by either the use of birth weight or gestational age (54). As birth weight is more reliably measured than gestational age, LBW (<2,500 g) was the more obvious choice to delineate a premature birth. Nevertheless, being born too small is conceptually distinct from being born too early. As discussed previously, LBW

Table 7.3 Risk factors and attributable risks for very low birth weight, United States, 1980–1999

	Very Low Birth Weight															
	1980–1984			1985–1989			1990–1994			1995–1999		
	% Total % Among VLBW %VLBW	OR	AR$_{total}$	% Total % Among VLBW % VLBW	OR	AR$_{total}$	% Total % Among VLBW % VLBW	OR	AR$_{total}$	% Total % Among VLBW % VLBW	OR	AR$_{total}$
Total % VLBW		1.20%			1.20%			1.30%			1.41%	
Teen	5.30% 9.50% 2.10%	1.16 (1.14–1.18)	4.30%	4.80% 8.10% 2.10%	1.04 (1.02–1.06)	3.20%	5.00% 8.10% 2.10%	1.1 (1.06–1.14)	3.10%	4.80% 7.10% 2.10%	1.04 (1.02–1.05)	2.80%
Old	5.20% 5.50% 1.20%	1.2 (1.18–1.23)	0%	7.50% 8.10% 1.30%	1.33 (1.31–1.35)	0.80%	9.90% 11.40% 1.50%	1.37 (1.33–1.42)	1.50%	12.50% 14.90% 1.70%	1.34 (1.32–1.35)	2.70%
High Education	34.30% 26.30% 0.90%	0.85 (0.84–0.86)	−11.80%	37.80% 29.10% 1.00%	0.85 (0.84–0.86)	−14.40%	37.90% 30.00% 1.00%	0.87 (0.85–0.89)	−13.30%	44.80% 39.10% 1.20%	0.86 (0.86–0.87)	−10.20%
Low Education	19.60% 26.50% 1.60%	1.18 (1.17–1.20)	8.50%	18.80% 24.90% 1.60%	1.15 (1.13–1.16)	7.20%	21.60% 26.00% 1.50%	1.06 (1.04–1.09)	5.60%	19.90% 21.60% 1.50%	1.03 (1.01–1.04)	2.20%
Unmarried	19.30% 35.80% 2.20%	1.47 (1.45–1.49)	20.50%	24.60% 42.70% 2.20%	1.52 (1.50–1.53)	24.20%	30.20% 48.10% 2.10%	1.46 (1.43–1.49)	25.40%	32.50% 46.10% 2.00%	1.27 (1.25–1.28)	19.90%
Primiparous	42.30% 44.80% 1.20%	1.33 (1.31–1.34)	4.30%	41.10% 42.90% 1.30%	1.33 (1.32–1.34)	3.20%	40.60% 42.90% 1.40%	1.3 (1.27–1.33)	3.90%	40.60% 44.0% 1.50%	1.44 (1.43–1.46)	5.70%
High Parity	3.60% 6.40% 2.10%	1.18 (1.16–1.21)	2.60%	3.40% 6.50% 2.40%	1.21 (1.18–1.23)	3.20%	3.80% 7.20% 2.50%	1.25 (1.20–1.30)	3.10%	3.40% 5.90% 2.50%	1.24 (1.22–1.26)	2.80%

Black	15.60%	33.90%	2.50%	2.15 (2.13–2.18)	21.40%	16.00%	36.40%	2.8	2.37 (2.35–2.40)	24.20%	16.40%	37.20%	3.00%	2.53 (2.47–2.58)	24.60%	15.40%	33.30%	3.00%	2.53 (2.50–2.55)	21.30%
Foreign-born	9.90%	8.60%	1.00%	0.97 (0.95–0.99)	−0.90%	13.10%	10.90%	1.00%	0.94 (0.92–0.95)	−2.40%	17.00%	13.70%	1.00%	0.98 (0.95–1.00)	−3.90%	19.40%	15.70%	1.10%	0.98 (0.97–0.99)	−5.00%
Multiple birth	2.00%	18.40%	10.80%	12.99 (12.8–13.2)	16.20%	2.20%	18.90%	10.70%	12.27 (12.12–12.43)	16.90%	2.50%	20.60%	11.00%	11.84 (11.55–12.13)	18.50%	2.90%	24.00%	11.80%	12.95 (12.82–13.08)	22.00%
Hypertension											3.40%	9.10%	3.50%	2.38 (2.30–2.46)	5.40%	4.30%	12.60%	4.10%	2.71 (2.68–2.74)	8.50%
Diabetes											2.40%	1.80%	1.00%	0.658 (0.61–0.71)	−0.80%	2.60%	2.60%	1.40%	0.83 (0.81–0.85)	0%
Smoking											12.40%	16.70%	1.80%	1.45 (1.42–1.49)	4.60%	10.70%	14.10%	1.90%	1.44 (1.42–1.46)	4.30%

Table 7.4 Risk factors and attributable risks for low birth weight, United States, 1980–1999

	1980–1984			1985–1989			1990–1994			1995–1999		
	% Total / % Among LBW / % LBW	OR	AR_total	% Total / % Among LBW / % LBW	OR	AR_total	% Total / % Among LBW / % LBW	OR	AR_total	% Total / % Among LBW / % LBW	OR	AR_total
Total % LBW	6.80%			6.90%			7.10%			7.50%		
Teen	5.30% / 8.30% / 10.80%	1.03 (1.02–1.04)	3.20%	4.80% / 7.20% / 10.40%	0.94 (0.93–0.94)	2.60%	5.00% / 7.20% / 10.40%	1.03 (1.02–1.05)	2.40%	4.80% / 6.70% / 10.40%	1.04 (1.03–1.04)	2.00%
Old	5.20% / 5.50% / 7.20%	1.23 (1.22–1.24)	0.30%	7.50% / 7.80% / 7.20%	1.29 (1.28–1.30)	0.40%	9.90% / 10.90% / 7.80%	1.32 (1.30–1.34)	1.10%	12.50% / 14.30% / 8.50%	1.31 (1.30–1.32)	2.00%
High Education	34.30% / 25.50% / 5.10%	0.79 (0.78–0.79)	−13.40%	37.80% / 28.50% / 5.30%	0.78 (0.77–0.78)	−15.00%	37.90% / 29.60% / 5.50%	0.83 (0.82–0.84)	−13.30%	44.80% / 38.40% / 6.40%	0.84 (0.83–0.84)	−11.00%
Low Education	19.60% / 28.20% / 9.90%	1.39 (1.38–1.40)	10.80%	18.80% / 26.40% / 9.80%	1.33 (1.32–1.33)	9.30%	21.60% / 27.40% / 8.90%	1.18 (1.16–1.19)	7.40%	19.90% / 23.40% / 8.80%	1.13 (1.12–1.14)	5.10%
Unmarried	19.30% / 32.70% / 11.50%	1.46 (1.45–1.47)	16.40%	24.60% / 39.20% / 11.00%	1.49 (1.49–1.50)	19.40%	30.20% / 44.20% / 10.40%	1.37 (1.35–1.38)	20.10%	32.50% / 43.70% / 10.00%	1.27 (1.26–1.27)	16.60%
Primiparous	42.30% / 44.20% / 7.10%	1.3 (1.30–1.31)	3.20%	41.10% / 42.60% / 7.10%	1.3 (1.30–1.31)	2.60%	40.60% / 42.10% / 7.40%	1.33 (1.31–1.34)	2.50%	40.60% / 43.00% / 7.90%	1.41 (1.40–1.41)	4.10%

High Parity	3.60%	5.60%	10.80%	1.16 (1.15–1.17)	2.10%	3.40%	5.50%	11.20%	1.19 (1.18–1.20)	2.20%	3.80%	6.20%	11.70%	1.21 (1.19–1.23)	2.50%	3.40%	5.30%	11.70%	1.26 (1.25–1.27)	2.00%
Black	15.60%	29.10%	12.70%	1.92 (1.91–1.93)	16.00%	16.00%	30.40%	13.10%	2 (2.00–2.02)	17.10%	16.40%	30.70%	13.30%	2.27 (2.24–2.29)	17.10%	15.40%	26.90%	13.10%	2.11 (2.10–2.12)	13.50%
Foreign-born	9.90%	8.80%	6.00%	0.92 (0.91–0.93)	−1.30%	13.10%	11.30%	5.90%	0.89 (0.88–0.90)	−2.00%	17.00%	14.30%	6.00%	1 (0.98–1.01)	−3.20%	19.40%	16.50%	6.30%	1.01 (1.00–1.01)	−3.20%
Multiple birth	2.00%	15.10%	51.50%	19.5 (19.3–19.6)	13.40%	2.20%	16.40%	51.30%	196 (19.4–19.7)	14.50%	2.50%	18.30%	53.30%	20.7 (20.4–21.0)	16.30%	2.90%	21.40%	56.20%	24.36 (24.2–24.5)	19.10%
Hypertension											3.40%	8.30%	17.20%	2.62 (2.58–2.67)	5.10%	4.30%	11.10%	19.30%	3.02 (3.00–3.04)	7.10%
Diabetes											2.40%	2.40%	7.10%	0.9 (0.88–0.93)	0%	2.60%	2.90%	8.30%	0.95 (0.94–0.96)	0.30%
Smoking											12.40%	20.20%	11.60%	1.95 (1.93–1.97)	9.00%	10.70%	17.20%	12.10%	1.98 (1.97–1.99)	7.40%

may result from an early birth but also from fetal growth restriction, i.e., being small for a given gestational age. As the etiologies of these distinct types of lower birth weight deliveries are different, it became more widely accepted to disaggregate prematurity into separate categories, i.e., either LBW or preterm. By current convention, preterm now refers to an early delivery and is defined by gestational age. LBW refers to the weight of the infant at delivery.

Relatedly, fetal growth refers to the birth weight of the infant for a specific gestational age. Small-for-gestational age (SGA), usually defined as less than the 10th percentile of birth weight for gestational age (54–56), is a commonly used indicator of fetal growth restriction. Although these indicators may overlap, i.e., a LBW infant may often be preterm; they are not interchangeable as each has distinct etiologies and separate risk factors (57, 58). Among LBW infants, approximately two-thirds are preterm, while less than 20% of small-for-gestational age infants are preterm.

Typically, preterm is defined as a delivery or birth at a gestational age less than 37 weeks. Other commonly used subcategories of preterm have been established to delineate moderate preterm (33–36 weeks), very preterm (<33 weeks), and extremely preterm (≤28 weeks). Table 7.5 provides recent data on all live births to US resident mothers for various gestational age, preterm, and fetal growth categories.

Measures: Preterm birth is an outcome defined by a single endpoint, i.e., being born prior to an established gestational age (37 weeks). Fundamentally, infants born preterm are assumed to have a certain added risk of death, disease, and disability, compared with normal term infants. However, although preterm births may be grouped together on the basis of having a higher risk of adverse outcomes, several distinct clinical categories of preterm delivery have been identified

Table 7.5 Proportions of live births by gestational age, fetal growth categories, and race, United States, 2001–2002

Gestational age categories	Overall	White	Black	Hispanic	Other
% Extremely preterm (<28 wks)	0.8	0.6	1.9	0.7	0.6
% Very preterm (<32 wks)	2.3	1.8	4.5	2.0	1.9
% Moderate preterm (33–36 wks)	9.5	8.8	12.7	9.2	8.8
% Preterm (<37 wks)	11.7	10.6	17.2	11.2	10.6
% Term (37–41 wks)	82.3	83.5	77.0	82.1	83.8
% Postterm (42+ wks)	6.1	5.9	5.8	6.8	5.6
% Small-for-gestational age (<10th percentile)	10.3	8.5	15.9	9.6	12.2
% Average-for-gestational age (10th–90th percentile)	79.7	79.7	77.9	80.6	80.3
% Large-for-gestational age (>90th percentile)	10.3	11.9	6.2	9.8	7.6
% SGA preterm	1.5	1.4	2.7	1.2	1.5
% SGA term	8.3	7.0	12.9	8.1	10.3

(59, 60). Preterm births have been classified into three separate subgroups according to clinical presentation:

- Births occurring after spontaneous premature labor, related to premature contractions (50% of cases)
- Spontaneous rupture of the membranes (roughly 30% of cases)
- Indicated delivery of a premature infant for the benefit of either infant or mother (about 20% of cases) (61, 62)

Although preterm birth may be defined as a delivery prior to what is considered the normal length of gestation, preterm birth is recognized as stemming from several etiologically distinct pathways. In essence, preterm birth is not a single entity but is the result of one or more distinct causal processes, each of which may result in a similar event: being born too soon. Although the subclassification of preterm birth by clinical presentation is a step forward toward separating preterm deliveries into more homogenous subgroups, there continues to be ongoing discussion regarding whether the widely used three-category classification truly defines separate preterm entities. The accurate classification of preterm birth subgroups is important to more exactly establish risk factors and to assure that interventions are targeted at those who are truly at risk. To the extent that the components of an intervention are focused on a specific etiological pathway for preterm birth but targeted broadly to all individuals at risk for preterm birth in general, the intervention may well appear to lack efficacy. Moreover, risk factors and predeterminants may differ by subgroup, further hindering research in establishing separate and distinct categories of preterm birth. Some researchers suggest combining spontaneous premature labor (contractions) and spontaneous rupture of the membranes as it has been noted that the risk factors for these categories are similar (59). Because of these findings, indicating that spontaneous rupture of membranes and spontaneous labor are the result of similar processes, there is an argument for combining these back together into one group. However, some researchers further suggest that there is more etiological overlap between spontaneous and indicated preterm birth than first suspected (59). For example, maternal hypertension and fetal intrauterine growth restriction are indications for preterm delivery and are also suspected to be risk factors for spontaneous preterm birth (59).

Intrauterine Growth Restriction

It is difficult to distinguish the etiologies of preterm birth. Prior to the 1960s, it was presumed that all babies born less than 2500 grams were "premature". However, Lubchenco and colleagues (63) recognized that there is a cohort of infants that do not achieve their normal growth potential, which can lead to an increased risk of perinatal mortality as well as short- and long-term morbidities, as noted in Chapter 5. Infants who are growth-restricted experience higher rates of fetal and infant death, birth asphyxia, hypothermia, hypoglycemia, meconium aspiration, and long-term neurological impairment (64, 65).

It is widely recognized that factors such as race, altitude, gender, and SES can influence fetal growth (63, 65, 66). However, it is important to recognize that intrauterine growth restriction (IUGR) is not a single disease but it is the result of many fetal and maternal disorders. Chromosomal abnormalities and congenital malformations are responsible for about 20% of IUGR fetuses (67–70). Maternal vascular disease, associated with a decreased placental blood flow, is believed to account for 25–30% of all IUGR (71). Other potential risk factors for IUGR include multiple gestations, infections, small placenta, extremes of under and/or malnutrition, thrombophylic disorders, drugs/lifestyle, and high altitude or hypoxic disorder. (67, 71–73). Ultrasound is the current standard for diagnosis of IUGR and obstetrical surveillance is paramount for management.

Notwithstanding, the value of identifying distinct etiological pathways that leads to preterm birth is evident. Limitations to the conceptualization of preterm birth and its various subtypes decidedly impact the advancement of our understanding of the causes and prevention of preterm birth. The research results of the investigation of poorly defined preterm etiologic categories may prove misleading in spite of impressive findings. Going hand in hand with research on prevention and intervention efforts is the ongoing development and refinement of a better conceptualization of preterm birth and the articulation of its numerous etiologic pathways that may intertwine in any given individual mother.

Data Sources: Birth certificate data compiled by state vital record offices are the basic source of population-based gestational age information in the United States. State vital record data are further compiled by NCHS and are made publicly available on CD-ROMS (16). Hospital-based perinatal data systems are increasingly being implemented and represent another source of gestational age information on regional, local, and hospital catchment populations.

Gestational Age Categories:

Extremely preterm: ≤ 28 weeks
Very preterm: ≤ 32 weeks
Moderately preterm: 33–36 weeks
Preterm: < 37 weeks
Term: 37–41 weeks
Postterm: 42+ weeks

Intrauterine/Fetal Growth:

Small-for-gestational age: Less than 10th percentile of birth weight for gestational age

Gestational Age Categories: In order to assess the risks associated with gestational age and fetal growth, subcategories have been developed.

Average-for-gestational age: 10th–90th percentile of birth weight for gestational age

Large-for-gestational age: Greater than 90th percentile of birth weight for gestational age

Small-for-gestational age term: 37–40 weeks gestation less than 10th percentile of birth weight for gestational age

Small-for-gestational age preterm: <37 weeks gestation less than 10th percentile of birth weight for gestational age

Measurement Issues: Beyond the classification of preterm etiological subcategories, the basic determination of whether a delivery was *too soon* depends in part on the measurement of gestational age (length of gestation). An accurate estimate of gestational age is essential not just for research on preterm birth but for the management of pregnancy and newborn infants (74, 75). Gestational age serves as a proxy measure for the extent of fetal development and the fetus' readiness for birth. As an indicator of newborn maturity, gestational age is closely associated with the newborn's chances for survival during the first year and the likelihood of developing neonatal complications. Moreover, knowledge of a preterm infant's gestational age is necessary for interpreting his or her neurodevelopmental examination and for assessing developmental progress. Gestational age is usually expressed as completed weeks of gestation. For example, a newborn resulting from a gestation of 37 weeks and 6 days would be referred to as having a gestational age of 37 weeks.

Gestational age is used to calculate a variety of statistical indicators that are used to monitor the health status of populations and assess the need for targeted public health interventions (75). Hence, preterm and very preterm percentages in populations may reflect the prevalence of a variety of insults, including infection, psychosocial and physical stress, poor nutrition and substance abuse. Small-for-gestational age percentages, based on knowledge of the population birth weight distribution for specific gestational age intervals, serve as an indicator of maternal nutritional deficits during pregnancy. Lastly, gestational age is used in conjunction with the month prenatal care began and the number of prenatal care visits to compute indices of adequacy of prenatal care utilization. These gestational age-based health status and health care utilization indices are useful on a population basis for assessing the need for services, targeting services to at-risk populations, and evaluating the efficacy of those interventions.

Gestational age has typically been defined as the length of time from the date of the last normal menses to the date of birth (76, 77). This definition overestimates the duration of pregnancy by approximately 2 weeks, which is the average interval from the beginning of the last menstrual cycle to the point of conception. The definition of gestational age, based on the last menstrual period (LMP), has several limitations (78–85). There is considerable individual variability (i.e., ~7–25 days) in the interval between onset of the LMP and the date of conception. Further errors in determining the date of LMP may occur due to irregular menses, bleeding early in pregnancy, and recall errors by mothers. Approximately 20% of live birth certificates in the United States have been reported to have a missing or incomplete date of LMP, and greater proportions of missing or implausible dates of LMP have

Vital Records and Gestational Age: Clinical Estimate or LMP?

Gestational age, as reported on the U.S. vital statistics records, traditionally has been determined by the interval calculated from the date of last menstrual period (LMP) to the date of delivery [86, 77, 87]. Numerous studies have reported on the measurement limitations of using LMP to establish the duration of pregnancy, observing biologically implausible gestational ages at certain birth weights and reporting errors or omissions occurring more often in women of low socioeconomic and educational status [88–94, 83, 79]. Accordingly, other approaches for estimating gestational age have been proposed, e.g., ultrasound, antenatal and postnatal assessments, although none are truly temporal measures of the duration of pregnancy [86, 96–101, 75]. Instead, these alternate measures estimate the length of pregnancy from indicators of fetal growth or development and report the estimate on a scale corresponding to weeks or days from LMP [101].

Although the LMP method of gestational age measurement has long served as the standard for vital statistics records, the clinical estimate (or physician's estimate) has been periodically collected on vital records [71, 102, 103]. However, concerns about its measurement validity have been raised [64, 71]. The clinical estimate (CE) may be derived from a variety of methods, such as ultrasound and obstetric (e.g., fundal height and fetal heart tones) measures. Neonatal assessments should not be included when determining the clinical estimate, although such assessments of the newborn have undoubtedly been used. Moreover, the availability and use of any of these methods vary among hospitals, making it difficult to determine the standard for derivation [75]. Certain methods used to obtain clinical estimates of gestational age may also lack consistent validity among population subgroups (e.g., validity may vary by the presence of maternal complications and characteristics, or across the gestational age range, or may be greater for term compared to preterm infants) [104–107].

Since the reintroduction of the clinical estimate on vital records in the late 1980s, it has been used to assess the accuracy of LMP-based gestational age and as a substitute for the LMP gestational age for cases with missing or perceived inaccurate LMP values. However, given there may not be perfect agreement between measures and agreement may vary among populations subgroups, the substitution of one measure for the other may result in systematic biases. Should these biases lead to an under-estimation of the risk of preterm birth or other adverse gestational age-related pregnancy outcomes in high-risk populations, e.g., African-Americans, there are potentially far-reaching consequences for any misinterpretation of population-based research investigations that might influence state and national needs assessments and resultant programs and policies.

been reported for women of lower socioeconomic status, who by virtue of higher preterm and small for gestational age percentages have the greatest need for an accurate estimate of gestational age.

The interval between the date of LMP and the date of birth has long served as the best available method or *gold standard* for determining the gestational age of the infant and, as such, has been used in validation studies of alternative gestational age estimation methods (108). Validity and reliability studies of alternative gestational age measures assess the degree to which the alternative measure consistently predicts, agrees with, or is correlated with the selected gold standard measure across the full range of gestational age values, while further looking for evidence of any systematic biases that might stem from examination procedures or study population characteristics. Because of the widely recognized limitations to the estimation of gestational age by LMP, a number of alternative prenatal and postnatal approaches to determining gestational age have been developed (108–110). The clinical estimate of gestational age is now included on the vital records certificate and is used in some analyses related to preterm birth and gestational age.

Table 7.6 provides a list of prenatal measures for estimating gestational age and further indicates the specific focus of the measure (75).

Obstetric measures of fetal heart tones, quickening and uterine fundal growth have often been used to confirm dates based on LMP, but are limited because of individual variability, confounding variables, e.g., polyhydramnios, and the requirement of an early initiation of prenatal care. Many view early prenatal ultrasound, e.g., in first or early second trimester, as the new gold standard for comparison with or validation of new gestational age measures, even though ultrasound methods were originally validated with LMP as the gold standard. Ultrasound estimates of gestational age are based on different measures of fetal size, e.g., crown-rump length, biparietal diameter, femur length, sacral length, foot length, jaw size, and abdominal, chest, and head circumference, and are most accurate early in gestation. As the pregnancy progresses beyond the second trimester, there is more individual variation in normal fetal growth and fetal growth is more vulnerable to individual and environmental factors, including uteroplacental insufficiency, maternal exposure to drugs or toxins, and congenital infections. Minority and impoverished women, often facing barriers to accessing prenatal care services, may be less likely to obtain early ultrasound. As such, ultrasound gestational age estimates may be less accurate for these groups. Further, ultrasound is not universally available, particularly in less developed

Table 7.6 Prenatal methods for determining gestational age

Method	Focus of measure
Last menstrual period[1]	Pregnancy duration
Fetal heart tones[2]	Physical and neurological maturity
Quickening[2]	Physical and neurological maturity
Uterus at umbilicus[2]	Fetal size
Uterine fundal height[2]	Fetal size
Presence of embryo sac[3]	Fetal size
Crown rump length[4]	Fetal size
Head circumference[4]	Fetal size
Biparietal diameter[4]	Fetal size
Femur length[4]	Fetal size
Sacral length	Fetal size
Foot length	Fetal size
Jaw size	Fetal size
Chest diameter	Fetal size
Abdominal circumference[5]	Fetal size

[1]Traditional measure of gestational age duration commonly employed in population-based, public health studies using vital records
[2]Typically monitored by obstetricians during prenatal care visits
[3]More recently developed ultrasound measure for clinical use
[4]Commonly used ultrasound measures for estimating gestational age
[5]More typically used to assess adequacy of growth for gestational age

countries. Finally, the quality of ultrasound equipment and the level of training of technicians may vary across sites of care and the reference populations used to validate the various ultrasound measures may differ.

Because accurate prenatal estimates are not universally available, postnatal assessments of gestational age have also been developed (75). Examining physical and neurological characteristics of the newborn, Dubowitz and coworkers devised a scoring system to estimate gestational age (108). It was later revised and shortened by Ballard et al., and other postnatal methods of determining gestational age have also been developed (109, 110). Concerns have been raised regarding the accuracy of these approaches, particularly for preterm and very preterm infants (82). Among these concerns are their ability to be universally applied to various subpopulations, including different racial groups (112). Table 7.7 details the postnatal approaches to determine gestational age. The specific trait being measured by each gestational age estimation method, e.g., pregnancy duration, fetal size, or physical and neurological maturity, is also provided (75).

There are distinct conceptual differences among the alternative strategies for estimating gestational age, and these differences have implications for preterm research. Gestational age based on LMP is a direct measure of the duration of the pregnancy and is thus a unit of time measure. Many of the prenatal measures (uterine fundal height and ultrasound) and the newborn measures (birth weight, length, head circumference, and foot length) are direct measures of fetal/infant size, and these utilize the extent of fetal growth as an indirect measure of duration of

Table 7.7 Postnatal methods for determining gestational age

Method	Focus of measure
Birth weight[1]	Infant size
Head circumference	Infant size
Foot length	Infant size
Crown-heel length	Infant size
Dubowitz[2]	Physical and neurological maturity
Ballard[3]	Physical and neurological maturity
Revised Ballard	Physical and neurological maturity
Lens vessels[4]	Physical maturity
Cranial ultrasound	Physical and neurological maturity
Nerve conduction velocities	Physical and neurological maturity

[1]Still used as a gross indicator of gestational age, although limitations are widely known. More typically used to assess adequacy of growth for gestational age and as a research method to impute missing gestational age values and to identify grossly inaccurate gestational age values
[2]Because of preference for the Ballard, this measure may have limited use in the United States
[3]Probably most commonly used newborn estimate of gestational age used in the United States
[4]Applicable only to a limited range of gestational ages

gestation. The remaining postnatal measures (Dubowitz, Ballard, lens vessels, nerve conduction velocities, and cranial ultrasound) evaluate different aspects of infant maturity using physical or neurological milestones that are believed to be attained by the average fetus or infant by developing for a specified length of time. All of the alternative measures of gestational age translate their findings to the same scale as gestational age from LMP (20–44-weeks gestation), even though weeks is strictly a measure of duration of time.

Underpinning these indirect measures of duration of gestational age are three assumptions: (1) normal growth and maturation occur in most infants at a similar pace during pregnancy, (2) that the normal rates of intrauterine growth and maturation are about the same, and (3) that readiness for birth is a direct function of time in utero. Although pregnancy duration, fetal size, and newborn physical and neurological maturation are clearly associated with one another and further associated with infant morbidity and mortality, it must be emphasized that all of these gestational age estimation measures are attempting to operationally define variations in the underlying biological conditions that correspond to an optimal point of readiness for birth. The relationships among the duration of pregnancy, the extent of fetal size, the degree of physical and neurological maturation, and the readiness for birth may well vary among populations and be influenced by a variety of factors. As such, the validity of these gestational age measures, as indicators of readiness for birth, is based on a set of assumptions that have proven more tenuous as our medical technology has extended the limits of viability to the extremes of gestational age.

There is growing evidence in the literature that these alternative measures of gestational age do not correspond with one another to the extent once believed, even within the basic prenatal and postnatal categories. Some gestational age measures may tend to underestimate or overestimate others and this may vary by gestational age (78–82). Further, some measures may not provide consistently valid estimates for specific subgroups (82). Herein lies the concerns for preterm research. Studies that change gestational age measures during their course may uncover trends in the rate or incidence of preterm birth that merely reflects the change in measurement approach. Such biased results may provide inaccurate assessments of the impact of interventions. Other studies using different gestational age measures more frequently for some population subgroups or geographic areas than others may artificially inflate or deflate the preterm rates for those comparison groups. This may lead to the inaccurate determination of cases of preterm birth and a biased establishment of risk characteristics and high-risk areas. Epidemiological studies of preterm birth in large populations, often using vital records, typically rely on LMP or, more recently, LMP and the clinical estimate as reported on the birth certificate to define gestational age. It is these studies that have typically established current national trends and international comparisons in preterm rates. Meanwhile, clinical studies may more typically have access to early ultrasound data, although their selected study populations may be less representative of the larger population at risk of preterm birth. These measurement issues hinder comparisons among study findings, limit the interpretation and generalizability of the results, and persist as an ever lurking potential bias to preterm research (79, 82).

7.3.2 Descriptive Epidemiology

Temporal Trends: During the last two decades of the twentieth century, among live born babies, preterm rates in the USA steadily increased. As depicted in Fig. 7.13, an approximate 30% and 36% increase was observed for very preterm and preterm rates, respectively, from 1980 to 2002. There was a steady decline of SGA births through the 1980s and 1990s; however, the rate of SGA has remained steady in the early 2000s.

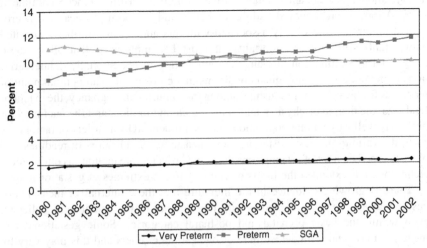

Fig. 7.13 Trends in maturity, United States, 1980–2002

Further examination of the gestational age distribution during the latter part of this period reveals a slight decrease in mean gestational age from 39.2 weeks in 1985–1988 to 38.7 weeks in 2001–2002. Additionally, there is an overall shift in the distribution resulting in greater percentages of preterm birth and decreases in the percentages of postterm (42+ weeks) births. These patterns are displayed in Figs. 7.14 and 7.15, which show the gestational age distribution of preterm live births to US resident mothers, using data from the NCHS linked live birth-infant death cohort files.

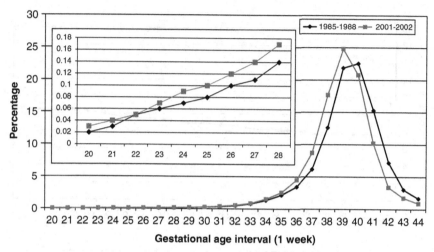

Fig. 7.14 Gestational age distribution, United States, 1985–1988 and 2001–2002

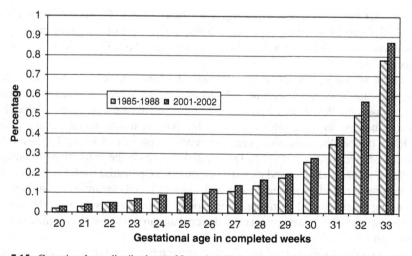

Fig. 7.15 Gestational age distribution (<33 weeks), United States, 1985–1988 and 2001–2002

Table 7.8 Proportion of live births to US resident mothers by gestational age category and year

Gestational age categories	1985–1988	2001–2002
% Extremely preterm (≤28 weeks)	0.66	0.81
% Very preterm (≤32 weeks)	1.9	2.3
% Moderate preterm (33–36 weeks)	7.7	9.5
% Preterm (<37 weeks)	9.7	11.7
% Term (37–41 weeks)	78.5	82.3
% Postterm (42+ weeks)	11.9	6.1

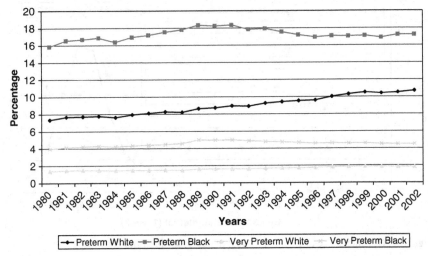

Fig. 7.16 Trends in maturity: very preterm and preterm by race, United States, 1980–2002

For the two time periods portrayed in these figures, for infants born alive, Table 7.8 provides the percentage of births for the various preterm categories. Between 1985–1988 and 2001–2002, the percentage of preterm births rose approximately 21%.

These increasing trends in preterm delivery have not been consistent among racial groups in the USA. Figure 7.16 provides trends in preterm and very preterm percentages for Whites and Blacks, based on reported race of mother. Although a steady increase in these rates is evident for Whites, this temporal pattern is not evident for blacks. This divergence in trends of preterm delivery has been the subject of investigation (27, 112). Differential changes in the proportion of multiple births of whites and older and unmarried mothers are potential contributors to these dissimilar trends in prematurity, as are changes in racial disparities in vital record reporting practice, e.g., more complete reporting of extremely preterm deliveries. Differentials in the measurement of gestational age among these groups may also be involved.

Geographic Variability: Considerable geographic variability in very preterm and preterm rates is evident in the United States. As shown in Figs. 7.17 and

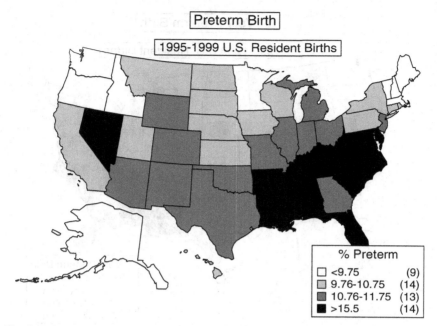

Fig. 7.17 State-specific preterm birth rates, United States, 1995–1999

7.18, higher preterm and very preterm rates are evident in the southeastern states. While the racial composition of states may partly underlie the observed geographic pattern, other factors are likely to be involved. Recent investigations have established that prevailing national trends in preterm births are not applicable to each state, and there is considerable state heterogeneity in both preterm rates and trends in preterm rates by racial groups, potentially reflecting reporting issues and other demographic, economic, social risk, and health care delivery and financing factors.

International comparisons of prematurity and intrauterine growth are problematic because of differences in reporting of live births and fetal deaths, affecting rates of preterm birth. Laws, procedures, and vital record reporting vary substantially. The U.S. preterm birth rate has been reported to be almost two-fold higher compared with European and other countries. However, it is important to note that these differences may be erroneous because of different methodologies in data collection (113).

Demographic Variability: Variations among racial and ethnic groups in gestational age and preterm percentages have long been observed (26, 114, 115). Fig. 7.19 presents the percent gestational age distribution for Whites, Blacks, Japanese, Asian Indian, and Samoan births, all to U.S. resident mothers. Although there is a similar mode for each group, important differences are evident in the very preterm tail with Blacks exhibiting the highest proportion of very preterm births (Fig. 7.20).

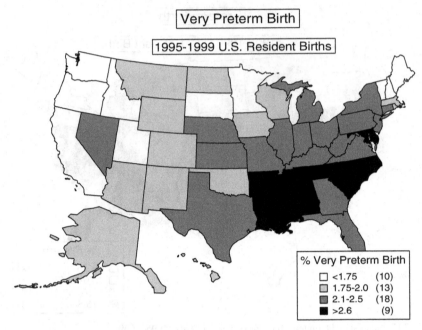

Fig. 7.18 State-specific very preterm birth rates, United States, 1995–1999

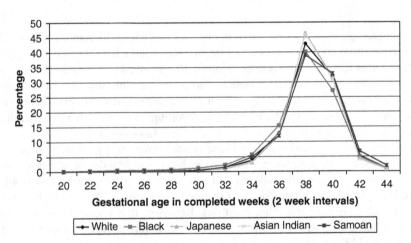

Fig. 7.19 Gestational age distribution of live births by race, United States, 2001–02

7.3.3   Factors Influencing Gestational Age and Fetal Growth

Risk Factors and Attributable Risks: A maternal morbidity may influence the gestational age distribution of women who have the condition. Some risk factors are detailed in Table 7.9 and include those that pre-date the pregnancy, e.g.,

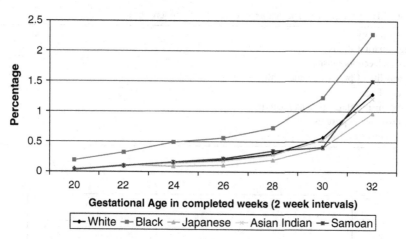

Fig. 7.20 Gestational age distribution (<32 weeks) by race, United States, 2001–2002

Table 7.9 Immutable medical risk factors associated with preterm birth

Previous low birth weight or preterm delivery*
Multiple 2nd trimester spontaneous abortion
Prior first trimester induced abortion
Familial and intergenerational factors
History of infertility
Nulliparity
Placental abnormalities
Cervical and uterine anomalies
Gestational bleeding
Intrauterine growth restriction
In utero diethylstilbestrol exposure
Multiple gestations*
Infant sex
Short stature
Low prepregnancy weight/low body mass index
Urogenital infections
Preeclampsia

*Among most predictive risk factors for preterm delivery

previous LBW or preterm delivery, multiple second trimester abortions, maternal stature and body mass, and history of infertility. Placental abnormalities, cervical/uterine anomalies, and preeclampsia are additional medical risk factors for prematurity that cannot be readily prevented. Finally, intrauterine infection remains in this category as research on the efficacy of antibiotic therapy for prevention of preterm delivery from these infections continues.

Demographic risks associated with preterm delivery include Black race, single marital status, low socioeconomic status, maternal age, and others (Table 7.10). While demographic factors cannot cause the premature expulsion of a fetus, these

Table 7.10 Demographic risk factors associated with preterm birth

Race/ethnicity
Single marital status
Low socioeconomic status
Seasonality of pregnancy and birth
Maternal age
Employment-related physical activity
Occupational exposures
Environment exposures

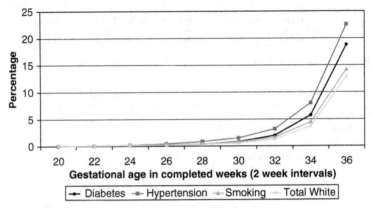

Fig. 7.21 Gestational age distribution of live births among U.S. resident White mothers by diabetes, hypertension, and smoking, 2001–2002

factors may antagonize some other deleterious factors. A meta-analysis of factors associated with preterm birth revealed that low socioeconomic status might correlate to other nutritional, toxic, anthropometric, or infectious factors that may themselves be causal (116).

Stress and maternal psychological factors have frequently been linked to pregnancy outcomes, and chronic stress has been related to low socioeconomic status (117–126). There have been difficulties in measuring stress of life events, but consistent associations have been reported between perceived stress and preterm birth. Chronic stressors may include financial insecurities, poor and crowded living conditions, unemployment, stressful working conditions, domestic violence, and unsatisfying marital relationships. Many of these risk factors are multifactorial and are deeply intertwined with social class, culture, race, and ethnicity. Continued research is needed in the area of stress and preterm birth to determine the capacity for prevention. Essential to the development of successful interventions in this area is the elucidation of biological pathways by which stressors influence preterm labor and the identification of biologic markers that are more specific indicators of risk than current measures of demographics and socioeconomic status.

As depicted in Figs. 7.21 and 7.22, which displays data for the infants of White and Black mothers only, the preterm tails of the gestational age distributions of births of hypertensive and diabetic mothers tend to be elevated, indicating higher proportions of preterm infants. In addition, women who smoke have a higher frequency of very preterm deliveries than women who do not smoke. Illicit drug use during pregnancy has been associated with a greater than two-fold increased risk of preterm birth or premature rupture of membrane (126).

The gestational age distribution varies markedly by the number at birth (127). As displayed in Fig. 7.23, the entire gestational age distribution for triplets and twins is shifted toward the preterm tail and the average gestational age of these multiples is 2–4 weeks shorter than that of singletons. The increase in multiple birth deliveries has been identified as a possible major contributor for the concurrent rise in preterm

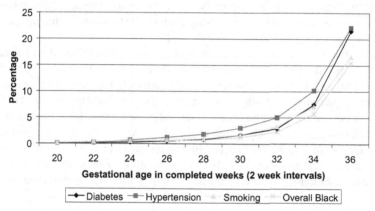

Fig. 7.22 Gestational age distribution of live births among U.S. resident Black mothers by diabetes, hypertension, and smoking, 2001–2002

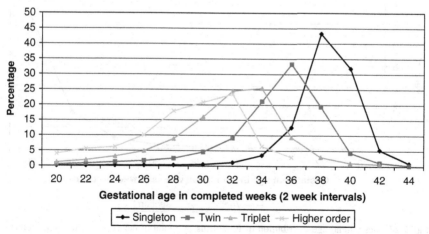

Fig. 7.23 Gestational age distribution of live births by plurality, United States, 2001–2002

births and has been related to changes in the use of ART (artificial reproductive technology) (128).

Variations in gestational age by mode of delivery have also been noted. Higher preterm and very preterm percentages are found for C-sectioned births. Although trends in the use of C-section have varied over the last two decades, there has been a general increase in the use of C-section for the delivery of preterm and LBW infants (129) (Fig. 7.24).

Table 7.11 describes selected risk factors for preterm birth by four time periods (1980–1984, 1985–1989, 1990–1994, and 1995–1999). The risk factors include age of mother, maternal education, marital status, parity, maternal race, maternal nativity status, maternal complications of diabetes and hypertension, maternal smoking, and multiple birth. For each risk factor, the table provides the percent of births with the characteristic, the percent of preterm births with the characteristic, and the percent preterm among births with the characteristic. Odds ratios are derived from a logistic regression using preterm birth as the outcome variable. The attributable risk fraction is also indicated.

During the 20-year interval, women aged ≥35 years contributed an increasing percentage of all live births (from 5.2% in 1980–1984 to 12.6% in 1995–1999). Initially 0.3% of all preterm deliveries could be attributed to these older women, but by the end of the interval, 1.6% of all preterm deliveries could be attributed to them. This increase occurred despite a stable odds ratio for preterm birth associated with older maternal age. A slightly different situation occurred for multiple births. The percentage of all live births that resulted from twins or higher-order gestations increased from 2% to almost 3%, but the odds ratio for preterm birth associated with these gestations (compared with singleton gestations) *also* increased from 8.6

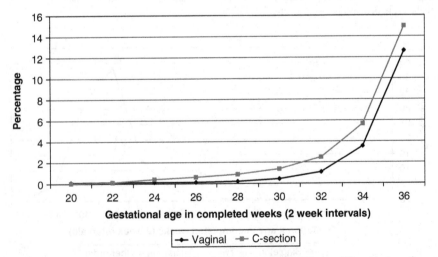

Fig. 7.24 Gestational age distribution of live births by mode of delivery, US resident mothers, 2001–2002

Table 7.11 Attributable risks to preterm births in 5-year intervals among live births to u.s. resident mothers

		Preterm Birth											
		1980–1984			1985–1989			1990–1994			1995–1999		
		% Total / % Among Preterm / % Preterm	OR	AR$_{total}$	% Total / % Among Preterm / % Preterm	OR	AR$_{total}$	% Total / % Among Preterm / % Preterm	OR	AR$_{total}$	% Total / % Among Preterm / % Preterm	OR	AR$_{total}$
Total % Preterm		9.10%			9.80%			10.60%			11.10%		
Teen	% Total	5.30%	1.3	3.90%	4.60%	1.2	3.20%	5.00%	1.21	2.60%	4.80%	1.17	1.80%
	% Among Preterm	8.70%	(1.29–1.31)		7.60%	(1.19–1.21)		7.30%	(1.19–1.23)		6.50%	(1.16–1.17)	
	% Preterm	15.80%			16.10%			15.70%			15.10%		
Old	% Total	5.20%	1.19	0.30%	7.60%	1.21	0.40%	9.90%	1.2	0.90%	12.60%	1.21	1.60%
	% Among Preterm	5.60%	(1.18–1.20)		7.90%	(1.21–1.22)		10.70%	(1.19–1.22)		14.00%	(1.20–1.21)	
	% Preterm	9.70%			10.20%			11.30%			12.40%		
High Education	% Total	34.30%	0.84	−11.90%	38.30%	0.84	−13.00%	37.90%	0.85	−12.10%	45.10%	0.87	−9.60%
	% Among Preterm	27.40%	(0.84–0.85)		30.30%	(0.83–0.84)		30.70%	(0.84–0.85)		39.90%	(0.86–0.87)	
	% Preterm	7.00%			7.80%			8.40%			9.80%		
Low Education	% Total	19.60%	1.26	8.90%	18.40%	1.21	7.80%	21.60%	1.16	7.00%	19.60%	1.11	4.20%
	% Among Preterm	26.10%	(1.26–1.27)		24.80%	(1.21–1.22)		26.90%	(1.15–1.17)		22.80%	(1.11–1.12)	
	% Preterm	12.40%			13.20%			13.10%			12.80%		
Unmarried	% Total	19.30%	1.42	14.80%	24.00%	1.43	16.80%	30.20%	1.35	16.20%	32.30%	1.23	12.10%
	% Among Preterm	30.70%	(1.42–1.43)		36.70%	(1.42–1.43)		41.30%	(1.34–1.36)		40.50%	(1.23–1.24)	
	% Preterm	15.00%			15.00%			14.60%			13.90%		
Primiparous	% Total	42.30%	1.1	0.30%	41.30%	1.08	−0.70%	40.60%	1.05	−1.80%	40.70%	1.07	−1.40%
	% Among Preterm	42.90%	(1.10–1.11)		40.90%	(1.07–1.08)		39.60%	(1.04–1.06)		39.80%	(1.07–1.08)	
	% Preterm	9.10%			9.70%			10.30%			10.90%		
High Parity	% Total	3.60%	1.2	2.10%	3.10%	1.23	2.10%	3.80%	1.25	2.40%	3.30%	1.27	1.90%
	% Among Preterm	5.30%	(1.19–1.22)		5.20%	(1.22–1.24)		6.00%	(1.23–1.27)		5.10%	(1.26–1.28)	
	% Preterm	15.00%			16.30%			17.40%			17.00%		
Black	% Total	15.60%	1.91	14.80%	15.80%	1.94	15.00%	16.40%	1.97	13.80%	15.40%	1.69	9.80%
	% Among Preterm	27.90%	(1.91–1.92)		28.50%	(1.93–1.95)		27.90%	(1.95–1.98)		23.60%	(1.68–1.70)	
	% Preterm	16.50%			17.60%			18.00%			17.10%		
Foreign-born	% Total	9.90%	1.03	0.22%	13.10%	1.01	−0.20%	17.00%	1.04	−1.20%	19.30%	0.99	−1.50%
	% Among Preterm	10.20%	(1.02–1.04)		12.90%	(1.00–1.01)		16.00%	(1.03–1.05)		17.90%	(0.995–1.00)	

					Estimate (CI)	
Multiple birth	9.20%	2.00%	9.30%	41.70%	8.55 (8.48–8.62)	7.40%
	9.60%	2.20%	10.30%	45.60%	9.28 (9.21–9.34)	8.40%
	9.90%	2.50%	12.10%	51.60%	9.88 (9.74–10.02)	9.90%
	10.30%	2.90%	14.80%	57.10%	13.14 (13.06–13.21)	12.30%
Hypertension	3.40%	6/3%	19.20%		1.84 (1.81–1.87)	2.90%
	4.30%	8.80%	22.50%		2.27 (2.26–2.29)	4.70%
Diabetes	2.40%	3.00%	13.20%		1.28 (1.25–1.31)	0.70%
	2.60%	3.60%	15.40%		1.37 (1.36–1.38)	1.10%
Smoking	12.40%	15.20%	12.90%		1.25 (1.24–1.26)	3.20%
	10.70%	13.10%	13.60%		1.26 (1.25–1.26)	2.60%

Table 7.12 Possibly mutable risk factors associated with preterm birth

No or inadequate prenatal care usage
Cigarette smoking
Use of marijuana and other illicit drugs
Cocaine use
Alcohol consumption
Caffeine intake
Maternal weight gain
Dietary intake
Sexual activity during late pregnancy
Leisure-time physical activities

to 13.1. The impact of increases in the odds ratio and increases in frequency of multiple gestation combined to produce a noticeable increase in the percentage of preterm births that can be attributed to multiple gestation (from 7.4% in 1980–1984 to 12.3% in 1995–1999).

Intervention: Little success has been achieved by numerous efforts to prevent preterm birth (130–134). Moreover, there has been only modest success in accurately identifying women at risk for preterm birth, although quite a number of risk factors have been identified (135). Unfortunately, many of the better established and more predictive risk factors are either immutable in the current pregnancy or, due to our present state of knowledge, pose significant challenges for either prevention or effective intervention (Tables 7.9 and 7.10).

Although often difficult to modify, a number of maternal behavioral risk factors for preterm delivery have been identified and are potentially mutable (Table 7.12). Among those that can be targeted for prevention include cigarette smoking, prenatal care utilization, and illicit drug use. However, the proportion of the pregnant population engaged in illicit drug use may be small and, to the extent that intervention efforts are effective in preventing drug use during pregnancy, the potentially attainable decrease in overall preterm birth rates from such intervention may be quite modest.

Conclusion: Throughout the latter half of this century, infant mortality rates have continued to decline in the United States (1, 114, 129, 136–140). The ongoing reduction in the risk of an infant death has largely been driven by improvements in birth weight- and gestational age-specific infant mortality rates, stemming from advancements in intensive medical care services and technology (27). However, as the decline in infant mortality rates has tapered off in recent years, and in some states has reversed, growing concerns have emerged about the direction of future trends in US infant mortality rates (115). These concerns are heightened by the simultaneous increases in LBW and preterm rates that have been observed for over two decades in the USA and elsewhere (129, 141–144). As it is unclear if yet another technological breakthrough in high-risk medical services will emerge to drive further reductions in infant death rates, the need to prevent premature births has been has become paramount (138, 145).

The importance of reducing the risk of LBW and preterm birth has long been recognized if for no other reason than the health care costs associated with an extremely small or early birth are many times higher than those of normal weight infants (146, 147). Lowering the risk of infant mortality through reductions in high-risk preterm births would likely be much more cost effective than the current reliance on improving their survival with high-risk intensive care services (147–149). But beyond the elevated newborn health care costs of premature infants, preterm births have an appreciable risk of long-term neurological impairment and developmental delay (150–152). The ongoing medical and support service needs of these infants and their families add to the overall health care system cost burden over time and emphasize the continuing health and developmental problems that some preterm infants face. Finally, the high preterm birth rates in the USA have been identified as a major contributor to this nation's relatively poor ranking in infant mortality among other developed countries (1). Although LBW has often received greater attention than preterm birth as the leading factor underlying poor pregnancy outcomes in the USA, it has been recognized that in order to successfully address these problems, the *key goal is prevention of preterm birth* (1).

Discussion Topics

1. Infants born to women with gestational diabetes have a higher risk of high birth weight. What are the possible causes and consequences?
2. Over the past few decades, neonatal and infant mortality have decreased because of birth-weight-specific improvements in infant mortality. Explain this phenomenon.
3. An investigator is trying to decide which measure of gestational age to use in an analysis – last menstrual period or clinical estimate. What are the pros and cons for each? Which one should be used?
4. You are the project manager for a preterm birth prevention program and must make a presentation to the Board of Health. What are some possible areas for intervention in the area of preterm birth?
5. Racial disparities in mortality exist between Whites and Blacks, but the disparities are not consistent across all birth weights and gestational ages. Describe this phenomenon and provide possible explanations.

Promising Areas of Research

1. Improvement of gestational age data collection and clarification of most appropriate measure (LMP or CE) to be used for population-based analyses

2. Exploration of the outcomes of infants born moderately preterm as these numbers are increasing
3. Research on the relationship between birth weight and preterm birth with stress and other contextual factors related to the health and well-being of the mother and infant

Abbreviations

ART	Assisted Reproductive Technology
ELBW	Extremely Low Birth Weight
IUGR	Intrauterine Growth Restriction
LMP	Last Menstrual Period
LBW	Low Birth Weight
MLBW	Moderately Low Birth Weight
NCHS	National Center for Health Statistics
SES	Socio-economic Status
SGA	Small-for-Gestational Age
VLBW	Very Low Birth Weight

References

1. Paneth NS. The problem of low birth weight. *The Future of Children,* 1995; 5(1): 19–34.
2. Kramer M. Determinants of low birth weight: Methodological assessment and meta-analysis. *Bulletin of the World Health Organization,* 1987; 65: 663–737.
3. Lunde A, Melve KK, Gjessing HK, Skjaerven R, Irgens LM. Genetic and environmental influences on birth weight, birth length, head circumference, and gestational age by use of population-based parent-offspring data. *American Journal of Epidemiology,* 2007; 165: 734–741.
4. World Health Organization. Manual of the International Statistical Classification of Diseases, Injuries, and Causes of Death, 6th edition (Adopted 1948). Geneva: WHO; 1948.
5. Dunham E, McAlenney P. A study of 244 prematurely born infant. *Journal of Pediatrics,* 1936; 91: 717–727.
6. Ylppö A. Zur physiologie, klinik und zum schicksal der frühgeborenen (physiology, clinical course, and outcome of premature infants). *Z Kinderheilkkd,* 1919; 24: 1–110.
7. Ylppö A. Pathologisch-anatomische studien bie frühgeborenen (pathological & anatomical studies of prematures). *Z Kinderheilkkd,* 1919; 24: 212–431.
8. Shiono PH, Behrman RE. Low birth weight: Analysis and recommendation. *The Future of Children,* 1995; 5(1): 4–17.
9. Boulet SL, Alexander GR, Salihu H, Pass MA. Macrosomic births in the United States: Determinants, outcomes, and proposed grades of risks. *American Journal of Obstetrics and Gynecology,* 2003; 188: 1372–1378.
10. Boulet SL, Alexander GR, Salihu H. Mode of delivery and the survival of macrosomic infants in the United States, 1995–1999. *Birth,* 2006; 33: 278–283.
11. McCormick M. The contribution of low birth weight to infant mortality and childhood morbidity. *New England Journal of Medicine* 1985; 312: 82–90.

12. Hogue C, Buehler J, Strauss L, Smith J. Overview of the National Infant Mortality Surveillance (NIMS) project – Design, methods, results. *Public Health Reports* 1987; 102: 126–138.
13. Fanaroff AA, Stoll BJ, Wright LL, et al. NICHD Neonatal Research Network. Trends in neonatal and morbidity and mortality for very low birthweight infants. *American Journal of Obstetrics and Gynecology* 2007; 196: 147.e1–147.e8.
14. Hack M, Fanaroff AA. Outcomes of children of extremely low birth weight and gestational age in the 1990s. *Seminars in Neonatology* 2000; 5: 89–106.
15. Vohr BR, Wright LL, Dusick AM. Neurodevelopmental and functional outcomes of extremely low birth weight infants in the National Institute of Child Health and Human Development Neonatal Research Network, 1993–1994. *Pediatrics* 2000; 105: 1216–1226.
16. National Center for Health Statistics. Technical appendix from Vital Statistics of the United States, 2004, Natality. US Department of Health and Human Services, Centers for Disease Control and Prevention, National Center for Health Statistics. Sept. 2006.
17. Parrish KM, Holt VL, Connell FA, Williams B, LoGerfo JP. Variations in the accuracy of obstetric procedures and diagnoses on birth records in Washington State, 1989. *American Journal of Epidemiology* 1993; 138: 119–127.
18. Piper JM, Mitchel EF Jr, Snowden M, Hall C, Adams M, Taylor P. Validation of 1989 Tennessee birth certificates using maternal and newborn hospital records. *American Journal of Epidemiology* 1993; 137: 758–768.
19. Kirby RS. Invited commentary: Using vital statistics databases for perinatal epidemiology: Does the quality go in before the name goes on? *American Journal of Epidemiology* 2000; 154: 889–890.
20. DiGiuseppe DL, Aron DC, Ranborn L, Harper DL, Rosenthal GE. Reliability of birth certificate data: A multi-hospital comparison to medical records information. *Maternal and Child Health Journal* 2002; 6: 169–179.
21. Ananth CV. Perinatal epidemiologic research with vital statistics data: Validity is the essential quality. *American Journal of Obstetrics and Gynecology* 2005; 193: 5–6.
22. David RJ. The quality and completeness of birthweight and gestational age data in computerized birth files. *American Journal of Public Health* 1980; 70: 964–973.
23. Petersen DJ, Alexander GR. Threats to accurate interpretation of secondary data. In: Kotch JB, ed. Maternal and Child Health: Programs, Problems, and Policy in Public Health. Gaithersburg, MD: Aspen; 1997: 395–404.
24. Wingate MS, Alexander GR. Racial and ethnic differences in perinatal mortality: The role of fetal death. *Annals of Epidemiology,* 2006; 16: 485–491.
25. Lee KS, Paneth N, Gartner LM, et al. Neonatal mortality: An analysis of the recent improvement in the United States. *American Journal of Public Health*, 1980; 70: 15–21.
26. Alexander GR, Tompkins ME, Allen MC, et al. Trends and racial differences in birth weight and related survival. *Maternal Child Health Journal*, 1999; 3: 71–79.
27. Allen MC, Alexander GR, Tompkns ME, et al. Racial differences in temporal changes in newborn viability and survival by gestational age. *Paediatric and Perinatal Epidemiology*, 2000; 14: 152–158.
28. United Nations Children's Fund and World Health Organization. Low Birthweight: Country, Regional and Global Estimates. New York: UNICEF; 2004.
29. Alexander GR, Kogan M. Ethnic differences in birth outcomes: The search for answers continues. *Birth*, 1998; 3: 210–213.
30. Kramer MS, Séguin L, Lydon J, Goulet L. Socio-economic disparities in pregnancy outcome: Why do the poor fare so poorly? *Paediatric and Perinatal Epidemiology*, 2000; 14: 194–210.
31. Shiono P, Rauh V, Park M, Lederman S, Zuskar D. Ethnic differences in birthweight: The role of lifestyle and other factors. *American Journal of Public Health*, 1997; 87: 787–793.
32. Pearl M, Braveman P, Abrams B. The relationship of neighborhood socioeconomic characteristics to birthweight among 5 ethnic groups in California. *American Journal of Public Health*, 2001; 91: 1808–1814.

33. Grady SC. Racial disparities in low birthweight and the contribution of residential segregation: A multilevel analysis. *Social Science and Medicine*, 2006; 63: 3013–3029.
34. Collins JW, Simon DM, Jackson TA, Drolet A. Advancing maternal age and infant low birth weight among urban African-American: The effects of neighborhood poverty. *Ethnicity and Disease*, 2006; 16: 180–186.
35. Savitz DA, Kaufman JS, Dole N, Siega-Riz AM, Thorpe JM Jr, Kaczor DT. Poverty, education, race, and pregnancy outcome. *Ethnicity and Disease*, 2004; 14: 322–329.
36. Perreira KM, Cortes KE. Race/ethnicity and nativity differences in alcohol and tobacco use during pregnancy. *American Journal of Public Health*, 2006; 96: 1629–1636.
37. Boyd ME, Usher RH, McClean FH. Fetal macrosomia: Prediction, risks, and proposed management. *Obstetrics and Gynecology*, 1983; 61: 715–722.
38. Spellacy WN, Miller S, Winegar A, Petersen PQ. Macrosomia: Maternal characteristics and infant complications. *Obstetrics and Gynecology*, 1985; 66: 258–261.
39. Meshari AA, DeSilva S, Rahman I. Fetal macrosomia: Maternal risks and fetal outcome. *International Journal of Gynecology and Obstetrics*, 1990; 32: 215–222.
40. ACOG Practice Bulletin No. 22. Washington, DC: American College of Obstetricians and Gynecologists; 2000.
41. Brunskill AJ, Rossing MA, Connell FA, Daling J. Antecedents of macrosomia. *Paediatric and Perinatal Epidemiology*, 1991; 5: 392–401.
42. Langer O. Fetal macrosomia: Etiologic factors. *Clinical Obstetrics and Gynecology*, 2000; 43: 283–297.
43. Lipscomb KR, Gregory K, Shaw K. The outcome of macrosomic infants weighing at least 4500 grams: Los Angeles County + University of Southern California experience. *Obstetric and Gynecology*, 1995; 85: 558–564.
44. Sacks DA, Chen W. Estimating fetal weight in the management of macrosomia. *Obstetrical and Gynecological Survey*, 2000; 55: 229–239.
45. Parks DG, Ziel HK. Macrosomia: A proposed indication for primary cesarean section. *Obstetrics and Gynecology* 1978; 52: 407–409.
46. Davis R, Woelk G, Mueller BA, Daling J. The role of previous birth weight on risk for macrosomia in a subsequent birth. *Epidemiology* 1995; 6: 607–611.
47. Bérard J, Dufour J, Vinatier D, Subtil D, Vanderstichèle S, Monnier JC, et al. Fetal macrosomia: Risk factors and outcome: A study of the outcome concerning 100 cases >4500g. *European Journal of Obstetrics, Gynecology, and Reproductive Biology*, 1998; 77: 51–59.
48. Mocanu EV, Greene RA, Byrne BM, Turner MJ. Obstetric and neonatal outcome of babies weighing more than 4.5 kg: An analysis by parity. *European Journal of Obstetrics, Gynecology, and Reproductive Biology*, 2000, 92: 229–233.
49. Xiong X, Demianczuk NN, Buekens P, Saunders L, Duncan MB. Association of preeclampsia with high birth weight for gestational age. *American Journal of Obstetrics and Gynecology*, 2000; 183: 148–155.
50. Hedderson MM, Weiss NS, Sacks DA, Pettitt DJ, Selby JV, Quesenberry CP, Ferrera A. Pregnancy weight gain and risk of neonatal complications: Macrosomia, hypoglycemia, and hyperbilirubinemia. *Obstetrics and Gynecology*, 2006; 108(5): 1153–1161.
51. Hill DE. Effect of insulin on fetal growth. *Seminars in Perinatology*, 1978; 2: 319–328
52. Grassi AE, Giuliano MA. The neonate with macrosomia. *Clinical Obstetrics and Gynecology*, 2000; 43(2): 340–348.
53. Hamilton BE, Minino AM, Martin JA, Kochanek KD, Strobino DM, Guyer B. Annual summary of vital statistics: 2005. *Pediatrics*, 2007; 119: 345–360.
54. Silverman WA. Nomenclature for duration of gestation, birth weight and intrauterine growth. *Pediatrics* 1967; 39: 935–939.
55. Battaglia F, Lubchenco LO. A practical classification of newborn infants by weight and gestational age. *Journal of Pediatrics*, 1967; 71: 159–163.

56. Wilcox AJ. On the importance – and the unimportance – of birthweight. *International Journal of Epidemiology,* 2001;30: 1233–1241.
57. Kramer MS. Preventing preterm birth: Are we making progress? *Prenatal and Neonatal Medicine,* 1998; 3: 10–12.
58. Kramer MS. Intrauterine growth and gestational duration determinants. *Pediatrics* 1987; 80 (4): 502–511.
59. Klebanoff MA. Conceptualizing categories of preterm birth. *Prenatal and Neonatal Medicine,* 1998; 3: 13–15.
60. Klebanoff MA, Shiono PA. Top down, bottom up, and inside out: Reflections on preterm birth. *Paediatric and Perinatal Epidemiology,* 1995; 9: 125–129.
61. Tucker JM, Goldenberg RL, Davis RO, et al. Etiologies of preterm birth in an indigent population: Is prevention a logical explanation? *Obstetrics and Gynecology* 1991; 77: 343–347.
62. Guinn DA, Goldenberg RL, Hauth CJ, et al. 1995. Risk factors for the development of preterm premature rupture of the membranes after arrest of preterm labor. *American Journal Obstetrics and Gynecology* 173: 310–315.
63. Lubchenco LO, Hansman C, Boyd E. Intrauterine growth as estimated from live born birth-weight data at 24–42 weeks of gestation. *Pediatrics* 1963; 32:793.
64. Creasy RK, Resnick R. Intrauterine growth restriction: In: Creasy RK, Resnick R, editors. Maternal-fetal medicine: principles and practice. 4th ed. Philadelphia: Saunders; 1998. p.569–84.
65. Williams RL, Creasy RK, Cunningham GC, Hawes WE, Norris FD, Tashiro M. Fetal growth and perinatal viability in California. *Obstet Gynecol* 1982; 59:624–32.
66. Zhang J, Bowes WA Jr. Birth-weight-for-gestational age patterns by race, sex, and parity in the United States population. *Obstet Gynecol* 1995; 86:200–8.
67. Resnik R. Intrauterine growth restriction. *Obstet Gynecol* 2002; 99:490–96.
68. Snijders RJM, Sherrod C, Gosden CM, Nicolaides KH. Fetal growth retardation: Associated malformations and chromosome abnormalities. *Am J Obstet Gynecol* 1993; 168:547–55.
69. Khoury MJ, Erickson D, Cordero JE, McCarthy BJ. Congenital malformations and intrauterine growth retardation: A population study. Pediatrics; 82:83–90.
70. Sickler GK, Nyberg DA, Sohaey R, Luthy DA. Polyhydraminos and fetal growth restriction: Ominous combination. J Ultrasound Med 1997; 16:609–14.
71. Odegard RA, Vatten LJ, Nilsen ST, Salvesen KA, Austgulen R. Preeclampsia and fetal growth. Obstet Gynecol 2000;96:950–5.
72. Ananth CV, Vinzileos AM. Maternal-fetal conditions necessitating a medical intervention resulting in preterm birth. Am J Obstet Gynecol 2006; 195:155–1563.
73. Heinonen S, Taipale P, Saarikoski S. Weights of placentae from small-for-gestational age infants revisited. Placenta 2001;22:399–404.
74. Allen MC, Amiel-Tison C, Alexander GR. Measurement of gestational age and maturity. *Prenatal and Neonatal Medicine,* 1998; 3: 56–59.
75. Alexander GR, Allen MC. Conceptualization, measurement, and use of gestational age. I. Clinical and public health practice. *Journal of Perinatology* 1996; 16(2): 53–59.
76. Reid J. On the duration of pregnancy in the human female. *Lancet* 1850; 2: 77–81.
77. Treloar AE, Behn BG, Cowan DW. Analysis of the gestational interval. *American Journal of Obstetrics and Gynecology* 1967; 99: 34–45.
78. Kramer MS, McLean FH, Boyd ME, Usher RH. The validity of gestational age estimation by menstrual dating in term, preterm, and postterm gestations. *JAMA,* 1988; 260: 3306–3308.
79. Wingate MS, Alexander GR, Buekens P, Vahratian A. Comparison of gestational age classifications: Date of last menstrual period vs. clinical estimate. *Annals of Epidemiology,* 2007; 17: 425–430.
80. Martin JA. United States vital statistics and the measurement of gestational age. *Paediatric and Perinatal Epidemiology,* 2007; 21 (Suppl 2): 13–21.
81. Ananth CV. Menstrual versus clinical estimate of gestational age dating in the United States: Temporal trends and variability in indices of perinatal outcomes. *Paediatric and Perinatal Epidemiology,* 2007; 21 (Suppl 2): 22–30.

82. Alexander GR, Tompkins ME, Hulsey TC, Petersen DJ, Mor JM. Discordance between LMP-based and clinically estimated gestational age: Implications for research, programs, and policy. *Public Health Reports*, 1995; 110: 395–402.

83. Alexander GR, Tompkins ME, Cornely DA. Gestational age reporting and preterm delivery. *Public Health Reports* 1990; 105(3): 267–275.

84. David RJ. The quality and completeness of birthweight and gestational age data in computerized data files. *American Journal of Public Health* 1980;70: 964–973.

85. Gjessing HK, Skjaerven R, Wilcox AJ. Errors in gestational age: Evidence of bleeding early in pregnancy. *American Journal of Public Health* 1999;89: 213–218.

86. Silverman WA. Nomenclature for duration of gestation, birth weight and intrauterine growth. *Pediatrics* 1967; 39: 935–939.

87. Taffel S, Johnson D, Heuser R. A method of imputing length of gestation on birth certificates. Vital and Health Statistics [2], DHHS Publication No. (PHS) 93. National Center for Health Statistics, *Hyattsville, MD*, 1982.

88. Frazier TM. Error in reported date of last menstrual period. Am J Obstet Gynecol 77: 915–918, 1959.

89. Schwartz S, West H. Potentialities and limitations of medical data of official birth certificates. *Am J Public Health* 50: 338–345, 1960.

90. Hammes LM, Treloar AE. Gestational interval from vital records. *Am J Public Health* 60: 1496–1505, 1970.

91. Wenner WH, Young EB. Nonspecific date of last menstrual period: an indication of poor reproductive outcome. *Am J Obstet Gynecol* 120: 1071–1079, 1974.

92. Buekens P, Delvoye P, Wollast E, Robyn C. Epidemiology of pregnancies with unknown last menstrual period. *J Epidem Comm Hlth* 1984; 38: 79–80.

93. Hall MN, Carr-Hill RA, Fraser C, et al. The extent and antecedents of uncertain gestation. *Brit J Obstet Gynaecol* 1985; 92: 445–51.

94. Hall MH, Carr-Hill RA. The significance of uncertain gestation for obstetric outcome. *Brit J Obstet Gynecol* 1985; 92: 452–460.

95. Parker JD, Schoendorf KC. Implications of cleaning gestational age data. *Paediatr Perinat Epidemiol* 2002; 16: 181–187.

96. Finnstrom O. Studies on maturity in newborn infants. VI. Comparison between different methods for maturity estimation. *Acta Paediat Scand* 1972; 61: 33–44.

97. Cappurro H, Konichesky S, Fonseca D, Caldeyro-Barcia R. A simplified score for diagnosis of gestational age in the newborn infant. *J Pediatr* 1978; 93(1): 120–2.

98. Jimenez JM, Tyson JE and Reisch JS. Clinical measures of gestational age in normal pregnancies. *Obstet Gynecol* 1983; 61(4): 438–443.

99. Campbell S, Warsof SL, Little D, et al. Routine ultrasound screening for the prediction of gestational age. *Obstet Gynecol* 1985; 65: 613–620.

100. Ott WJ. Accurate gestational dating. *Obstet Gynecol* 66: 311–315, 1985.

101. Ballard JL, Khoury JC, Wedig K, et al. New Ballard Score, expanded to include extremely premature infants. *J Pediatr* 1991; 119(3): 417–423.

102. Alexander GR, Petersen DJ, Powell-Griner E, Tompkins ME. A comparison of gestational age reporting methods based on physician estimate and date of last normal menses from fetal death reports. *Am J Public Health* 1989; 79: 600–602.

103. Petersen DJ, Alexander GR, Powell-Griner E, Tompkins ME. Variations in the reporting of gestational age at induced termination of pregnancy. *Am J Public Health* 79: 603–606, 1989.

104. Spinnato JA, Sibai BM, Shaver DC, Anderson GD, et al. Inaccuracy of Dubowitz gestational age in low birth weight infants. *Obstet Gynecol* 1984; 63(4): 491–5.

105. Shukla H, Atakent YS, Ferrara A, Topsis J, Antoine C. Postnatal overestimation of gestational age in preterm infants. *JDC* 1987; 141: 1106–7.

106. Alexander GR, Hulsey TC, Smeriglio VL, Comfort M, Levkoff A. Factors influencing the relationship between a newborn assessment of gestational maturity and the gestational interval. *Paediatr Perinat Epidem* 1990; 4: 133–46.

107. Alexander, GR, de Caunes F, Hulsey TC, Tompkins ME, Allen MC. Ethnic variation in postnatal assessments of gestational age: a reappraisal. *Paediatr Perinat Epidemiol* 1992; 6: 423–433.

108. Dubowitz LMS, Dubowitz V, Goldberg C. Clinical assessment of gestational age in the newborn infant. *Journal of Pediatrics* 1970; 77(1): 1–10.

109. Ballard JL, Novak KK, Driver M. A simplified score for assessment of fetal maturation of newly born infants. *Journal of Pediatrics* 1979; 95(5, Part 1): 769–774.

110. Ballard PL. Scientific rationale for the use of antenatal glucocorticoids to promote fetal development. *Pediatric Review*, 2000; 1(5): E83–E90.

111. Papiernik É, Alexander GR. Discrepancy between gestational age and fetal maturity among ethnic groups. In: Chervenak F, editor. Fetus as a Patient. Carnforth, UK: Parthenon; 1999.

112. Centers for Disease Control and Prevention. State-specific changes in singleton preterm births among black and white women – United States, 1990 and 1997. *Morbidity and Mortality Weekly Report* 2000; 49: 837–840.

113. Institute of Medicine. Preterm Birth: Causes, Consequences, and Prevention (Behrman RE, Butler AS, eds). States Committee on understanding premature birth and assuring healthy outcomes, Board on health sciences policy; 2007.

114. Demissie K, Rhoads GG, Ananth CV, Alexander GR, Kramer MS, Kogan MD, Joseph KS. Trends in preterm birth and neonatal mortality among Blacks and Whites in the United States from 1989 to 1997. *American Journal of Epidemiology,* 2001;154: 307–315.

115. Centers for Disease Control and Prevention. State Infant Mortality Initiative. Atlanta, GA: Centers for Disease Control and Prevention; 2006.

116. Berkowitz GS, Lapinski RH. Relative and attributable risk estimates for preterm birth. *Prenatal and Neonatal Medicine*, 1998; 3: 53–55.

117. Berkowitz GS, Papiernik E. Epidemiology of preterm birth. *Epidemiologic Review*, 1993; 15: 414–443.

118. Copper RL, Goldenberg RL, Elder N, et al. The preterm prediction study: Maternal stress is associated with spontaneous preterm birth at less than thirty-five weeks' gestation. *American Journal of Obstetrics and Gynecology,* 1996; 175: 1286–1292.

119. Holtzman C, Paneth N, Fisher R, et al. Rethinking the concept of risk factors for preterm delivery: Antecedents, markers and mediators. *Prenatal and Neonatal Medicine* 1998; 3: 47–52.

120. Kogan MD, Alexander GR. Social and behavioral factors in preterm birth. *Prenatal and Neonatal Medicine,* 1998; 3: 29–31.

121. Kramer MS, Goulet L, Lydon J, et al. Socio-economic disparities in preterm birth: Causal pathways and mechanisms. *Paediatric and Perinatal Epidemiology*, 2001; 15 (Suppl 2): 104–123.

122. McCauley J, Kern DE, Kolodner K, et al. The 'battering syndrome': Prevalence and clinical characteristics of domestic violence in primary care internal medical practices. *Annals of Internal Medicine*, 1995; 123: 737–746.

123. Muhajarine N, D'Arcy C. Physical abuse during pregnancy: Prevalence and risk factors. *Canadian Medical Association*, 1999; 160: 1007–1011.

124. Nordentoft M, Lou HC, Hansen D, et al. Intrauterine growth retardation and premature delivery: The influence of maternal smoking and psychosocial factors. *American Journal of Public Health*, 1996; 86: 347–354.

125. Peacock JL, Bland M, Anderson HR. Preterm delivery: Effects of socioeconomic factors, psychological stress, smoking, alcohol, and caffeine. *British Medical Journal*, 1995; 311: 531–536.

126. Dew PC, Guillory VJ, Okah FA, Cai J, Hoff GL. The effect of compromising behaviors on preterm birth. *Maternal and Child Health Journal*, 2007; 11: 227–233.

127. Blondel B, Kogan MD, Alexander GR, et al. The impact of the increasing number of multiple births on the rates of preterm birth and low birth weight: An international study. *American Journal of Public Health*, 2002; 92: 1323–1330.

128. Anonymous. Contribution of assisted reproductive technology and ovulation-inducing drugs to triplet and higher-order multiple births – United States, 1980–1997. MMWR 2000; 49: 535–539.

129. Martin JA, Hamilton BE, Sutton PD, Ventura SJ, Menacker F, Kirmeyer S, Munson ML. Births: Final Data for 2005. National vital statistics report, vol. 56, no. 6. Hyattsville, MD: National Center for Health Statistics; 2007.

130. Alexander GR, Weiss J, Hulsey TC, et al. Preterm birth prevention: An evaluation of programs in the United States. Birth 1991; 18: 160–169.

131. Goldenberg RL, Andrews WW. Editorial: Intrauterine infection and why preterm prevention programs have failed. American Journal of Public Health 1996; 86: 781–783.

132. Goldenberg RL, Rouse DJ. Prevention of premature birth. New England Journal of Medicine, 1998; 339(5): 313–320.

133. Goldenberg RL. The prevention of low birth weight and its sequela. Preventive Medicine, 1994; 23: 627–631.

134. Copper RL, Goldenberg RL, Creasy RK, et al. A multicenter study of preterm birth weight and gestational age-specific neonatal mortality. American Journal of Obstetrics and Gynecology, 1993; 168(1): 78–84.

135. Institute of Medicine. Preventing Low Birth Weight. Washington, DC: National Academy Press, 1985.

136. Centers for Disease Control and Prevention. Infant mortality and low birth weight among black and white infants-United States, 1980–2000. Morbidity and Mortality Weekly Report, 2002; 51: 589–592.

137. Carmichael SL, Iyasu S. Changes in the black-white infant mortality gap from 1983 to 1991 in the United States. American Journal of Preventive Medicine 1998; 15(3): 220–227.

138. Lee KS, Paneth N, Gartner LM, et al. Neonatal mortality: An analysis of the recent improvement in the United States. American Journal of Public Health, 1980; 70(1): 15–21.

139. Philip AGS. Neonatal mortality rate: Is further improvement possible? Journal of Pediatrics, 1995; 126(3): 427–432.

140. Alexander GR, Wingate MS, Bader D, Kogan MD. The increasing racial disparity in infant mortality rates: composition and contributors to recent U.S. trends. American Journal of Obstetrics and Gynecology, 2008; 198: 51e1–51e9.

141. Alexander GR, Slay M. Prematurity at birth: Trends, racial disparities, and epidemiology. Mental retardation and developmental disabilities research reviews, 2002; 8: 215–220.

142. Centers for Disease Control and Prevention. Preterm singleton births-United States, 1989–96. Morbidity and Mortality Weekly Report, 1999; 48 (9): 185–189.

143. Joseph KS, Kramer MS, Marcoux S, et al. Determinants of preterm birth rates in Canada from 1981 through 1994. New England Journal of Medicine, 1998; 339: 1434–1439.

144. Sepowitz S. Why infant very low birth weight rates have failed to decline in the United States vital statistics. International Journal of Epidemiology 1994; 23(2): 321–326.

145. Paneth NS. Technology at birth. American Journal of Public Health, 1990; 80: 791–792.

146. Levit EM, Baker LS, Corman H, Shiono PH. The direct cost of low birth weight. Future of Children 1995; 5(1):35–56.

147. Rogowski JA. The economics of preterm delivery. Prenatal and Neonatal Medicine, 1998; 3: 16–20.

148. Johnston RB, Williams MA, Hogue CJR, et al. Overview: New perspectives on the stubborn challenge of preterm birth. Paediatric and Perinatal Epidemiology, 2001; 15 (Suppl 2): 3–6.

149. Mattison DR, Damus K, Fiore E, et al. Preterm delivery: A public health perspective. Paediatric and Perinatal Epidemiology, 2001; 15 (Suppl 2): 7–17.

150. McCormick MC. The contribution of low birth weight to infant mortality and childhood morbidity. New England Journal of Medicine, 1985; 312: 82–89.

151. Hack M, Taylor HG, Klein N, et al. School-age outcomes in children with birth weights under 750 g. New England Journal of Medicine, 1994; 331: 753–759.

152. Saigal S, Hoult LA, Streiner DL, et al. 2000. School difficulties at adolescence in a regional cohort of children who were extremely low birth weight. Pediatrics, 2000; 105: 325–331

Chapter 8
Conclusion

In this text, we have sought to provide a framework for studying perinatal epidemiology in its public health context. Our subject often is overlooked in an era of miracle drugs to treat chronic diseases, a *war* on cancer that may soon rival the Hundred Years' War of the seventeenth century, daily reports on genetics discoveries, and the omnipresent focus on HIV and other infectious diseases. Our media continually confront us with images of human suffering and tragedy, often in developing nations, but sometimes much closer to home. In the face of these other pressing concerns, why should we care about perinatal epidemiology?

Perinatal epidemiology provides the evidence base for the organization and delivery of clinical services and public health programs to ensure optimal pregnancy outcomes for women and their infants. Health care services for labor and delivery represent one of the largest sectors of hospitalization. The ever-rising rates of cesarean delivery make it one of the most common surgeries involving an inpatient hospital stay in the USA.

Perinatal epidemiology emphasizes the reproductive health of women. We must view pregnancy and child-rearing within the context of the life cycle of women and their families. Women contribute to overall levels of well-being in our society. Their optimal health before, during, and after pregnancy enhances their abilities physically, mentally, socially, and materially. Our children and our children's children are our future – which are more than sufficient justification for a scientific focus on the field of perinatal epidemiology.

Research in perinatal epidemiology will continue to evolve. Some of the patterns, trends, and generalizations reported in this text may change. Preventive interventions may have different outcomes in some populations. Researchers and program managers will devise new approaches to promote health, reduce risk factors, and manage adverse outcomes that may result in future changes in the magnitude of observed rates and ratios as well as strength of associations. Rather than providing definitive answers to specific questions in the field of perinatal epidemiology, we have sought to develop and explicate a model that can be used to assess and understand new research findings as they appear. Most of our empirical generalizations can be expected to persist, even if the specific magnitudes of observed associations change over time.

M.M. Adams et al., *Perinatal Epidemiology for Public Health Practice.*
doi: 10.1007/978-0-387-09439-7_8; © Springer Science + Business Media, LLC 2009

In preparing the text, we considered the depth and breadth of our subject. We needed to select topics to include in the text. Our primary objective was to provide a broad portrait of women's reproductive health and maternal morbidity and mortality as well as fetal growth and infant morbidity and mortality. We chose not to cover many topics, because we deemed them ancillary to this primary objective. Among the important topics that we could not address and that warrant focused treatment are prenatal care, maternal smoking, and infant exposure to environmental tobacco smoke, as well as multiple birth and its effects on maternal morbidity and fetal and infant well-being. Although breastfeeding and infant immunizations have clear benefits for babies, both of these topics warrant a direct focus, which did not mesh with the structure of our text. Maternal weight and maternal weight gain are also important topics and fertile ground for current research. The text addresses them only as they relate directly to maternal and infant outcomes. As perinatal researchers and public health professionals consider these topics, we hope that our general approach will apply to their thinking.

In writing this text, we sought to provide a general reference and a practical information source for students, clinicians, and public health professionals. We present standard definitions for terms commonly used in perinatal epidemiology and describe recent patterns and trends for the most common indicators and measures in perinatal epidemiology. We describe the etiologies for many common maternal and infant morbidities, and associated mortality. Throughout the text we discuss evidence-based preventive interventions that can be implemented by public health practitioners. We hope, therefore, that this text will introduce students and trainees to perinatal epidemiology and maternal and child health. We also want it to become a reference for those seeking a single source for information on perinatal rates, measures, risk factors, and preventive interventions for women of reproductive age, women during pregnancy and the postpartum period, and their newborns during the first year of life. Lastly, we intend for it to be a starting point for empirical research to identify modifiable risk factors and new interventions to improve perinatal outcomes for mothers and their babies.

We dedicate this book to the memory of our dearly beloved colleague, Greg R. Alexander. For Greg, we want this book to improve – even in a small way – the lives of mothers and their infants through better understanding of the processes that promote optimal pregnancy outcomes and infant health status. As Greg served as a lifelong inspiration to his colleagues, his students, his mentees and all who had the opportunity to know or work with him, may this text inspire the next cohort of public health professionals and perinatal practitioners to continue and expand on his legacy.

Appendix U.S. Model Vital Records

U.S. STANDARD REPORT OF FETAL DEATH

LOCAL FILE NO. STATE FILE NUMBER:

MOTHER

1. NAME OF FETUS (optional-at the discretion of the parents)	2. TIME OF DELIVERY (24hr)	3. SEX (M/F/Unk)	4. DATE OF DELIVERY (Mo/Day/Yr)

5a. CITY, TOWN, OR LOCATION OF DELIVERY	7. PLACE WHERE DELIVERY OCCURRED (Check one)	8. FACILITY NAME (If not institution, give street and number)
5b. ZIP CODE OF DELIVERY	• Hospital • Freestanding birthing center • Home Delivery: Planned to deliver at home? • • Yes • No	
6. COUNTY OF DELIVERY	• Clinic/Doctor's office • Other (Specify)	9. FACILITY ID. (NPI)

10a. MOTHER'S CURRENT LEGAL NAME (First, Middle, Last, Suffix)	10b. DATE OF BIRTH (Mo/Day/Yr)
10c. MOTHER'S NAME PRIOR TO FIRST MARRIAGE (First, Middle, Last, Suffix)	10d. BIRTHPLACE (State, Territory, or Foreign Country)

11a. RESIDENCE OF MOTHER-STATE	11b. COUNTY	11c. CITY, TOWN, OR LOCATION
11d. STREET AND NUMBER	11e. APT. NO.	11f. ZIP CODE	11g. INSIDE CITY LIMITS? • Yes • No

FATHER

12a. FATHER'S CURRENT LEGAL NAME (First, Middle, Last, Suffix)	12b. DATE OF BIRTH (Mo/Day/Yr)	12c. BIRTHPLACE (State, Territory, or Foreign Country)

DISPOSITION

13. METHOD OF DISPOSITION:
• Burial • • Cremation • • Hospital Disposition • • Donation • • Removal from State • • Other (Specify)_____

ATTENDANT AND REGISTRATION INFORMATION

14. ATTENDANT'S NAME, TITLE, AND NPI NAME: _____ NPI: _____ TITLE: • MD • DO • CNM/CM • OTHER MIDWIFE • OTHER (Specify)_____	15. NAME AND TITLE OF PERSON COMPLETING REPORT Name _____ Title _____	16. DATE REPORT COMPLETED MM / DD / YYYY	17. DATE RECEIVED BY REGISTRAR MM / DD / YYYY

18. CAUSE/CONDITIONS CONTRIBUTING TO FETAL DEATH

CAUSE OF FETAL DEATH

18a. INITIATING CAUSE/CONDITION	18b. OTHER SIGNIFICANT CAUSES OR CONDITIONS
(AMONG THE CHOICES BELOW, PLEASE SELECT THE ONE WHICH MOST LIKELY BEGAN THE SEQUENCE OF EVENTS RESULTING IN THE DEATH OF THE FETUS)	(SELECT OR SPECIFY ALL OTHER CONDITIONS CONTRIBUTING TO DEATH IN ITEM 18b)

18a column:

Maternal Conditions/Diseases (Specify)_____

Complications of Placenta, Cord, or Membranes
• • Rupture of membranes prior to onset of labor
• • Abruptio placenta
• • Placental insufficiency
• • Prolapsed cord
• • Chorioamnionitis
• • Other (Specify)_____

Other Obstetrical or Pregnancy Complications (Specify)_____

Fetal Anomaly (Specify)_____

Fetal Injury (Specify)_____

Fetal Infection (Specify)_____

Other Fetal Conditions/Disorders (Specify)_____

• • Unknown

18b column:

Maternal Conditions/Diseases (Specify)_____

Complications of Placenta, Cord, or Membranes
• • Rupture of membranes prior to onset of labor
• • Abruptio placenta
• • Placental insufficiency
• • Prolapsed cord
• • Chorioamnionitis
• • Other (Specify)_____

Other Obstetrical or Pregnancy Complications (Specify)_____

Fetal Anomaly (Specify)_____

Fetal Injury (Specify)_____

Fetal Infection (Specify)_____

Other Fetal Conditions/Disorders (Specify)_____

• • Unknown

18c. WEIGHT OF FETUS (grams preferred, specify unit) _____ • • grams • lb/oz 18d. OBSTETRIC ESTIMATE OF GESTATION AT DELIVERY _____ (completed weeks)	18e. ESTIMATED TIME OF FETAL DEATH • • Dead at time of first assessment, no labor ongoing • • Dead at time of first assessment, labor ongoing • • Died during labor, after first assessment • • Unknown time of fetal death	18f. WAS AN AUTOPSY PERFORMED? • Yes • No • Planned 18g. WAS A HISTOLOGICAL PLACENTAL EXAMINATION PERFORMED? • Yes • No • Planned 18h. WERE AUTOPSY OR HISTOLOGICAL PLACENTAL EXAMINATION RESULTS USED IN DETERMINING THE CAUSE OF FETAL DEATH? • Yes • No

Mother's Name Mother's Medical Record No. _____

REV. 11/2003

MOTHER

19. MOTHER'S EDUCATION (Check the box that best describes the highest degree or level of school completed at the time of delivery)	20. MOTHER OF HISPANIC ORIGIN? (Check the box that best describes whether the mother is Spanish/Hispanic/Latina. Check the "No" box if mother is not Spanish/Hispanic/Latina)	21. MOTHER'S RACE (Check one or more races to indicate what the mother considers herself to be)
• • 8th grade or less	• • No, not Spanish/Hispanic/Latina	• • White
• • 9th - 12th grade, no diploma	• • Yes, Mexican, Mexican American, Chicana	• • Black or African American
• • High school graduate or GED completed	• • Yes, Puerto Rican	• • American Indian or Alaska Native (Name of the enrolled or principal tribe)_____
• • Some college credit but no degree	• • Yes, Cuban	• • Asian Indian
	• • Yes, other Spanish/Hispanic/Latina	• • Chinese
• • Associate degree (e.g., AA, AS)	(Specify)_____	• • Filipino
• • Bachelor's degree (e.g., BA, AB, BS)		• • Japanese
• • Master's degree (e.g., MA, MS, MEng, MEd, MSW, MBA)		• • Korean
		• • Vietnamese
• • Doctorate (e.g., PhD, EdD) or Professional degree (e.g., MD, DDS, DVM, LLB, JD)		• • Other Asian (Specify)_____
		• • Native Hawaiian
		• • Guamanian or Chamorro
		• • Samoan
		• • Other Pacific Islander (Specify)_____
		• • Other (Specify)_____

22. MOTHER MARRIED? (At delivery, conception, or anytime between) • • Yes • • No	23a. DATE OF FIRST PRENATAL CARE VISIT ___/___/___ MM DD YYYY • No Prenatal Care	23b. DATE OF LAST PRENATAL CARE VISIT ___/___/___ MM DD YYYY	24. TOTAL NUMBER OF PRENATAL VISITS FOR THIS PREGNANCY (If none, enter "0".) ____

25. MOTHER'S HEIGHT ____ (feet/inches)	26. MOTHER'S PREPREGNANCY WEIGHT ____ (pounds)	27. MOTHER'S WEIGHT AT DELIVERY ____ (pounds)	28. DID MOTHER GET WIC FOOD FOR HERSELF DURING THIS PREGNANCY? • • Yes • • No

29. NUMBER OF PREVIOUS LIVE BIRTHS	30. NUMBER OF OTHER PREGNANCY OUTCOMES (spontaneous or induced losses or ectopic pregnancies)	31. CIGARETTE SMOKING BEFORE AND DURING PREGNANCY For each time period, enter either the number of cigarettes or the number of packs of cigarettes smoked. IF NONE, ENTER "0".

29a. Now Living Number ____ • None	29b. Now Dead Number ____ • None	30a. Other Outcomes Number (Do not include this fetus) ____ • None	Average number of cigarettes or packs of cigarettes smoked per day. # of cigarettes OR # of packs Three Months Before Pregnancy ____ OR ____ First Three Months of Pregnancy ____ OR ____ Second Three Months of Pregnancy ____ OR ____ Third Trimester of Pregnancy ____ OR ____

29c. DATE OF LAST LIVE BIRTH ___/___ MM YYYY	30b. DATE OF LAST OTHER PREGNANCY OUTCOME ___/___ MM YYYY	32. DATE LAST NORMAL MENSES BEGAN ___/___/___ MM DD YYYY	33. PLURALITY - Single, Twin, Triplet, etc. (Specify)_____	34. IF NOT SINGLE BIRTH - Born First, Second, Third, etc. (Specify)_____

35. MOTHER TRANSFERRED FOR MATERNAL MEDICAL OR FETAL INDICATIONS FOR DELIVERY? • • Yes • • No
IF YES, ENTER NAME OF FACILITY MOTHER TRANSFERRED FROM:_____

MEDICAL AND HEALTH INFORMATION

36. RISK FACTORS IN THIS PREGNANCY (Check all that apply):	37. INFECTIONS PRESENT AND/OR TREATED
Diabetes	DURING THIS PREGNANCY (Check all that apply)
• • Prepregnancy (Diagnosis prior to this pregnancy)	• • Gonorrhea
• • Gestational (Diagnosis in this pregnancy)	• • Syphilis
Hypertension	• • Chlamydia
• • Prepregnancy (Chronic)	• • Listeria
• • Gestational (PIH, preeclampsia)	• • Group B Streptococcus
• • Eclampsia	• • Cytomegalovirus
• • Previous preterm birth	• • Parvovirus
• • Other previous poor pregnancy outcome (includes perinatal death, small-for-gestational age/intrauterine growth restricted birth)	• • Toxoplasmosis
• • Pregnancy resulted from infertility treatment-If yes, check all that apply:	• • None of the above
• • Fertility-enhancing drugs, Artificial insemination or intrauterine insemination	• • Other (Specify)_____
• • Assisted reproductive technology (e.g., in vitro fertilization (IVF), gamete intrafallopian transfer (GIFT))	
• • Mother had a previous cesarean delivery If yes, how many ____	
• • None of the above	

38. METHOD OF DELIVERY	39. MATERNAL MORBIDITY (Check all that apply) (Complications associated with labor and delivery)	40. CONGENITAL ANOMALIES OF THE FETUS (Check all that apply)
A. Was delivery with forceps attempted but unsuccessful? • • Yes • • No	• • Maternal transfusion	• • Anencephaly
B. Was delivery with vacuum extraction attempted but unsuccessful? • • Yes • • No	• • Third or fourth degree perineal laceration	• • Meningomyelocele/Spina bifida
C. Fetal presentation at delivery	• • Ruptured uterus	• • Cyanotic congenital heart disease
• • Cephalic	• • Unplanned hysterectomy	• • Congenital diaphragmatic hernia
• • Breech	• • Admission to intensive care unit	• • Omphalocele
• • Other	• • Unplanned operating room procedure following delivery	• • Gastroschisis
D. Final route and method of delivery (Check one)	• • None of the above	• • Limb reduction defect (excluding congenital amputation and dwarfing syndromes)
• Vaginal/Spontaneous		• • Cleft Lip with or without Cleft Palate
• Vaginal/Forceps		• • Cleft Palate alone
• Vaginal/Vacuum		• • Down Syndrome
• Cesarean		• • Karyotype confirmed
If cesarean, was a trial of labor attempted?		• • Karyotype pending
• Yes		• • Suspected chromosomal disorder
• No		• • Karyotype confirmed
E. Hysterotomy/Hysterectomy		• • Karyotype pending
• • Yes • • No		• • Hypospadias
		• • None of the anomalies listed above

Mother's Name _____   Mother's Medical Record No. _____

REV. 11/2003

NOTE: This recommended standard fetal death report is the result of an extensive evaluation process.
Information on the process and resulting recommendations as well as plans for future activities is available on the Internet at: http://www.cdc.gov/nchs/vital_certs_rev.htm.

U.S. STANDARD CERTIFICATE OF LIVE BIRTH

LOCAL FILE NO.   BIRTH NUMBER:

CHILD	1. CHILD'S NAME (First, Middle, Last, Suffix)		2. TIME OF BIRTH (24hr)	3. SEX	4. DATE OF BIRTH (Mo/Day/Yr)
	5. FACILITY NAME (If not institution, give street and number)	6. CITY, TOWN, OR LOCATION OF BIRTH		7. COUNTY OF BIRTH	

MOTHER	8a. MOTHER'S CURRENT LEGAL NAME (First, Middle, Last, Suffix)	8b. DATE OF BIRTH (Mo/Day/Yr)
	8c. MOTHER'S NAME PRIOR TO FIRST MARRIAGE (First, Middle, Last, Suffix)	8d. BIRTHPLACE (State, Territory, or Foreign Country)

9a. RESIDENCE OF MOTHER-STATE	9b. COUNTY	9c. CITY, TOWN, OR LOCATION
9d. STREET AND NUMBER	9e. APT. NO. 9f. ZIP CODE	9g. INSIDE CITY LIMITS? • •Yes • •No

FATHER	10a. FATHER'S CURRENT LEGAL NAME (First, Middle, Last, Suffix)	10b. DATE OF BIRTH (Mo/Day/Yr)	10c. BIRTHPLACE (State, Territory, or Foreign Country)

CERTIFIER	11. CERTIFIER'S NAME:	12. DATE CERTIFIED	13. DATE FILED BY REGISTRAR
	TITLE: • •MD • •DO • •HOSPITAL ADMIN. • •CNM/CM • •OTHER MIDWIFE • • OTHER (Specify)	MM DD YYYY	MM DD YYYY

INFORMATION FOR ADMINISTRATIVE USE

MOTHER	14. MOTHER'S MAILING ADDRESS: • •Same as residence, or: State:	City, Town, or Location:
	Street & Number:	Apartment No.: Zip Code:

15. MOTHER MARRIED? (At birth, conception, or any time between) • •Yes • •No	16. SOCIAL SECURITY NUMBER REQUESTED	17. FACILITY ID. (NPI)
IF NO, HAS PATERNITY ACKNOWLEDGMENT BEEN SIGNED IN THE HOSPITAL? • •Yes • •No	FOR CHILD? • •Yes • •No	
18. MOTHER'S SOCIAL SECURITY NUMBER:	19. FATHER'S SOCIAL SECURITY NUMBER:	

INFORMATION FOR MEDICAL AND HEALTH PURPOSES ONLY

MOTHER	20. MOTHER'S EDUCATION (Check the box that best describes the highest degree or level of school completed at the time of delivery)	21. MOTHER OF HISPANIC ORIGIN? (Check the box that best describes whether the mother is Spanish/Hispanic/Latina. Check the "No" box if mother is not Spanish/Hispanic/Latina)	22. MOTHER'S RACE (Check one or more races to indicate what the mother considers herself to be)
	• • 8th grade or less	• • No, not Spanish/Hispanic/Latina	• • White
	• • 9th - 12th grade, no diploma		• • Black or African American
	• • High school graduate or GED completed	• • Yes, Mexican, Mexican American, Chicana	• • American Indian or Alaska Native (Name of the enrolled or principal tribe)
	• • Some college credit but no degree	• • Yes, Puerto Rican	• • Asian Indian
	• • Associate degree (e.g., AA, AS)		• •Chinese
	• • Bachelor's degree (e.g., BA, AB, BS)	• • Yes, Cuban	• •Filipino
	• •Master's degree (e.g., MA, MS, MEng, MEd, MSW, MBA)	• • Yes, other Spanish/Hispanic/Latina (Specify)	• •Japanese
	• •Doctorate (e.g., PhD, EdD) or Professional degree (e.g., MD, DDS, DVM, LLB, JD)		• •Korean • •Vietnamese • •Other Asian (Specify) • •Native Hawaiian • •Guamanian or Chamorro • •Samoan • •Other Pacific Islander (Specify) • •Other (Specify)

FATHER	23. FATHER'S EDUCATION (Check the box that best describes the highest degree or level of school completed at the time of delivery)	24. FATHER OF HISPANIC ORIGIN? (Check the box that best describes whether the father is Spanish/Hispanic/Latino. Check the "No" box if father is not Spanish/Hispanic/Latino)	25. FATHER'S RACE (Check one or more races to indicate what the father considers himself to be)
	• • 8th grade or less	• • No, not Spanish/Hispanic/Latino	• • White
	• • 9th - 12th grade, no diploma		• • Black or African American
	• • High school graduate or GED completed	• • Yes, Mexican, Mexican American, Chicano	• • American Indian or Alaska Native (Name of the enrolled or principal tribe)
	• • Some college credit but no degree	• • Yes, Puerto Rican	• • Asian Indian
	• • Associate degree (e.g., AA, AS)		• •Chinese
	• • Bachelor's degree (e.g., BA, AB, BS)	• • Yes, Cuban	• •Filipino
	• •Master's degree (e.g., MA, MS, MEng, MEd, MSW, MBA)	• • Yes, other Spanish/Hispanic/Latino (Specify)	• •Japanese
	• •Doctorate (e.g., PhD, EdD) or Professional degree (e.g., MD, DDS, DVM, LLB, JD)		• •Korean • •Vietnamese • •Other Asian (Specify) • •Native Hawaiian • •Guamanian or Chamorro • •Samoan • •Other Pacific Islander (Specify) • •Other (Specify)

Mother's Name ___
Mother's Medical Record No. ___

26. PLACE WHERE BIRTH OCCURRED (Check one)	27. ATTENDANT'S NAME, TITLE, AND NPI	28. MOTHER TRANSFERRED FOR MATERNAL MEDICAL OR FETAL INDICATIONS FOR DELIVERY? • •Yes • •No
• •Hospital	NAME: _____ NPI: _____	IF YES, ENTER NAME OF FACILITY MOTHER TRANSFERRED FROM:
• •Freestanding birthing center	TITLE: • •MD • •DO • •CNM/CM • •OTHER MIDWIFE	
• •Home Birth: Planned to deliver at home? • •Yes • •No	• •OTHER (Specify)	
• •Clinic/Doctor's office		
• •Other (Specify)		

REV. 11/2003

MOTHER

29a. DATE OF FIRST PRENATAL CARE VISIT	29b. DATE OF LAST PRENATAL CARE VISIT	30. TOTAL NUMBER OF PRENATAL VISITS FOR THIS PREGNANCY
___/___/___ • No Prenatal Care MM DD YYYY	___/___/___ MM DD YYYY	(If none, enter "0".)

31. MOTHER'S HEIGHT	32. MOTHER'S PREPREGNANCY WEIGHT	33. MOTHER'S WEIGHT AT DELIVERY	34. DID MOTHER GET WIC FOOD FOR HERSELF DURING THIS PREGNANCY? • •Yes • •No
_____ (feet/inches)	_____ (pounds)	_____ (pounds)	

35. NUMBER OF PREVIOUS LIVE BIRTHS (Do not include this child)	36. NUMBER OF OTHER PREGNANCY OUTCOMES (spontaneous or induced losses or ectopic pregnancies)	37. CIGARETTE SMOKING BEFORE AND DURING PREGNANCY For each time period, enter either the number of cigarettes or the number of packs of cigarettes smoked. IF NONE, ENTER '0'. Average number of cigarettes or packs of cigarettes smoked per day.	38. PRINCIPAL SOURCE OF PAYMENT FOR THIS DELIVERY

35a. Now Living	35b. Now Dead	36a. Other Outcomes		# of cigarettes		# of packs	• •Private Insurance
Number _____	Number _____	Number _____	Three Months Before Pregnancy	_____	OR	_____	• •Medicaid
• •None	• •None	• •None	First Three Months of Pregnancy	_____	OR	_____	• •Self-pay
			Second Three Months of Pregnancy	_____	OR	_____	• •Other (Specify) _____
			Third Trimester of Pregnancy	_____	OR	_____	

35c. DATE OF LAST LIVE BIRTH	36b. DATE OF LAST OTHER PREGNANCY OUTCOME	39. DATE LAST NORMAL MENSES BEGAN	40. MOTHER'S MEDICAL RECORD NUMBER
___/___ MM YYYY	___/___ MM YYYY	___/___/___ M M D D YYYY	

MEDICAL AND HEALTH INFORMATION

41. RISK FACTORS IN THIS PREGNANCY (Check all that apply)	43. OBSTETRIC PROCEDURES (Check all that apply)	46. METHOD OF DELIVERY

41. RISK FACTORS IN THIS PREGNANCY (Check all that apply)

Diabetes
- • • Prepregnancy (Diagnosis prior to this pregnancy)
- • • Gestational (Diagnosis in this pregnancy)

Hypertension
- • • Prepregnancy (Chronic)
- • • Gestational (PIH, preeclampsia)
- • • Eclampsia

- • • Previous preterm birth

- • • Other previous poor pregnancy outcome (includes perinatal death, small-for-gestational age/intrauterine growth restricted birth)

- • • Pregnancy resulted from infertility treatment-If yes, check all that apply:
  - • • Fertility-enhancing drugs, Artificial insemination or Intrauterine insemination
  - • • Assisted reproductive technology (e.g., In vitro fertilization (IVF), gamete intrafallopian transfer (GIFT))
- • • Mother had a previous cesarean delivery If yes, how many _____
- • • None of the above

42. INFECTIONS PRESENT AND/OR TREATED DURING THIS PREGNANCY (Check all that apply)
- • • Gonorrhea
- • • Syphilis
- • • Chlamydia
- • • Hepatitis B
- • • Hepatitis C
- • • None of the above

43. OBSTETRIC PROCEDURES (Check all that apply)
- • • Cervical cerclage
- • • Tocolysis

External cephalic version:
- • Successful
- • Failed
- • None of the above

44. ONSET OF LABOR (Check all that apply)
- • • Premature Rupture of the Membranes (prolonged, ≥12 hrs.)
- • • Precipitous Labor (<3 hrs.)
- • • Prolonged Labor (≥20 hrs.)
- • • None of the above

45. CHARACTERISTICS OF LABOR AND DELIVERY (Check all that apply)
- • • Induction of labor
- • • Augmentation of labor
- • • Non-vertex presentation
- • • Steroids (glucocorticoids) for fetal lung maturation received by the mother prior to delivery
- • • Antibiotics received by the mother during labor
- • • Clinical chorioamnionitis diagnosed during labor or maternal temperature ≥38°C (100.4°F)
- • • Moderate/heavy meconium staining of the amniotic fluid
- • • Fetal intolerance of labor such that one or more of the following actions was taken: in-utero resuscitative measures, further fetal assessment, or operative delivery
- • • Epidural or spinal anesthesia during labor
- • • None of the above

46. METHOD OF DELIVERY

A. Was delivery with forceps attempted but unsuccessful?
- • •Yes • • No

B. Was delivery with vacuum extraction attempted but unsuccessful?
- • •Yes • • No

C. Fetal presentation at birth
- • • Cephalic
- • • Breech
- • • Other

D. Final route and method of delivery (Check one)
- • Vaginal/Spontaneous
- • Vaginal/Forceps
- • Vaginal/Vacuum
- • Cesarean
  If cesarean, was a trial of labor attempted?
  - • Yes
  - • No

47. MATERNAL MORBIDITY (Check all that apply) (Complications associated with labor and delivery)
- • • Maternal transfusion
- • • Third or fourth degree perineal laceration
- • • Ruptured uterus
- • • Unplanned hysterectomy
- • • Admission to intensive care unit
- • • Unplanned operating room procedure following delivery
- • • None of the above

NEWBORN INFORMATION

NEWBORN

48. NEWBORN MEDICAL RECORD NUMBER:

49. BIRTHWEIGHT (grams preferred, specify unit)
- • •grams • •lb/oz

50. OBSTETRIC ESTIMATE OF GESTATION:
_____ (completed weeks)

51. APGAR SCORE:
Score at 5 minutes:_____
If 5 minute score is less than 6,
Score at 10 minutes:_____

52. PLURALITY - Single, Twin, Triplet, etc.
(Specify)_____

53. IF NOT SINGLE BIRTH - Born First, Second, Third, etc. (Specify)_____

54. ABNORMAL CONDITIONS OF THE NEWBORN (Check all that apply)
- • • Assisted ventilation required immediately following delivery
- • • Assisted ventilation required for more than six hours
- • • NICU admission
- • • Newborn given surfactant replacement therapy
- • • Antibiotics received by the newborn for suspected neonatal sepsis
- • • Seizure or serious neurologic dysfunction
- • • Significant birth injury (skeletal fracture(s), peripheral nerve injury, and/or soft tissue/solid organ hemorrhage which requires intervention)
- • •None of the above

55. CONGENITAL ANOMALIES OF THE NEWBORN (Check all that apply)
- • • Anencephaly
- • • Meningomyelocele/Spina bifida
- • • Cyanotic congenital heart disease
- • • Congenital diaphragmatic hernia
- • • Omphalocele
- • • Gastroschisis
- • • Limb reduction defect (excluding congenital amputation and dwarfing syndromes)
- • • Cleft Lip with or without Cleft Palate
- • • Cleft Palate alone
- • • Down Syndrome
  - • • Karyotype confirmed
  - • • Karyotype pending
- • • Suspected chromosomal disorder
  - • • Karyotype confirmed
  - • • Karyotype pending
- • • Hypospadias
- • • None of the anomalies listed above

Mother's Name _____   Mother's Medical Record No. _____

56. WAS INFANT TRANSFERRED WITHIN 24 HOURS OF DELIVERY? • • Yes • • No IF YES, NAME OF FACILITY INFANT TRANSFERRED TO:_____	57. IS INFANT LIVING AT TIME OF REPORT? • •Yes • •No • •Infant transferred, status unknown	58. IS THE INFANT BEING BREASTFED AT DISCHARGE? • • Yes • • No

REV. 11/2003

NOTE: This recommended standard birth certificate is the result of an extensive evaluation process. Information on the process and resulting recommendations as well as plans for future activities is available on the Internet at: http://www.cdc.gov/nchs/vital_certs_rev.htm.

U.S. STANDARD CERTIFICATE OF DEATH

LOCAL FILE NO.   STATE FILE NO.

NAME OF DECEDENT
For use by physician or institution

To Be Completed/Verified By: FUNERAL DIRECTOR

1. DECEDENT'S LEGAL NAME (Include AKA's if any) (First, Middle, Last)			2. SEX	3. SOCIAL SECURITY NUMBER

4a. AGE-Last Birthday (Years)	4b. UNDER 1 YEAR		4c. UNDER 1 DAY		5. DATE OF BIRTH (Mo/Day/Yr)	6. BIRTHPLACE (City and State or Foreign Country)
	Months	Days	Hours	Minutes		

7a. RESIDENCE-STATE	7b. COUNTY	7c. CITY OR TOWN

7d. STREET AND NUMBER	7e. APT. NO.	7f. ZIP CODE	7g. INSIDE CITY LIMITS? • Yes • No

8. EVER IN US ARMED FORCES? • Yes • No	9. MARITAL STATUS AT TIME OF DEATH • Married • Married, but separated • Widowed • Divorced • Never Married • Unknown	10. SURVIVING SPOUSE'S NAME (If wife, give name prior to first marriage)

11. FATHER'S NAME (First, Middle, Last)	12. MOTHER'S NAME PRIOR TO FIRST MARRIAGE (First, Middle, Last)

13a. INFORMANT'S NAME	13b. RELATIONSHIP TO DECEDENT	13c. MAILING ADDRESS (Street and Number, City, State, Zip Code)

14. PLACE OF DEATH (Check only one, see instructions)

IF DEATH OCCURRED IN A HOSPITAL: • Inpatient • Emergency Room/Outpatient • Dead on Arrival	IF DEATH OCCURRED SOMEWHERE OTHER THAN A HOSPITAL: • Hospice facility • Nursing home/Long term care facility • Decedent's home • Other (Specify):

15. FACILITY NAME (If not institution, give street & number)	16. CITY OR TOWN, STATE, AND ZIP CODE	17. COUNTY OF DEATH

18. METHOD OF DISPOSITION: • Burial • Cremation • Donation • Entombment • Removal from State • Other (Specify):	19. PLACE OF DISPOSITION (Name of cemetery, crematory, other place)

20. LOCATION-CITY, TOWN, AND STATE	21. NAME AND COMPLETE ADDRESS OF FUNERAL FACILITY

22. SIGNATURE OF FUNERAL SERVICE LICENSEE OR OTHER AGENT	23. LICENSE NUMBER (Of Licensee)

To Be Completed By: MEDICAL CERTIFIER

ITEMS 24-28 MUST BE COMPLETED BY PERSON WHO PRONOUNCES OR CERTIFIES DEATH	24. DATE PRONOUNCED DEAD (Mo/Day/Yr)	25. TIME PRONOUNCED DEAD

26. SIGNATURE OF PERSON PRONOUNCING DEATH (Only when applicable)	27. LICENSE NUMBER	28. DATE SIGNED (Mo/Day/Yr)

29. ACTUAL OR PRESUMED DATE OF DEATH (Mo/Day/Yr) (Spell Month)	30. ACTUAL OR PRESUMED TIME OF DEATH	31. WAS MEDICAL EXAMINER OR CORONER CONTACTED? • Yes • No

CAUSE OF DEATH (See instructions and examples)   Approximate interval: Onset to death

32. PART I. Enter the chain of events—diseases, injuries, or complications—that directly caused the death. DO NOT enter terminal events such as cardiac arrest, respiratory arrest, or ventricular fibrillation without showing the etiology. DO NOT ABBREVIATE. Enter only one cause on a line. Add additional lines if necessary.

IMMEDIATE CAUSE (Final disease or condition resulting in death) ——→ a. _____
Due to (or as a consequence of): _____

Sequentially list conditions, if any, leading to the cause listed on line a. Enter the UNDERLYING CAUSE (disease or injury that initiated the events resulting in death) LAST

b. _____
Due to (or as a consequence of): _____

c. _____
Due to (or as a consequence of): _____

d. _____

PART II. Enter other significant conditions contributing to death but not resulting in the underlying cause given in PART I.	33. WAS AN AUTOPSY PERFORMED? • Yes • No
	34. WERE AUTOPSY FINDINGS AVAILABLE TO COMPLETE THE CAUSE OF DEATH? • Yes • No

35. DID TOBACCO USE CONTRIBUTE TO DEATH? • Yes • Probably • No • Unknown	36. IF FEMALE: • Not pregnant within past year • Pregnant at time of death • Not pregnant, but pregnant within 42 days of death • Not pregnant, but pregnant 43 days to 1 year before death • Unknown if pregnant within the past year	37. MANNER OF DEATH • Natural • Homicide • Accident • Pending Investigation • Suicide • Could not be determined

38. DATE OF INJURY (Mo/Day/Yr) (Spell Month)	39. TIME OF INJURY	40. PLACE OF INJURY (e.g., Decedent's home; construction site; restaurant; wooded area)	41. INJURY AT WORK? • Yes • No

42. LOCATION OF INJURY: State:	City or Town:	
Street & Number:	Apartment No.:	Zip Code:

43. DESCRIBE HOW INJURY OCCURRED:	44. IF TRANSPORTATION INJURY, SPECIFY: • Driver/Operator • Passenger • Pedestrian • Other (Specify)

45. CERTIFIER (Check only one):
• Certifying physician-To the best of my knowledge, death occurred due to the cause(s) and manner stated.
• Pronouncing & Certifying physician-To the best of my knowledge, death occurred at the time, date, and place, and due to the cause(s) and manner stated.
• Medical Examiner/Coroner-On the basis of examination, and/or investigation, in my opinion, death occurred at the time, date, and place, and due to the cause(s) and manner stated.

Signature of certifier: _____

46. NAME, ADDRESS, AND ZIP CODE OF PERSON COMPLETING CAUSE OF DEATH (Item 32)

47. TITLE OF CERTIFIER	48. LICENSE NUMBER	49. DATE CERTIFIED (Mo/Day/Yr)	50. FOR REGISTRAR ONLY- DATE FILED (Mo/Day/Yr)

To Be Completed By: FUNERAL DIRECTOR

51. DECEDENT'S EDUCATION-Check the box that best describes the highest degree or level of school completed at the time of death.	52. DECEDENT OF HISPANIC ORIGIN? Check the box that best describes whether the decedent is Spanish/Hispanic/Latino. Check the "No" box if decedent is not Spanish/Hispanic/Latino.	53. DECEDENT'S RACE (Check one or more races to indicate what the decedent considered himself or herself to be)
• 8th grade or less	• No, not Spanish/Hispanic/Latino	• White • Black or African American • American Indian or Alaska Native (Name of the enrolled or principal tribe)
• 9th - 12th grade; no diploma		
• High school graduate or GED completed	• Yes, Mexican, Mexican American, Chicano	• Asian Indian • Chinese
• Some college credit, but no degree	• Yes, Puerto Rican	• Filipino • Japanese
• Associate degree (e.g. AA, AS)		• Korean • Vietnamese
• Bachelor's degree (e.g. BA, AB, BS)	• Yes, Cuban	• Other Asian (Specify)_____
• Master's degree (e.g. MA, MS, MEng, MEd, MSW, MBA)	• Yes, other Spanish/Hispanic/Latino (Specify) _____	• Native Hawaiian • Guamanian or Chamorro
• Doctorate (e.g., PhD, EdD) or Professional degree (e.g. MD, DDS, DVM, LLB, JD)		• Samoan • Other Pacific Islander (Specify)_____ • Other (Specify)_____

54. DECEDENT'S USUAL OCCUPATION (Indicate type of work done during most of working life. DO NOT USE RETIRED).

55. KIND OF BUSINESS/INDUSTRY

REV. 11/2003

MEDICAL CERTIFIER INSTRUCTIONS for selected items on U.S. Standard Certificate of Death
(See Physicians' Handbook or Medical Examiner/Coroner Handbook on Death Registration for instructions on all items)

ITEMS ON WHEN DEATH OCCURRED
Items 24-25 and 29-31 should always be completed. If the facility uses a separate pronouncer or other person to indicate that death has taken place with another person more familiar with the case completing the remainder of the medical portion of the death certificate, the pronouncer completes Items 24-28. If a certifier completes Items 24-25 as well as items 29-49, Items 26-28 may be left blank.

ITEMS 24-25, 29-30 – DATE AND TIME OF DEATH
Spell out the name of the month. If the exact date of death is unknown, enter the **approximate** date. If the date cannot be approximated, enter the date the body is found and identify as **date found**. Date pronounced and actual date may be the same. Enter the exact hour and minutes according to a 24-hour clock; estimates may be provided with "Approx." placed before the time.

ITEM 32 – CAUSE OF DEATH (See attached examples)
Take care to make the entry legible. Use a computer printer with high resolution, typewriter with good black ribbon and clean keys, or print legibly using permanent **black** ink in completing the CAUSE OF DEATH Section. **Do not abbreviate** conditions entered in section.

Part I (Chain of events leading directly to death)
•Only **one** cause should be entered on each line. Line (a) MUST ALWAYS have an entry. DO NOT leave blank. Additional lines may be added if necessary.
•If the condition on Line (a) resulted from an underlying condition, put the underlying condition on Line (b), and so on, until the full sequence is reported. **ALWAYS** enter the **underlying cause of death** on the lowest used line in Part I.
  •For each cause indicate the best estimate of the interval between the presumed onset and the date of death. The terms "unknown" or "approximately" may be used. General terms, such as minutes, hours, or days, are acceptable, if necessary. **DO NOT** leave blank.
  •The terminal event (for example, cardiac arrest or respiratory arrest) should not be used. If a mechanism of death seems most appropriate to you for line (a), then you must always list its cause(s) on the line(s) below it (for example, cardiac arrest **due to** coronary artery atherosclerosis or cardiac arrest **due to** blunt impact to chest).
• If an organ system failure such as congestive heart failure, hepatic failure, renal failure, or respiratory failure is listed as a cause of death, always report its etiology on the line(s) beneath it (for example, renal failure **due to** Type I diabetes mellitus).
•When indicating neoplasms as a cause of death, include the following: 1) primary site or that the primary site is unknown, 2) benign or malignant, 3) cell type or that the cell type is unknown, 4) grade of neoplasm, and 5) part or lobe of organ affected. (For example, a primary well-differentiated squamous cell carcinoma, lung, left upper lobe.)
•Always report the fatal injury (for example, stab wound of chest), the trauma (for example, transection of subclavian vein), and impairment of function (for example, air embolism).

PART II (Other significant conditions)
•Enter all diseases or conditions contributing to death that were not reported in the chain of events in Part I and that did not result in the **underlying cause of death.** See attached examples.
•If two or more possible sequences resulted in death, or if two conditions seem to have added together, report in Part I the one that, in your opinion, most directly caused death. Report in Part II the other conditions or diseases.

CHANGES TO CAUSE OF DEATH
Should additional medical information or autopsy findings become available that would change the cause of death originally reported, the original death certificate should be amended by the certifying physician by **immediately** reporting the revised cause of death to the State Vital Records Office.

ITEMS 33-34 - AUTOPSY
•33 - Enter "Yes" if either a partial or full autopsy was performed. Otherwise enter "No."
•34 - Enter "Yes" if autopsy findings were available to complete the cause of death; otherwise enter "No". Leave item blank if no autopsy was performed.

ITEM 35 - DID TOBACCO USE CONTRIBUTE TO DEATH?
Check "yes" if, in your opinion, the use of tobacco contributed to death. Tobacco use may contribute to deaths due to a wide variety of diseases; for example, tobacco use contributes to many deaths due to emphysema or lung cancer and some heart disease and cancers of the head and neck. Check "no" if, in your clinical judgment, tobacco use did not contribute to this particular death.

ITEM 36 - IF FEMALE, WAS DECEDENT PREGNANT AT TIME OF DEATH OR WITHIN PAST YEAR?
This information is important in determining pregnancy-related mortality.

ITEM 37 - MANNER OF DEATH
•Always check Manner of Death, which is important: 1) in determining accurate causes of death; 2) in processing insurance claims; and 3) in statistical studies of injuries and death.
•Indicate "Pending investigation" if the manner of death cannot be determined whether due to an accident, suicide, or homicide within the statutory time limit for filing the death certificate. This should be changed later to one of the other terms.
•Indicate "Could not be Determined" **ONLY** when it is impossible to determine the manner of death.

ITEMS 38-44 - ACCIDENT OR INJURY – to be filled out in all cases of deaths due to injury or poisoning.
•38 - Enter the exact month, day, and year of injury. Spell out the name of the month. **DO NOT** use a number for the month. (Remember, the date of injury may differ from the date of death.) Estimates may be provided with "Approx." placed before the date.
•39 - Enter the exact hour and minutes of injury or use your best estimate. Use a 24-hour clock.
•40 - Enter the general place (such as restaurant, vacant lot, or home) where the injury occurred. **DO NOT** enter firm or organization names. (For example, enter "factory", **not** "Standard Manufacturing, Inc.")
•41 - Complete if anything other than natural disease is mentioned in Part I or Part II of the medical certification, including homicides, suicides, and accidents. This includes all motor vehicle deaths. The item **must** be completed for decedents ages 14 years or over and may be completed for those less than 14 years of age if warranted. Enter "Yes" if the injury occurred at work. Otherwise enter "No". An injury may occur at work regardless of whether the injury occurred in the course of the decedent's "usual" occupation. Examples of injury at work and injury not at work follow:

Injury at work	Injury not at work
Injury while working or in vocational training on job premises	Injury while engaged in personal recreational activity on job premises
Injury while on break or at lunch or in parking lot on job premises	Injury while a visitor (not on official work business) to job premises
Injury while working for pay or compensation, including at home	Homemaker working at homemaking activities
Injury while working as a volunteer law enforcement official etc.	Student in school
Injury while traveling on business, including to/from business contacts	Working for self for no profit (mowing yard, repairing own roof, hobby)
	Commuting to or from work

•42 - Enter the complete address where the injury occurred including zip code.
•43 - Enter a brief but specific and clear description of how the injury occurred. Explain the circumstances or cause of the injury. Specify **type of gun** or **type of vehicle** (e.g., car, bulldozer, train, etc.) when relevant to circumstances. Indicate if more than one vehicle involved; specify type of vehicle decedent was in.
•44 -Specify role of decedent (e.g. driver, passenger). Driver/operator and passenger should be designated for modes other than motor vehicles such as bicycles. Other applies to watercraft, aircraft, animal, or people attached to outside of vehicles (e.g. surfers).

Rationale: Motor vehicle accidents are a major cause of unintentional deaths; details will help determine effectiveness of current safety features and laws.
REFERENCES
For more information on how to complete the medical certification section of the death certificate, refer to tutorial at http://www.TheNAME.org and resources including instructions and handbooks available by request from NCHS, Room 7318, 3311 Toledo Road, Hyattsville, Maryland 20782-2003 or at www.cdc.gov/nchs/about/major/dvs/handbk.htm

Cause-of-death – Background, Examples, and Common Problems

Accurate cause of death information is important
•to the public health community in evaluating and improving the health of all citizens, and
•often to the family, now and in the future, and to the person settling the decedent's estate.

The cause-of-death section consists of two parts. **Part I** is for reporting a chain of events leading directly to death, with the **immediate cause** of death (the final disease, injury, or complication directly causing death) on line a and the **underlying cause** of death (the disease or injury that initiated the chain of events that led directly and inevitably to death) on the lowest used line. **Part I** is for reporting all other significant diseases, conditions, or injuries that contributed to death but which did not result in the underlying cause of death given in Part I. The cause-of-death information should be **YOUR best medical OPINION**. A condition can be listed as "probable" even if it has not been definitively diagnosed.

Examples of properly completed medical certifications:

32. PART I. Enter the chain of events—diseases, injuries, or complications—that directly caused the death. DO NOT enter terminal events such as cardiac arrest, respiratory arrest, or ventricular fibrillation without showing the etiology. DO NOT ABBREVIATE. Enter only one cause on a line. Add additional lines if necessary.	CAUSE OF DEATH (See instructions and examples)	Approximate interval: Onset to death
IMMEDIATE CAUSE (Final disease or condition ----> resulting in death)	a. Rupture of myocardium Due to (or as a consequence of):	Minutes
Sequentially list conditions, if any, leading to the cause listed on line a. Enter the **UNDERLYING CAUSE** (disease or injury that initiated the events resulting in death) LAST	b. Acute myocardial infarction Due to (or as a consequence of): c. Coronary artery thrombosis Due to (or as a consequence of): d. Atherosclerotic coronary artery disease	6 days 5 years 7 years

PART II. Enter other significant conditions contributing to death but not resulting in the underlying cause given in PART I. Diabetes, Chronic obstructive pulmonary disease, smoking	33. WAS AN AUTOPSY PERFORMED? • •Yes • •No
	34. WERE AUTOPSY FINDINGS AVAILABLE TO COMPLETE THE CAUSE OF DEATH? • •Yes • •No

35. DID TOBACCO USE CONTRIBUTE TO DEATH? • • Yes • • Probably • • No • • Unknown	36. IF FEMALE: • •Not pregnant within past year • •Pregnant at time of death • •Not pregnant, but pregnant within 42 days of death • •Not pregnant, but pregnant 43 days to 1 year before death • •Unknown if pregnant within the past year	37. MANNER OF DEATH • •Natural • •Homicide • •Accident • •Pending Investigation • •Suicide • •Could not be determined

32. PART I. Enter the chain of events—diseases, injuries, or complications—that directly caused the death. DO NOT enter terminal events such as cardiac arrest, respiratory arrest, or ventricular fibrillation without showing the etiology. DO NOT ABBREVIATE. Enter only one cause on a line. Add additional lines if necessary.	CAUSE OF DEATH (See instructions and examples)	Approximate interval: Onset to death
IMMEDIATE CAUSE (Final disease or condition ----> resulting in death)	a. Aspiration pneumonia Due to (or as a consequence of):	2 Days
Sequentially list conditions, if any, leading to the cause listed on line a. Enter the **UNDERLYING CAUSE** (disease or injury that initiated the events resulting in death) LAST	b. Complications of coma Due to (or as a consequence of): c. Blunt force injuries Due to (or as a consequence of): d. Motor vehicle accident	7 weeks 7 weeks 7 weeks

PART II. Enter other significant conditions contributing to death but not resulting in the underlying cause given in PART I.	33. WAS AN AUTOPSY PERFORMED? • •Yes • •No
	34. WERE AUTOPSY FINDINGS AVAILABLE TO COMPLETE THE CAUSE OF DEATH? • •Yes • •No

35. DID TOBACCO USE CONTRIBUTE TO DEATH? • • Yes • • Probably • • No • • Unknown	36. IF FEMALE: • •Not pregnant within past year • •Pregnant at time of death • •Not pregnant, but pregnant within 42 days of death • •Not pregnant, but pregnant 43 days to 1 year before death • •Unknown if pregnant within the past year	37. MANNER OF DEATH • •Natural • •Homicide • •Accident • •Pending Investigation • •Suicide • •Could not be determined

38. DATE OF INJURY (Mo/Day/Yr) (Spell Month) August 16, 2003	39. TIME OF INJURY Approx. 2320	40. PLACE OF INJURY (e.g., Decedent's home; construction site; restaurant; wooded area) road side near state highway	41. INJURY AT WORK? • •Yes • •No

42. LOCATION OF INJURY: State: Missouri		City or Town: near Alexandria	
Street & Number: mile marker 17 on state route 46a	Apartment No.:		Zip Code:

43. DESCRIBE HOW INJURY OCCURRED: Decedent driver of van, ran off road into tree	44. IF TRANSPORTATION INJURY, SPECIFY: • • Driver/Operator • • Passenger • • Pedestrian • • Other (Specify)

Common problems in death certification

The **elderly decedent** should have a clear and distinct etiological sequence for cause of death, if possible. Terms such as senescence, infirmity, old age, and advanced age have little value for public health or medical research. Age is recorded elsewhere on the certificate. When a number of conditions resulted in death, the physician should choose the single sequence that, in his or her opinion, best describes the process leading to death, and place any other pertinent conditions in Part II. If after careful consideration the physician cannot determine a sequence that ends in death, then the medical examiner or coroner should be consulted about conducting an investigation or providing assistance in completing the cause of death.

The **infant decedent** should have a clear and distinct etiological sequence for cause of death, if possible. "Prematurity" should not be entered without explaining the etiology of prematurity. Maternal conditions may have initiated or affected the sequence that resulted in infant death, and such maternal causes should be reported in addition to the infant causes on the infant's death certificate (e.g. Hyaline membrane disease **due to** prematurity, 28 weeks **due to** placental abruption **due to** blunt trauma to mother's abdomen).

When **SIDS** is suspected, a complete investigation should be conducted, typically by a medical examiner or coroner. If the infant is under 1 year of age, no cause of death is determined after scene investigation, clinical history is reviewed, and a complete autopsy is performed, then the death can be reported as Sudden Infant Death Syndrome.

When processes such as the following are reported, additional information about the etiology should be reported:

Abscess	Carcinomatosis	Disseminated intra vascular	Hyponatremia	Pulmonary arrest
Abdominal hemorrhage	Cardiac arrest	coagulopathy	Hypotension	Pulmonary edema
Adhesions	Cardiac dysrhythmia	Dysrhythmia	Immunosuppression	Pulmonary embolism
Adult respiratory distress syndrome	Cardiomyopathy	End-stage liver disease	Increased intra cranial pressure	Pulmonary insufficiency
Acute myocardial infarction	Cardiopulmonary arrest	End-stage renal disease	Intra cranial hemorrhage	Renal failure
Altered mental status	Cellulitis	Epidural hematoma	Malnutrition	Respiratory arrest
Anemia	Cerebral edema	Exsanguination	Metabolic encephalopathy	Seizures
Anoxia	Cerebrovascular accident	Failure to thrive	Multi-organ failure	Sepsis
Anoxic encephalopathy	Cerebellar tonsillar herniation	Fracture	Multi-system organ failure	Septic shock
Arrhythmia	Chronic bedridden state	Gangrene	Myocardial infarction	Shock
Ascites	Cirrhosis	Gastrointestinal hemorrhage	Necrotizing soft-tissue infection	Starvation
Aspiration	Coagulopathy	Heart failure	Old age	Subdural hematoma
Atrial fibrillation	Compression fracture	Hemothorax	Open (or closed) head injury	Subarachnoid hemorrhage
Bacteremia	Congestive heart failure	Hepatic failure	Paralysis	Sudden death
Bedridden	Convulsions	Hepatitis	Pancytopenia	Thrombocytopenia
Biliary obstruction	Decubiti	Hepatorenal syndrome	Perforated gallbladder	Uncal herniation
Bowel obstruction	Dehydration	Hyperglycemia	Peritonitis	Urinary tract infection
Brain injury	Dementia (when not	Hyperkalemia	Pleural effusions	Ventricular fibrillation
Brain stem herniation	otherwise specified)	Hypovolemic shock	Pneumonia	Ventricular tachycardia
Carcinogenesis	Diarrhea			Volume depletion

If the certifier is unable to determine the etiology of a process such as those shown above, the process must be qualified as being of an unknown, undetermined, probable, presumed, or unspecified etiology so it is clear that a distinct etiology was not inadvertently or carelessly omitted.

The following conditions and types of death might seem to be specific or natural but when the medical history is examined further may be found to be complications of an injury or poisoning (possibly occurring long ago). Such cases should be reported to the medical examiner/coroner.

Asphyxia	Epidural hematoma	Hip fracture	Pulmonary emboli	
Bolus	Exsanguination	Hyperthermia	Seizure disorder	Subdural hematoma
Choking	Fall	Hypothermia	Sepsis	Surgery
Drug or alcohol overdose/drug or alcohol abuse	Fracture	Open reduction of fracture	Subarachnoid hemorrhage	Thermal burns/chemical burns

REV. 11/2003

FUNERAL DIRECTOR INSTRUCTIONS for selected items on U.S.

Standard Certificate of Death (For additional information concerning all items on certificate see Funeral Directors' Handbook on Death Registration)

ITEM 1. DECEDENT'S LEGAL NAME
Include any other names used by decedent, if substantially different from the legal name, after the abbreviation AKA (also known as) e.g. Samuel Langhorne Clemens AKA Mark Twain, **but not** Jonathon Doe AKA John Doe

ITEM 5. DATE OF BIRTH
Enter the full name of the month (January, February, March etc.) Do not use a number or abbreviation to designate the month.

ITEM 7A-G. RESIDENCE OF DECEDENT (information divided into seven categories)
Residence of decedent is the place where the decedent actually resided. The place of residence is not necessarily the same as "home state" or "legal residence". Never enter a temporary residence such as one used during a visit, business trip, or vacation. Place of residence during a tour of military duty or during attendance at college is considered permanent and should be entered as the place of residence. If the decedent had been living in a facility where an individual usually resides for a long period of time, such as a group home, mental institution, nursing home, penitentiary, or hospital for the chronically ill, report the location of that facility in item 7. If the decedent was an infant who never resided at home, the place of residence is that of the parent(s) or legal guardian. **Never** use an acute care hospital's location as the place of residence for any infant. If Canadian residence, please specify Province instead of State.

ITEM 10. SURVIVING SPOUSE'S NAME
If the decedent was married at the time of death, enter the full name of the surviving spouse. If the surviving spouse is the wife, enter her name prior to first marriage. This item is used in establishing proper insurance settlements and other survivor benefits.

ITEM 12. MOTHER'S NAME PRIOR TO FIRST MARRIAGE
Enter the name used prior to first marriage, commonly known as the maiden name. This name is useful because it remains constant throughout life.

ITEM 14. PLACE OF DEATH
The place where death is pronounced should be considered the place where death occurred. If the place of death is unknown but the body is found in your State, the certificate of death should be completed and filed in accordance with the laws of your State. Enter the place where the body is found as the place of death.

ITEM 51. DECEDENT'S EDUCATION *(Check appropriate box on death certificate)*
Check the box that corresponds to the highest level of education that the decedent completed. **Information in this section will not appear on the certified copy of the death certificate. This information is used to study the relationship between mortality and education (which roughly corresponds with socioeconomic status). This information is valuable in medical studies of causes of death and in programs to prevent illness and death.**

ITEM 52. WAS DECEDENT OF HISPANIC ORIGIN? *(Check "No" or appropriate "Yes" box)*
Check "No" or check the "Yes" box that best corresponds with the decedent's ethnic Spanish identity as given by the informant. Note that "Hispanic" is not a race and item 53 must also be completed. Do not leave this item blank. With respect to this item, "Hispanic" refers to people whose origins are from Spain, Mexico, or the Spanish-speaking Caribbean Islands or countries of Central or South America. Origin includes ancestry, nationality, and lineage. There is no set rule about how many generations are to be taken into account in determining Hispanic origin; it may be based on the country of origin of a parent, grandparent, or some far-removed ancestor. Although the prompts include the major Hispanic groups, other groups may be specified under "other". "Other" may also be used for decedents of multiple Hispanic origin (e.g. Mexican-Puerto Rican). **Information in this section will not appear on the certified copy of the death certificate. This information is needed to identify health problems in a large minority population in the United States. Identifying health problems will make it possible to target public health resources to this important segment of our population.**

ITEM 53. RACE *(Check appropriate box or boxes on death certificate)*
Enter the race of the decedent as stated by the informant. Hispanic is not a race; information on Hispanic ethnicity is collected separately in item 52. American Indian and Alaska Native refer only to those native to North and South America (including Central America) and does not include Asian Indian. Please specify the name of enrolled or principal tribe (e.g., Navajo, Cheyenne, etc.) for the American Indian or Alaska Native. For Asians check Asian Indian, Chinese, Filipino, Japanese, Korean, Vietnamese, or specify other Asian group; for Pacific Islanders check Guamanian or Chamorro, Samoan, or specify other Pacific Island group. If the decedent was of mixed race, enter each race (e.g., Samoan-Chinese-Filipino or White, American Indian). **Information in this section will not appear on the certified copy of the death certificate. Race is essential for identifying specific mortality patterns and leading causes of death among different racial groups. It is also used to determine if specific health programs are needed in particular areas and to make population estimates.**

ITEMS 54 AND 55. OCCUPATION AND INDUSTRY
Questions concerning occupation and industry must be completed for all decedents 14 years of age or older. This information is useful in studying deaths related to jobs and in identifying any new risks. For example, the link between lung disease and lung cancer and asbestos exposure in jobs such as shipbuilding or construction was made possible by this sort of information on death certificates. **Information in this section will not appear on the certified copy of the death certificate.**

ITEM 54. DECEDENT'S USUAL OCCUPATION
Enter the usual occupation of the decedent. This is not necessarily the last occupation of the decedent. Never enter "retired". Give kind of work decedent did during most of his or her working life, such as claim adjuster, farmhand, coal miner, janitor, store manager, college professor, or civil engineer. If the decedent was a homemaker at the time of death but had worked outside the household during his or her working life, enter that occupation. If the decedent was a homemaker during most of his or her working life, and never worked outside the household, enter "homemaker". Enter "student" if the decedent was a student at the time of death and was never regularly employed or employed full time during his or her working life. **Information in this section will not appear on the certified copy of the death certificate.**

ITEM 55. KIND OF BUSINESS/INDUSTRY
Kind of business to which occupation in item 54 is related, such as insurance, farming, coal mining, hardware store, retail clothing, university, or government. DO NOT enter firm or organization names. If decedent was a homemaker as indicated in item 54, then enter either "own home" or "someone else's home" as appropriate. If decedent was a student as indicated in item 54, then enter type of school, such as high school or college, in item 55. **Information in this section will not appear on the certified copy of the death certificate.**

NOTE: This recommended standard death certificate is the result of an extensive evaluation process. Information on the process and resulting recommendations as well as plans for future activities is available on the Internet at: http://www.cdc.gov/nchs/vital_certs_rev.htm.

Glossary

Adverse event (outcome) Any disease, injury, or death.

Age-specific fertility rate The rate of fertility among women of a specific age.

Antepartum fetal death Fetal death occurring before the initiation of labor.

ART Assisted reproductive technology refers to interventions to assist couples to conceive.

Association A term signifying a relationship between two or more events or variables. Events are said to be associated when they occur more frequently together than one would expect by chance. Association does not imply a causal relationship. Statistical significance testing enables a researcher to determine the likelihood of observing the sample relationship by chance if in fact no association exists in the population that was sampled. The terms *association* and *relationship* are often used interchangeably.

Birth certificate Official, legal document recording details of a live birth, usually comprising name, date, place, identity of parents, and sometimes additional information such as birth weight. It provides the basis for the vital statistics of birth and birthrates in a political or administrative jurisdiction and the denominator for infant mortality and certain other vital statistics.

Birth cohort prevalence rate In developmental disabilities surveillance, the prevalence of a specific disorder in a geographic area, among children of a specific age who were born in that geographic area, within a specified time interval.

Birth defect A structural abnormality present at birth.

Birth interval The length of time between termination of one pregnancy and the termination of a second.

Birth order The ordinal number of a given live birth in relation to all previous live births of the same woman.

Birth rate A summary rate based on the number of live births in a population over a given time period, usually one year.

Birth weight Infant's weight recorded at birth, and in some countries, entered on the birth certificate.

Birth weight-specific mortality rate The number of infant deaths that occurred among live births in a specific birth weight category in a calendar year divided by the total number of live births that occurred in that category in that year. To express the rate per 1,000 live births, multiply the result by 1,000.

Case ascertainment Identification of cases of an exposure or health outcome in public health surveillance, usually according to a specific case definition.

Causality Relating causes to the effects they produce. Most of epidemiology concerns causality, and several types of causes can be distinguished. A cause is termed *necessary* when a particular variable must always precede an effect. This effect need not be the sole result of the one variable. A cause is termed "sufficient" when a particular variable inevitably initiates or produces an effect. Any given cause may be necessary, sufficient, neither, or both.

Cause-of-death Defined by the World Health Organization as the underlying cause of death, which is recorded on the death certificate. The cause of death is (a) the disease or injury that initiated the train of morbid events leading directly to death or (b) the circumstances of the accident or violence that produced the fatal injury.

Cohort fertility The fertility of cohort of women who were born during a specified interval and followed through their reproductive years.

Cohort infant mortality rate The number of infant deaths that occurred among live births in a calendar year, divided by the total number of live births that year. To express the rate per 1,000 infants per year, multiply the result by 1,000.

Confidence interval A range of values for a variable of interest, constructed statistically so that this range has a specified probability of including the true value of the variable (1).

Contraceptive failure rate The average probability of having an unintended pregnancy during a year of using a specific contraceptive method.

Crude birth rate The rate of live births in a defined population during 1 year. The denominator is the average or mid-year population during that year.

Crude fertility rate Rate of live births during 1 year in a defined population of women aged 15–44 years. The denominator is the mid-year female population aged 15–44 years.

Cumulative birth rate The total number of births to women who were born during a specified interval until they reach a specified age.

Death certificate A vital record signed by a licensed physician or by another designated health worker that includes cause of death, decedent's name, sex, birth data, places of residence and of death, and whether the deceased had been medically attended before death. Occupation, birthplace, and other information may be included. Immediate cause of death is recorded on the first line, followed by conditions giving rise to the immediate cause; the underlying cause is entered last.

Death rate An estimate of the proportion of a population that dies during a specified period. The numerator is the number of persons dying during the period; the denominator is the number in the population. For the death rate per year, the denominator often is estimated as mid-year population.

Disease May be defined as a failure of the adaptive mechanisms of an organism to counteract adequately, normally, or appropriately noxious stimuli or infectious pathogen, to which it is subjected, resulting in a disturbance in the function or structure of some part of the organism. This definition emphasizes that disease is multifactorial and may be prevented or treated by changing any factor or a combination of the factors. Disease is a very elusive and difficult concept to define, being largely socially defined. Thus, criminality and drug dependence are presently seen by some as diseases, when they were previously considered to be moral or legal problems.

Epidemiology The study of the patterns of determinants and antecedents of disease in human populations. Epidemiology utilizes biology, clinical medicine, and statistics in an effort to understand the etiology (causes) of illness and/or disease. The ultimate goal of the epidemiologist is not merely to identify underlying causes of a disease but to apply findings to disease prevention and health promotion.

Exposure A general term used to describe contact with a risk factor. An exposure can be a physical agent (e.g., radiation) or a behavior (e.g., excessive drinking).

Fertility The actual production of live offspring. Stillbirths, fetal deaths, and abortions are not included in the measurement of fertility.

Fertility rate The rate of live births per 1,000 women aged 15–44 years.

Fertility ratio The rate of children aged <5 years per 1,000 women aged 15–44 years.

Fetal death Defined by the World Health Organization as "death prior to the complete expulsion or extraction from its mother of a product of conception, irrespective of the duration of pregnancy. The death is indicated by the fact that after such separation, the fetus does not breathe or show any other evidence of life such as beating of the heart, pulsation of the umbilical cord, or definite movement of voluntary muscles." This definition includes the following as fetal deaths: stillbirths, spontaneous abortions, and miscarriages.

Fetal mortality rate The number of fetal deaths divided by the sum of the number of live births plus the number of fetal deaths in a specified time period. To express the rate per 1,000 births per year, multiply the result by 1,000.

Fetal mortality ratio The ratio of the number of fetal deaths to live births in a specified period. To express the rate per 1,000 live births per year, multiply the result by 1,000.

Final data Complete data from vital records (such as birth and death certificates and fetal death reports) that have been reviewed by the National Center for Health Statistics for validity and consistency. Usually available by 2 years after the close of a data year.

General fertility rate The rate of live births during a year in a defined population of women aged 15–44 years during that year.

Gestational age The gestational age of a fetus is the elapsed time since conception. However, the moment when conception occurred is rarely known precisely, the duration of gestation is measured from the first day of the last normal menstrual period. Gestational age is measured in completed days or completed weeks.

Gestational weight gain Maternal weight gain during pregnancy.

Gross reproduction rate A hypothetical rate that represents the average number of daughters born to a cohort of women if the following conditions apply: (a) women in the cohort experienced the age-specific birthrates observed in a given year and (b) none of the cohort died during her childbearing years.

Health The state of complete physical, mental, and social well-being and not merely the absence of disease or infirmity. Health has many dimensions (anatomical, physiological, and mental) and is largely culturally defined. The relative importance of various disabilities will differ depending upon the cultural milieu and the role of the affected individual in that culture. Most attempts at measurement have been assessed in terms of morbidity and mortality.

HP2010 Healthy People 2010. It refers to health objectives for the United States.

Impaired fecundity In the National Survey of Family Growth, the status of a woman who (a) is part of an infertile couple or (b) reports that it is physically difficult or impossible to conceive or deliver a baby, or (c) has been told by a physician that pregnancy would pose a danger to her or the baby.

Incidence In epidemiology, the number of cases of disease, infection, or some other event having their onset during a prescribed period of time in relation to the unit of population in which they occur. Incidence measures morbidity or other events as they happen during an interval of time. Examples include the number of accidents occurring in a manufacturing plant during a year in relation to the number of employees in the plant, or the number of cases of mumps occurring in a school during a month in relation to the number of pupils enrolled in the school. It usually refers only to the number of new cases, particularly of chronic diseases.

Infant mortality The death of a live-born infant before its first birthday.

Infertile The status of a married couple who is not surgically sterilized, has not used contraception, and has not become pregnant after at least 12 months of intercourse.

Intrapartum fetal death Fetal death occurring after the initiation of labor and before delivery.

IVF In vitro fertilization: A reproductive technology that refers to fertilization of an embryo outside of the mother's body.

Kessner index A classification of prenatal care developed by the Institute of Medicine in 1973 that adjusts the timing and quantity of prenatal care for the length of gestation to determine levels of adequate, inadequate, and intermediate prenatal care. David Kessner was the first author of the Institute of Medicine's report on use of prenatal care.

Legal induced abortion An abortion conducted by a licensed health provider under conditions consistent with the legal requirements of the state.

Live birth "...the complete expulsion or extraction from its mother of a product of conception, regardless of the duration of pregnancy, which, after such separation, breathes or shows any evidence of life, such as beating of the heart, pulsation of the umbilical cord, or definite movement of voluntary muscles, whether or not the umbilical cord has been cut or the placenta is attached; each product of such a birth is considered liveborn." (1)

Low birth weight Birth weight less than 2,500 g.

Maternal death Death of a woman while pregnant or within 42 days of termination of pregnancy, irrespective of the duration and the site of pregnancy, from any cause related to or aggravated by the pregnancy or its management but not from accidental or incidental causes.

Maternal mortality The risk of dying from causes associated with childbirth. The numerator is the deaths arising during pregnancy or from puerperal causes, i.e., deaths occurring because of deliveries, complications of pregnancy, childbirth, and the puerperium.

Mistimed pregnancy According to questions included in the National Survey of Family Growth, a pregnancy that was intended but occurred sooner than the mother would have liked.

Morbidity The extent of illness, injury, or disability in a defined population. It is usually expressed in general or cause-specific rates of incidence or prevalence.

Mortality Death. Used to describe the relation of deaths to the population in which they occur. The mortality rate (death rate) expresses the number of deaths in a unit of population within a prescribed time and may be expressed as crude death rates (e.g., total deaths in relation to total population during a year) or as death rates specific for diseases and, sometimes, for age, sex, or other attributes (e.g., number of deaths from cancer in White males in relation to the White male population during a given year).

NCHS National Center for Health Statistics.

Neonatal death Death of a live-born infant from birth to 27 days after delivery.

Net pregnancy weight gain Total weight gain of the mother during pregnancy after the birth weight of the infant is subtracted.

NSFG National Survey of Family Growth.

Nulligravida A woman who has never been pregnant.

Obstetrics The branch of medicine dealing with pregnancy and the delivery of babies.

Parity The total number of times a woman delivered a living baby.

Periconceptional Occurring around the time of conception.

Perinatal period Defined by the ICD-10 as the period from 22 weeks of gestation through 7 completed days after delivery.

Perinatal mortality rate The numerator is the number of stillbirths and neonatal deaths in a specified time period. The denominator is the number of live births and stillbirths in the same time period. The WHO's definition, more appropriate in nations with less-well-established systems for vital records, is the number of stillbirths after 22 or more completed weeks of gestation and infant deaths occurring during 7 days after delivery divided by the number of live births and stillbirths in the same time period.

Period infant mortality rates The number of infant deaths occurring in a calendar year per the number of live births occurring during the same period. To express the rate per 1,000 live births per year, multiply the result by 1,000.

Postneonatal death Death of a live-born infant from 28 through 365 days after delivery.

Postterm Forty-two or more completed weeks of gestation

Preterm Less than 37 completed weeks of gestation

PRAMS Pregnancy Risk Assessment Monitoring System: A population-based surveillance program in the United States that collects information from new mothers about their pregnancies and the first few months after their deliveries.

Preconception care An organized and comprehensive program of health care that identifies and reduces a woman's risk before conception through risk assessment, health promotion, and interventions. Preconception care programs may be designed to include the male partner by providing counseling and educational information in preparation for fatherhood, such as genetic counseling and testing, financial and family planning, etc. May refer to prospective father or mother.

Pregnancy-associated mortality The death of a woman from any cause while pregnant or within 12 months after the termination of pregnancy, regardless of the duration and site of pregnancy.

Pregnancy mortality rate The number of pregnancy-related maternal deaths per 100,000 pregnancies, usually expressed per year.

Pregnancy mortality ratio The number of pregnancy-related deaths per 100,000 live births.

Pregnancy-related mortality A pregnancy-associated death resulting from (1) complications of the pregnancy itself, (2) the chain of events initiated by the pregnancy, that led to death, or (3) aggravation of an unrelated condition by the physiologic or pharmacologic effects of the pregnancy that subsequently caused death.

Pregnancy intention The desirability of conception.

Prenatal care Monitoring and management of the woman during pregnancy to prevent complications of pregnancy and to promote a healthy outcome for the mother and infant.

Preterm delivery Termination of pregnancy before the 37th completed week of gestation.

Prevalence The number of persons with a health condition in a specified population at a designated time.

Prevention (primary, secondary, tertiary)

Primary prevention: Implementing an intervention before the evidence of a disease or injury. This strategy can reduce or eliminate causative risk factors (risk reduction).

Secondary prevention: Implementing an intervention after a disease has begun, but before it is symptomatic (screening and treatment).

Tertiary prevention: Implementing an intervention after a disease or injury is established. This strategy can prevent sequelae.

Primary infertility The status of an infertile couple who has not previously conceived.

Probability (*p* value) The likelihood that an event will occur. When looking at differences between data samples, statistical techniques are used to determine if the differences are likely to reflect real differences in the whole group from which the sample is drawn or if they are simply the result of random variation in the samples. For example, a probability (or *p* value) of 0.01 indicates that the differences observed would have occurred by chance in one out of a hundred samples drawn from the same data.

Provisional data Limited, early data from filed death certificates. Provisional data on infant mortality are provided by the National Center for Health Statistics 3–4 months after the death certificates are filed in the states. These data include estimates of the number of infant deaths and selected causes of death.

Public health

1. The science dealing with the protection and improvement of community health by organized community effort. Public health activities are generally those that are less amenable to being undertaken by individuals or that are less effective when undertaken on an individual basis. Public health activities and typically do not include direct personal health services. Public health activities include immunizations; sanitation; preventive medicine, quarantine, and other disease control activities; occupational health and safety programs; assurance of the healthfulness of air, water, and food; health education; epidemiology; and others.

2. Application of scientific and technical knowledge to address community health needs, thereby preventing disease and promoting health. Core functions include collecting and analyzing data, developing comprehensive policies for entire populations, and assuring that appropriate services are delivered to all.

Rate A measure of the frequency of occurrence of an event during a defined time interval. For example, the annual mortality rate equals the number who die in 1 year divided by the number at risk of dying during that year. Rates are usually expressed using a standard denominator such as 1,000 or 100,000 persons.

Rate ratio The ratio of two rates expressed in epidemiology as the ratio of the rate of a health outcome in an exposed population to the rate in the unexposed population.

Risk or risk factor Risk is a term used by epidemiologists to quantify the likelihood that something will occur. A risk factor is something that either increases or decreases an individual's likelihood of developing a disease.

Screening The use of quick procedures to differentiate apparently well persons who have a disease or a high risk of disease from those who probably do not have the disease. It is used to identify high-risk individuals for more definitive study or follow-up. Multiple screening (or multiphasic screening) is the combination of a battery of screening tests for specific diseases. This screening is performed by technicians under medical direction and applied to large groups of apparently well persons.

Secondary infertility The status of an infertile couple who has had one or more previous conceptions.

Specialist A physician, dentist, or other health professional who is specially trained in a certain branch of medicine or dentistry related to specific services or procedures (e.g., surgery, radiology, pathology); certain age categories of patients (e.g., pediatrics, geriatrics); certain body systems (e.g., dermatology, orthopedics, cardiology); or certain types of diseases (e.g., allergy, psychiatry, periodontics). Specialists usually have advanced education and training related to their specialties.

Spontaneous abortion Spontaneous death prior to the complete expulsion or extraction from its mother of a product of conception. In some surveillance systems, this term indicates such deaths at gestational age less than 20 weeks.

Stillbirth Death prior to the complete expulsion or extraction from its mother of a product of conception. In some surveillance systems, this term indicates such deaths at gestational age of 20 weeks or more.

Survey An investigation in which information is collected systematically. A population survey may be conducted by face-to-face inquiry, by self-completed questionnaires, by telephone, by postal service, or in some other way. Each method has its advantages and disadvantages. The generalizability of results depends upon the extent to which those surveyed are representative of the entire population.

Teratogen An exposure that causes birth defects.

Term From 37 through less than 42 weeks completed gestation.

Total fertility rate A hypothetical rate computed by summing the age-specific fertility rates in a given period for a hypothetical cohort of women. It shows the potential impact of current fertility patterns on the total rate of births delivered by a cohort of women.

Unintended pregnancy According to questions included in the National Survey of Family Growth, a pregnancy identified as either unwanted or mistimed.

Unwanted pregnancy According to questions included in the National Survey of Family Growth, a pregnancy occurring when the mother reported that she did not want a child at the time of conception or any time in the future.

Vital statistics Statistics relating to births (natality), deaths (mortality), marriages, health, and disease (morbidity). Vital statistics for the United States are published by the National Center for Health Statistics.

WHO

World Health Organization.

Reference

1. Kramer MS, Platt RW, Yang H, Haglund B, Cnattingius S, Bergsjo P. Registration artifacts in international comparisons of infant mortality. Paediatr Perinat Epidemiol 2002; 16(1):16–22.

Index